AF540111

# HIV/AIDS
## ISSUES AND CHALLENGES

INTERNATIONAL ENCYCLOPAEDIA OF AIDS-2

# HIV/AIDS
# ISSUES AND CHALLENGES
## Part-II

Editor
**Dr. Digumarti Bhaskara Rao**
*M.Sc., M.A., M.A., M.Ed., Ph.D.*
*R. V. R. College of Education*
*Guntur–522 006*
*Andhra Pradesh. (INDIA)*

**2000**
**DISCOVERY PUBLISHING HOUSE**
NEW DELHI-110 002

First Published-2000

ISBN 81-7141-524-5 (Set)



*Published by:*
DISCOVERY PUBLISHING HOUSE
4831/24, Ansari Road, Prahlad Street,
Darya Ganj, New Delhi-110 002 (*INDIA)*
Phone: 3279245
Fax: 91-11-3253475

*Printed at:*
Arora Offset Press
Laxmi Nagar, Delhi 110 092.

# Preface

The HIV/AIDS is a new phenomenon in the human society. HIV destroys the immune system of human individuals, producing a defenselessness fatal state known as AIDS. The World Health Organisation has estimated that already one in every two hundred and fifty adults in the world is infected with Human Immunodeficiency Virus and according to WHO's projections a total of forty million men women and children worldwide will have been infected with HIV by the turn of this twentieth century. Visualising the devastating effects of the HIV/AIDS epidemic within our life times and beyond is difficult. Probably, no other disease in recent times has had the impact on human society generated by HIV/AIDS.

The HIV/AIDS epidemic has brought into focus many health related ethical, legal and human rights issues. This epidemic requires immediate and effective responses in new programming areas: attitudinal and behavioural changes, community-based care and support initiatives, and the maintenance of human development in the face of increasing rates of illness and deaths. At this point, education enters the scene as it can alter the HIV/AIDS situation since it brings change in the behaviour of the people.

This *International Encyclopaedia of AIDS* presents the worldwide information about HIV/AIDS, issues and challenges, reports and reviews, ethics laws and human rights, and educational activities and programmes to keep the policy makers, planners, professionals, activists, researchers, educationists, teachers and students well informed of the epidemic.

Dr. Digumarti Bhaskara Rao<br>
26 January 1999<br>
The Republic Day of India

# Acknowledgements

I am thankful to the World Health Organisation and its associated offices for using their material namely School Health Education to prevent AIDS and STD: A Resource Package for Curriculum Planners-Handbook for Curriculum Planners. Student's Activities, Teachers' Guide, Global Programme on AIDS-HIV Prevention and Care: Teaching Modules for Nurses and Midwives, Global Programme on AIDS. Community HIV Prevention Handbook; STD care Management-workbooks 1-7, Facing the Challenge of HIV/AIDS STDs: A Gender-based Response; HIV/AIDS and STD surveillance Data Management and Use-Report, Bangkok, 1995; Carrying out HIV Sentinal Surveillance-A Guide for Programme Managers, AIDS Prevention and Care in the workplace: Enhancing the Role of Private Sector; HIV Testing Policies and Gidelines; Carrying out HIV Sentinel surveillance; AIDS Prevention; Understanding and Living with AIDS; AIDS: A Modern Epidemic; HIV/AIDS in South-East Asia: IXth meeting of the National Programme Managers, New Delhi, 1993; Information, Education and Communication: A Guide for AIDS Programme Managers, Handbook on AIDS Home Care; HIV/AIDS in South-East Asia: A Pictorial summary; etc.

I am thankful to the United Nations Development Programme, UNDP's HIV and Development Programme, and UNDP's Regional Projects on HIV and Development for using their material namely Economic Implications of AIDS in Asia; Socio Economic Implications of the Epidemic; NGOs Working with Sex workers; NGO Responses to HIV/AIDS in Asia-Case Studies; HIV in the Workplace: Dealing with the Issues-Role Plays, Development and the HIV Epidemic, Law Ethics and HIV; HIV Law and Law Reform; Issue Papers; Study Papers; Working Papers; etc.

I am thankful to the Health and Nutrition Centre, Republic of Philippines for using its material namely sourcebook on HIV/AIDS Prevention Education for Tertiary Educational Institutions.

I am thankful to the Curriculum Development Programme, Ministry of Education, Government of Thailand for using its material namely Institutional Modules for AIDS Education.

I am thankful to US Department of Health and Human Services: Whitman-Walker Clinic, Inc., USA; East-West Centre, USA; National AIDS Control Organisation, Government of India; Academy of Culture Communication Education Science and Service, Guntur, United Nations and its agencies for using their material.

I am grateful to Bhaskar Bhattacharji; V. Alexeev, Geeta Sethi, Elizabeth Reid, Mina Mauerstein-Bail, A. A. Trinidad, Palomi Cuchi, D. Pushpa Latha for their kind co-operation.

Dr. Digumarti Bhaskara Rao,
Secretary
ACCESS
D-43, S.V. N. Colony,
Guntur-522 006

# Contents

# 30

# Lost Souls

**Ms. Elizabeth Reid**
UNDP, New York

William James in *The Moral Philosopher and the Moral Life* explores the hypothesis a world in which millions can live full and happy lives on one simple condition: that a certain lost soul on the far-off edge of things should lead a life of lonely torment.

Except for this one person, people in this world lead lives of happiness, of unthreatened well-being. More than that, it is only because of the isolated torment of this lost soul that their happiness can exist and continue. The suffering of that one person creates the possibility of their serenity. Without this suffering, their utopia could not be.

James implicitly poses the question: could one accept happiness under such conditions?

It seems to me that two questions can be distinguished. Firstly, if faced with such a situation, could we accept happiness at this cost? Secondly, what would happen to us if we did if we were prepared to pay this price for happiness?

The second question is addressed by Ursula Le Guin in a short story entitled "The Ones Who Walk Away From Omelas" (*The Wind's Twelve Quarters*, Bantam Books, 1976). She describes the city of Omelas, bright-towered by a sparkling sea. The people are gifted, creative happy in their relationships and their work. But they all know one thing: the tenderness of the friendships, the wisdom of their scholars, the health of their children and even the abundance of their harvest wholly depend on one child's abominable misery.

This child lives in a windowless basement under one of their beautiful buildings. The child and the circumstances that it lives in are a sickening and a shocking sight. It has not always lived there. It can remember sunlight and its mother's voice.

All young people as they reach an age of maturily are told about the child and most go to see it. They feel disgust, anger, outrage, impotence. They would like to do something for to child, but if the child were brought out into the sunlight, out of that vile place, then their way of living, its lack of cares, its untrammelled joys would, in that moment, wither away. These are the terms: if the child is even spoken to, the world as they know it would cease to exist. The terms are absolute.

The children rage and brood. But then they begin to rationalism even if the child could be released, it is now too degraded and deprived to be able to know any real joy:

> "it has been afraid too long ever to be tree ot fear. Its habits are too uncouth for it lo respond to humane treatment. Indeed, after so long it would probably be wretched without walls about it to protect it, and darkness for its eyes, and its own excrement to sit in."

They begin to see, and accept, a terrible justice in reality. Just as we have: we accept poverty, extreme poverty, in our midst, for example. For us, it rarely has a human face.

But let us return to the first question, the one William James poses and the question that might allow us to understand better how such lost souls come about: could we accept happiness at such a price?

James acknowledges human frailty. An impulse would arise within us, he feels, to clutch at the happiness so offered. However, he argues, it would be immediately suppressed by the knowledge of how hideous would be its enjoyment when deliberately accepted as the fruit of such a bargain. In James world, there must be no lost souls to degrade us.

A similar fundamental moral dilemma faces the world with the coming of the HIVepidemic: would we accept the ability to continue our past way of life at such an inhuman cost, the cost of quarantining, isolating and rejecting those infected with HIV? Are we as morally decent as William James? Or would we find such a cost acceptable? Will the Lost Souls of the epidemic be those we push away from ourselves so that we can continue to live as we were living before this epidemic, those we reject, imprison, repudiate?

Our past way of life has its roots in a world that has fundamentally changed. The HIV virus is now in our midst. In a social setting, we cannot tell where it is, whom it has infected. Potentially therefore, each and every act of unprotected sexual intercourse can be an occasion for its further transmission.

There is a widespread reluctance to change, to act in the present in a way that is consistently protective. This should not cause much surprise. Sexual behaviour has consistently and throughout history been marked by a widespread refusal to take responsibility for these acts and a refusal in particular to take precautionary and protective measures. The consequences of this refusal have included unwanted pregnancies and the trauma of abortion or birth in such circumstances, widespread infertility, shame and significant morbidity, including that of sexual partners and children. To this list are now added all of the tragic con sequences of HIV infection.

We know how to protect ourselves from HIV infection. However, the means to prevent the spread of HIV. unlike many other pathogens, depends not just on the impersonal application of technology but on human attributes, ultimately on both self-love and altruism. Changes are required not only to human behaviour, but to the very way that our society is structured and to our social values. The spread of the virus is much harder to slow down in conditions of social alienation, of poverty, even of wealth.

One change has occurred: the consequences of HIV infection are more feared than the consequences of other diseases that can be sexually transmitted. This fear could be a motivating force for each of us to make the required protective changes. Or it could reinforce the past refusal to accept responsibility for our conduct. In the latter case, the demand will be that the protection of the majority requires stringent measures to be taken against those infected. There will be pressure to shift the focus of HIV policy away from behaviour change in the whole community to identification, surveillance and isolating of those already infected. Emphasis will be placed, perhaps exclusively, on compulsory contact tracing, on the quarantining or sexual emasculation of those considered by the authorities to be unresponsive. In this way, the community's refusal to change its past ways of behaving, to act in a morally responsible way, will create our own lost souls, forced to pay the price for us all.

This has been recognised in national HIV policies in which one of the most important guiding principles has been that each person must take responsibility for preventing himself or herself from becoming infected sexually or through needle sharing. This responsibility cannot be thrust upon the infected and their cares. The nature of transmission and infection is such that each person in our community, not just the infected, must carry this responsibility. Those infected need the space and the support to learn how to live full and responsible lives knowing that they are infected; the whole community needs the knowledge, the means and the support to protect themselves .

The way a community responds to the HIV epidemic seems to be influenced by at least two factors. The first lies in the boundaries communities draw to define themselves: who is one of us and who is not. HIV policy responses to infection among drug users differ according to whether drug users are seen by the State or the community as enemies or as victims. New York and Edinburgh exemplify the first, and the HIV policy response has been a punitive mobilisation of the law rather than the setting in place of protective measures such as programmes for needle distribution and disposal. A similar distinction can be drawn between policy responses with regard to homosexuals, where the HIV policy alternatives have been either gross and culpable neglect along with calls for quarantining or tattooing or, alternatively, supportive measures which have assisted the gay community to develop an effective response.

Policy responses are more humane and supportive where those infected are accepted as an integral part of the community. There may be alienation, discrimination and stigma but nevertheless the community struggles to encompass and include the differences. Where the infected are ostracized, seen as enemies of the people, the policy responses mirror this perception. The implicit message is that the infected are expendable, their lives of little or no value to the community. The result is inevitably violation, violence and murder.

A second influencing factor seems to be leadership style. A recent study of eight us communities and their reactions to a HIV-infected school child in their midst (*Learning by Heart* David L, Kirp, Rutgers UP, 1989) shows that each community that responded with compassion and humanity had a leadership that created the conditions for arriving at a decision rather than imposing decisions on the community. Without this leadership, communities were adrift, reacting too often with bigotry, hatred and violence.

This leadership style has béen adopted in too few countries. Public statements by leaders, policy discussion papers and public hearings, discussions and debates are important means to significantly broaden community knowledge of these complex issues and to increase community participation in the processes of decision making.

Resistance to change is a human characteristic. But this tendency must be struggled against for the price of resisting change is now too high. To ensure that our response to the epidemic does not lead to the underpinning of our way of life by the torment of lost souls will require at least the following:

- that we continue to struggle to encompass and include everyone within the bounds of our community;
- that we continue with a participatory, inclusive and open style of leadership and decision making;
- that our protection and prevention policies continue to be directed at the whole community; and
- that we begin to conceptually explore and understand the high moral cost of doing otherwise.

The creation of lost souls can destroy the mogul-fabric of a society. There were some who walked away from Omelas. But they were few.

# 31

# Towards an Ethical Response to the HIV Epidemic

**Ms. Elizabeth Reid**
UNDP, New York

Here in Africa, as elsewhere in the world, the HIV virus is not infiltrating a benign world.

The realities of which we are a part include:

— the brutal and seemingly senseless slaughter taking place in Rwanda, and which has taken place in Angola, Liberia and elsewhere;

— the purposeless disintegration of a once proud and homogenous nation state in Somalia which has parallels to Zaire:

— the degradation of life in the slums of Abijan, or Nairobi, or Lagos, or Soweto, and elsewhere;

— the pervasive corruption of the educated elite and the consequent rarity of a courageous and altruistic leadership;

— the swelling ranks of the disinherited: men without occupation, youth without education, the hungry, the landless, the lawless and the rootless;

— the increasing presence of eroded fields, discarded plastic bags, unpassable roads, crumbling makeshift shelters and disease; and

— the often base motives of the intervening powers, be they former colonial powers, other nation states, international organizations, the drug cartels or multinational corporations.

Another way of looking at these realities is to note that we are living in a world where increasingly:

- the concept of nation states, and so of national boundaries, are, in many instances, becoming irrelevant;
- the reach of national governments is shrinking and larger and larger tracts of land or expanses of dwellings are ungoverned and ungovernable by national authorities;
- legal systems are becoming marginalized or irrelevant and their place taken by military and paramilitary forces, vigilante groups, private security services, bandits and criminals, with the resulting summary executions, necklacing, roadblocks, ambushes, extortion and terror; and
- the delicate balance which must hold between the government, the military and the people for governance and participation to be possible is no longer in equilibrium.

These are not the only realities and, even where they hold sway, they may not be irreversible but they are realities very relevant to the HIV epidemic.

In the shanty towns and slums, wherever the military move, along the new drug routes in Africa and amongst the educated elites, the virus is spreading with a rapidity difficult to conceive. Its spread is directly linked to the economic, cultural, strategic and political conditions which are fueling widespread social and moral disintegration.

In turn, as it spreads, it itself is contributing to the creation of poverty, crime, alcoholism, economic disintegration, landlessness and hopelessness, with thc despair and deaths of those concerned. This is especially true where the epidemic remains wrapped in silence, where people live in fear that they might be infected but cannot find out, where sexual partners do not talk to each other and parents do not ensure that someone, be it they themselves or someone else, continues to talk to their children. Perhaps the most culpably silent are those to whom people turn as role models, for counsel or for leadership.

Furthermore, the response in Africa to date has been based on the concept of nation states. It has assumed an effective reach of centralized bureaucracies and formal institutions, including the law. There has been no acknowledgement of their limitations because the epidemic and its response has been seen as addressable from outside by technological interventions—a drug, a condom, a test kit. There has been little thought given to the limit of governmental action in attitudinal and behavioural change, in getting people to talk amongst themselves and to care for and about each other. Yet these latter lie at the heart of an effective response.

These issues are too important not to question their impact on the epidemic and not to accept that these realities are as relevant to our understanding of HIV as is a surveillance system or an anti-discrimination law. Those who have more chance of surviving this epidemic, whether adults, adolescents or children, may well live in slums or shanty towns. The difference between those communities which will survive and those that will not will lie in the values to which the community subscribes and, most importantly, those by which it strives to act.

A basic question thus becomes what sort of communities are those which have a chance of surviving and how can they be enabled to overcome all of the influences that are sapping and undermining their moral and social vitality? Just as people must want to create a community within a slum, within a village or of a nation in which they can live without fear and with hope for the future, with respect for each other and with the gift of life for their children, without crime, assault, filth and poverty, so too must people want to create a world within which we can co-exist peacefully with this virus, within which we do not pass it on, in the living of our lives from one to another.

Hence the work that UNDP has been associated with in the creation and stimulation of the African Network on Ethics, Law and HIV. The most notable thing about the epidemic, and the basis for hope for a future, lies in the remarkable fact that, somehow or other, this epidemic can bring out, not the worst, but the best in people: courage, compassion. concern for self and others. Hope for the future is grounded in the courage and behaviour of those most deeply affected, the people living with HIV and AIDS, many of whom are with us here today. Strikingly, these are not often those in whom their families and their nations have invested, the highly educated of this continent, nor are they usually those in whom the people have placed their trust, the politicians and leaders, religious, traditional or otherwise. They come, very often, from the same living conditions which drive others to crime or alcohol or violence. The courageous in this movement are mostly drawn from the villages, the slums, from lives marked by poverty or hardship, from humbler occupations and vocations. The vast majority of them will never attend a meeting on HIV except with their neighbours.

UNDP believes that this initiative will contributing significantly to ensuring that this courage and commitment to a better world for self and others is not lost. For people to continue to speak out and be engaged and for their individual actions to form the basis of a mass movement for social change, there must be an enabling and empowering ethical and legal environment. This will require a critical mass of courageous, informed and engaged people in each country who will speak out, advocate, lobby, advise, draft and defend to this end. These individuals could be more effective and supportive to each other when linked together into a national network. Thus a process was begun two years ago which has now resulted in national networks coming into existence in nine of the ten countries participitating in the process. The tenth country, South Africa, has established its networks independently and is now joining this regional effort.

By means of a Planning Meeting, held in Accra last October, and this Inter-Country Consultation, the process is now underway of linking these national networks into an African Network on Ethics, Law and HIV through which experiences can be exchanged, strategies discussed and shared to address common problems and a regional strategy developed. As resources allow, these networks will be expanded and more countries included.

This initiative, to be effective, must lead to a world where those most affected, those who live their daily lives within the confines of this epidemic, must be able to speak and act for the good of their societies, without recrimination, without retaliation, without repudiation. But it must also lead to a greater understanding of and impetus towards the kind of society in which people will be able to survive this epidemic and an identification of the value system or systems which will foster this. This, I have argued, cannot be done in isolation from the social and economic conditions which determine the pattern and speed of its spread.

Fortunately, I believe, although this must be tested in the crucible of reality, that the principles required to address this epidemic and those required to address the complex reality of the world on which it is feeding overlap.

There is a need, often overlooked, to distinguish two types of principles:

- those that must guide and shape the actions of those working to overcome this epidemic, and your presence here today bears witness to the fact that we all of us fall into that category; and
- those that will enable a community to survive through the tragedy in which we are already living and which is to come.

I will not attempt to give an exhaustive list of such principles but only an indicative one. Let me first start with the first type for they are less frequently discussed. These are the principles required to guide the actions of those working to assist others, as well as themselves, to respond to the epidemic, be they doctors, leaders, lawyers, researchers, development workers, counsellors, or whatever, those one might simply call the outsiders: those outside of a family, village or nation working with it.

The principle of being informed: each person engaged in or a part of the response to the epidemic needs actively in an ongoing manner to continue the quest to understand this epidemic in all its complexity and as it unfolds and changes. This principle is a prerequisite for the conceptual and programmatic flexibility demanded by the epidemic.

The principle of association: to work within this epidemic is to work in partnership with those living the virus. Those who do not know them as partners and confidants, who do not spend time in their company, should not represent them, speak for them, speak about them, attend conference on the subject, be employed as consultants, receive research grants or project financing, or head national programmes. If this principle is not respected, we run the risk of setting false priorities and designing irrelevant or infective programmes.

The principle of engagement: since each of us is affected, that is, there is no Them and Us within this epidemic, then each of us is and must be engaged, not just as actors, but active in our own interest and in the interests of those we love and care for. What we are facing can not be used as a situation of gain, nor as a situation of being employed, for the good of others or otherwise, nor as a situation of exploitation. To work, to be available, to volunteer, to spend one's time, to contribute one's talents is the engagement that this epidemic draws, and demands, from each person. Linked to this principle is the principle of language. It is equally important that the language used not divide the world into Them and Us, that it not strip those infected of their dignity nor define their identity as a human being in terms of their infection.

The principle of empowerment: this principle marks the manner in which we must work: as equals, in partnership, each bringing their own experience and skills to the partnership in a process of mutual capacity building. This is a difficult process. The experience of UNDP in working in partnership has led us to believe that one can only enter into true partnerships with people with similar value systems, in particular with those who are engaged. There may well be a diversity of beliefs, experiences, capacities, ways of thinking or working, disciplines and cultures; the critical value required for partnership is engagement. Furthermore, we have discovered that true partnership can only occur between or among equals, where all concerned are secure in their identities, their self-esteem and their place in the world.

Paradoxically, perhaps, it has often been easiest for UNDP to enter into partnership with those living with HIV and AIDS, those closest to them, and those working with them in the art of living. Perhaps it is because they have made the transition from knowing that they are infected to being able to take up their daily lives once more as someone living with the virus. This seems to create a will to live that they have to live and the determination that life be worth living which themselves produce the required self-esteem and security in their identity required for a partnership of mutual capacity building.

The principle of consensus-building: by its nature, this epidemic requires each person to face up to its realities. It is not a matter of some knowing and then providing direction to others and organizing them to carry out their directives. Rather, on the base of each couple, each family, each community, a process of consensus building must be catalysed so that all are involved in the discussions and in the decision making.

Turning briefly to those principles which will enable communities to survive and overcome this epidemic. These have been better mapped in the papers for this meeting and in the emerging discussion and literature on the nature of a community-based response, although there is still much work to do. These could include, as basic principles from which other more specific principles and directives for action can be derived, the following.

The principle of knowledge: that each person has the right to be able to determine their infection status in conditions of confidentiality and with counselling, and that this service must be voluntary, accessible and affordable. This principle is an essential prerequisite of the principle of openness, the imperative of this epidemic that the silence be shattered, the fear and the denital confronted and that each person be actively encouraged to talk about and decide upon this reality in all aspects of their life.

The principle of human dignity: that the essential human dignity of each person be respected in all aspects of their lives. This principle is ceaselessly and unrelentingly transgressed in the daily lives of women, a reality shared by the swelling ranks of the disinherited. Those most directly affected by this epidemic, who have been able to take up again their daily lives are now challenging us to honour it in principle and practice, to refind in our lives an unwavering commitment to mutual respect and trust as the basic values of human life.

The principle of protection: that all means of protecting themselves from infection or reinfection, both the technology, including condoms, and information, be available, affordable and accessible to each person who, reflecting on his or her life situation, sexuality, beliefs and values, has taken a decision to so protect themselves.

The principle of inclusion: that those most directly affected by the epidemic remain an integral part of their communities, with the right of access to all benefits available to others: education, training, employment, health and legal services, social support and benefits, sport, marriage etc. This principle is thus associated with the principle of non-discrimination and its behavioural imperatives against rejection, neglect, repudiation and stigmatization.

The principle of representation: that those most directly affected by the epidemic, living its realities in their daily lives, should participate in all discussions, activities and decision-making with respect to the epidemic.

The principle of compassion: this is the acknowledgement that each person is linked by relations of kinship, love, neighbourliness, empathy, dependency, respect or solidarity. To change and sustain the required changes, to be cared for, to be sheltered and provided for requires others. They cannot be achieved in isolation for they are not solitary or individual activities. Compassion is the ethical reflection of this interdependence.

The challenge facing this meeting lies in contributing to a process of better understanding the complex dynamics of the epidemic in its African setting, in reflecting on how one can create, catalyze and facilitate the building of consensus around the value systems or principles by which communities wish to live and nations to govern, and in adopting a set of principles, individually and collectively, which can guide our behaviour as activists in our struggle to bring about a world in which we wish to live and within which we can continue to live.

# 32

# TB/HIV Connection: What Health Care Workers Should Know

US Department of Health
and Human Sciences
Atlanta Georgia 30333

Tuberculosis (TB) is seen with increasing frequency among persons infected with the human immunodeficiency virus (HIV), the virus that causes acquired immunodeficiency syndrome (AIDS). HIV infection is one of the strongest known risk factors for the progression of TB from infection to disease. However, of the diseases associated with HIV infection, TB is one of the few that is transmissible, treatable, and preventable.

Patients who have active. infectious TB pose a potential occupational hazard to health care workers (HCWs) if the disease is not promptly diagnosed and eftectively treated. This booklet presents information about diagnosing, managing, and preventing TB in persons with HIV infection and preventing and treating TB in health care workers.

## TB AND HIV IN THE UNITED STATES

- An estimated l.0 million persons in the United States are infected with HIV.
- An estimated 10 to 15 million persons in the United States are infected with *Mycobacterium tuberculosis,* the organism that causes TB.
- In 1990, approximately 5per cent of all AIDS patients also had TB. In some areas, as many as 58 per cent of persons with TB are HIV seropositive.

# FACTS ABOUT HIV INFECTION

## Mode of Transmission

HIV is not spread by casual contact. It is spread primarily through sexual contact or through sharing needles used to inject drugs. HIV can also be spread from pregnant women to their unborn children or from women to children through breast-feeding. In addition, HIV has been transmitted to persons who received HIV-infected blood products or transfusions of HIV-infected blood. Since July 1985, however, all blood donations have been tested for HIV infection, and those tound to contain HIV antibodies are discarded. Now the risk of infection from blood products or blood transfusions is very low. In a few instances, HIV has been transmitted to HCWs through unintentional needle-stick exposures to HIV-intected blood.

## Pathogenesis

HIV is a retrovirus consisting of a central ribonucleic acid (RNA) surrounded by coats of virus-specific protein. In HIV-infected persons, the immune system recognizes the virus protein as foreign material and produces antibodies that are directed against this material. This is accomplished through complex mechanisms involving the white blood cells and the virus.

One important type of white blood cell is the lymphocyte, of which there are two types: B lymphocytes (B cells) and T lymphocytes (T cells). T cells include helper (CD4+) T cells and suppressor (CD8+) T cells. In persons infected with HIV, the total number of helper T cells is decreased because the virus infects the cells, reproduces within them, and then destroys them. As a result, immune defense mechanisms are impaired.

The helper (CD4+) T cell is the primary target for HIV infection because the virus is attracted to the CD4+ surface marker. Because the CD4+ T cell co-ordinates a number of immunologic functions, a loss of these cells leads to a progressive impairment of the immune response.[1] For example, low CD4+ counts are associated with anergy, the inability to mount a response to delayed-type hypersensitivity skin test antigens. Therefore, some HIV-infected persons with CD4+ counts of less than 200 who are cointected with M. tuberculosis may have a false-negative reaction to the tuberculin skin test..[2]

In addition as the number of CD4+ T cells decrease, the risk and severity of opportunistic diseases increases.[1] Some of the common opportunistic diseases experienced by persons infected with HIV are *Pneumocystis carinii* pneumonia, Kaposi's sarcoma, esophageal or bronchial candidiasis, extrapulmonary cryptococcosis, disseminated *Mycobacterium avium* complex, cytomegalovirus, HIV wasting syndrome, severe herpes simplex, toxoplasmosis of the brain, pulmonary TB, extrapulmonary TB, and other disseminated mycobacterial diseases.[3]

When people who are intected with HIV become ill with opportunistic diseases and intections, have CD4+ counts of less than 200, or have a CD4+ percentage of total lymphocytes of less than 14 per cent, they are generally said to have AIDS. As of January 1, 1993, pulmonary tuberculosis is an AIDS-defining disease in the expanded surveillance case definition for AIDS among adolescents and adults.[1]

## High-Risk Behaviours for HIV Infection

Current or past behaviours that put persons at high risk for HIV infection include

# injection drug use
# sexual activity between men
# sexual activity with someone who is infected with HIV
# sexual activity with someone who has practiced any of the above behaviours.

Other factors which increase the risk for HIV infection include:

# sexual activity with someone whose drug use or history of sexual behaviour is unknown (especially persons with multiple partners)
# receipt of blood products or blood transfusions between 1978 and 1985.

# FACTS ABOUT HIV-RELATED TB

## Mode of Transmission

TB is a communicable disease caused by the bacterium *Mycobacterium tuberculosis,* often called the tubercle bacillus. It is spread from person to person through the inhalation of airborne particles containing *M. tuberculosis.* These particles, also called droplet nuclei, are produced when a person with infectious TB of the lung or larynx forcefully exhales, such as when coughing, sneezing, speaking, or singing. These infectious particles can remain suspended in the air and inhaled by someone sharing the same air. TB is transmitted in closed areas where ventilation is poor. The risk of transmission increases when susceptible persons share air for prolonged periods with a person who has untreated pulmonary

TB. Persons who have TB in extrapulmonary sites (not including laryngeal TB) are usually not considered infectious to other people. However, under unusual circumstances, TB has been transmitted to HCWs from patients with extrapulmonary TB.[4,5]

## Pathogenesis

TB infection may occur when droplet nuclei are inhaled through the nose and mouth and then move down the trachea into the lungs and along the branches of the airways (the bronchi) until they reach the small air sacs of the lung (the alveoli). TB infection usually begins in the alveoli, where tubercle bacilli are initially able to multiply. During the first few weeks after infection, tubercle bacilli can spread from their initial location in the lungs (usually in the lower portions), to the lymph nodes in the center of the chest, and then to other parts of the body by way of the bloodstream. Tubercle bacilli can reach all areas of the body, but they often travel to the areas that are most susceptible to TB disease, such as the upper portions of the lungs, the kidneys, the brain and the bones. Within 2 to 10 weeks, the hody's immunologic response to the tubercle bacilli usually prevents the bacteria from multiplying and spreading more.

## TB Infection and Disease

TB infection in a person who does not have active disease is not considered a case of TB. Persons with TB infection who do not have disease:

- # cannot infect others;
- # usually have a positive reaction to the tuberculin skin test;
- # usually have a negative chest radiograph and no clinical symptoms of TB;
- # have tubercle bacilli in their bodies. Although contained, these bacilli remain viable (and capable of producing active disease at any time.

TB disease does not develop in everyone who is infected. In the United States, about 90 per cent of infected persons remain infected for life and never develop symptoms of TB. But in about 5 per cent of infected persons, disease develops in the first or second year after infection. and in another 5 per cent it develops later in life (this varies with age and immunologic status). The risk that active TB will develop in a person coinfected with TB and HIV is about 86 per year. In contrast, the risk that it will develop in a person infected only with TB is 5 per cent to 10 per cent, during a lifetime.

Most cases of TB (approximately 85per cent) occur in the lungs (pulmonary TB). But disease may occur at any site in the body, such as the larynx the lymph nodes, the brain, the kidneys, or the bones (extrapulmonary TB). Extrapulmonary TB and unusual presentations of pulmonary TB are more common among HIV-infected persons than among persons not infected with HIV.

The signs and symptoms of TB vary according to the location of the disease. General signs and symptoms may include fatigue, feeling ill, loss of appetite, weight loss, fever, and night sweats. In addition to the general signs and symptoms, pulmonary TB usually causes cough, chest pain, coughing up sputum, and sometimes coughing up blood (hemoptysis); TB of the spine may cause pain in the back; and TB of the kidney may cause blood in the urine. Table 32.1 summarizes selected clinical characteristics of persons with TB infection, active pulmonary TB, or extrapulmonary TB.

The development of HIV-related TB disease can follow either of two courses. First, if a person who has latent TB infection becomes coinfected with HIV, active TB may develop as HIV weakens the person's immune system. Second, if a person who has preexisting HIV infection becomes infected with TB,TB infection may progress rapidly to disease .

TABLE 32.1
Selected Clinical Characteristics of Persons with Tuberculosis Infection, Active Pulmonary Tuberculosis, or Extrapulmonary Tuberculosis

| | TB Infection | Active Pulmonary TB | Extra Pulmonary TB |
|---|---|---|---|
| Skin Test Result | usually positive | usually positive | usually positive |
| Signs and Symptoms | none | cough, hemoptysis, fever, night sweats, weight loss, fatigue, chest pain, and anorexia | depends on site in body affected<br><br>general signs and symptoms: fever, night sweats, weight loss, fatigue, feeling ill, and loss of appetite |
| Infected | yes | yes | yes |
| Infectious | no | usually (before effective treatment) | usually not |

## Risk Factors for TB

Anyone who has shared airspace with a person who has infectious TB is at risk for TB. Some persons are considered to be at high risk for TB infection and disease because they are more likely than others to be exposed to someone with TB: foreign-born persons from areas with a high prevalence of TB; residents and employees of long-term care facilities and correctional facilities; and medically underserved populations, including the poor, the homeless, high-risk racial and ethnic minority groups, and injection drug users (IDUs). Other persons are at high risk for TB disease once they are infected with TB: immunocompromised persons (especially HIV-intected persons), persons with other medical risk factors (such as diabetes, end-stage renal disease, and being 10 per cent or more below ideal body weight), and IDUs.

## Screening for TB Infection

The Mantoux tuberculin skin test is the recommended method of skin testing to determine whether a person is infected with *M. tuterculosis.* Multiple-puncture tests should not be used because the results are less reliable. The Mantoux skin test is performed by injecting 0.1 ml of 5 tuberculin units (TU) of purified protein derivative (PPD) intradermally, usually on the forearm. The patient's arm is examined 48 to 72 hours later for induration (palpable swelling) around the site of injection. The diameter of the indurated area across the forearm is measured. The area of erythema (redness) around the indurated area does not indicate infection with *M. tuberculosis* and should not be measured. A positive reaction to the tuberculin test usually means the patient has been infected with *M. tuberculosis.* For HIV-infected persons, a tuberculin skin test reaction of 5 or more millimeters of induration is considered positive.

All persons known to have or suspected of having HIV infection should be given a PPD tuberculin skin test. Persons coinfected with TB and HIV may have a false-negative skin test reaction because of anergy. Anergy is the inability to mount a delayed-type hypersensitivity (DTH) response to skin test antigens because of immunosuppression, which can be caused by certain medical conditions (e.g. HIV infection) or drugs. According to recent studies, HIV infection can depress tuberculin reactions even before the signs and symptoms of HIV infection develop.[2]

## Testing for Anergy

Because persons with HIV infection are more likely to have

an anergic response to a tuberculin skin test, these persons should be evaluated for DTH anergy at the time of tuberculin testing. The likelihood of a false-negative skin test result increases as the CD4+ T-cell count decreases. For this reason, a previous positive skin test result should be considered evidence of TB infection, even if the current skin test result is negative.

For anergy testing, Mantoux tuberculin testing should be accompanied by Mantoux testing with two DTH antigens (i.e., *Candida,* mumps or tetanus toxoid). The reactions should be measured 48 to 72 hours after the test is administered. Induration of 3 or more millimeters to any of the antigens is considered evidence of DTH responsiveness; failure to respond to all of the antigens is considered anergy. In general, persons who respond to DTH antigens but who have a negative reaction to tuberculin are not considered infected with *M. tuberculosis.* HIV-infected persons who are anergic (and thus tuberculin skin test negative) and who are at increased risk for TB should be considered for preventive therapy. Anergic persons who are at increased risk for TB but who choose not to take preventive therapy should be informed about the signs and symptoms of TB and instructed to report promptly for medical evaluation if any of these develop.

## Tuberculin Skin Test Reaction in Persons Vaccinated with BCG

Outside the United States, many countries use Bacille Calmette-Guerin (BCG) vaccination as part of their TB control activities, especially for infants. The size of tuberculin skin test reactions caused by BCG vaccination varies by the strain and the dose of the vaccine the age and the nutritional status at vaccination, the number of years since vaccination, and the frequency of tuberculin testing. Alter BCG vaccination, it is usually impossible to distinguish between a tuberculin skin test reaction caused by mycobacterial infection or by vaccination. However, BCG-induced tuberculin skin test reactivity wanes over time. Also, because BCG is used more often in countries where the prevalence of TB is high, BCG-vaccinated persons are more likely to have been exposed to TB. Therefore, these persons should be considered infected with *M. tuberculosis* if they have a positive reaction to 5 TU of PPD tuberculin. They also should be evaluated for TB disease and managed accordingly.

## Preventive Therapy for TB Infection

Taken correctly by infected persons. preventive therapy can reduce the risk of TB by more than 90 per cent,. The recommended preventive therapy regimen is isoniazid (INH) at a dosage of 5 mg/kg daily for adults and 10 mg/kg daily for children to a maximum of 300 mg, for at least 6 continuous months for adults and 9 continuous months for children. For HIV-infected persons, preventive therapy is recommended for at least 12 months. Patients given preventive therapy should be monitored monthly for adherence to therapy and for drug side effects, especially the signs and symptoms of hepatitis.

## Diagnosis of TB Disease

The key to diagnosing TB in HIV-intected persons is to suspect it for persons with signs or symptoms suggestive of the disease: coughing up sputum or blood, weight loss, fatigues night sweats, and fever.

Persons who have a positive skin test result and persons with TB symptoms (regardless of the skin test result) should be evaluated with a chest radiograph to rule out pulmonary TB. Health care workers must be aware that TB may present in unusual ways in HIV-infected persons. For example, it may cause infiltrates in any lung zone with no cavities, or it may cause mediastinal or hilar lymphadenopathy. Almost any abnormality on a chest radiograph may indicate TB. The radiograph may even appear entirely normal, while sputum or lung fluid specimens are culture positive for *M. tuberculosis.*

Patients who have abnormal chest radiographs should have sputum specimens collected for acid-fast bacilli (AFB) examination. For this examination the specimen is smeared onto a glass slide and stained with a fluorochrome stain or a conventional stain (e.g., Ziehl-Neelsen or Kinyoun). Laboratory personnel use the microscope to look for AFB on the smear. AFB are bacteria that remain stained even after they have been washed in an acid solution. Tubercle bacilli are one kind of AFB. Fluorochrome stains offer two advantages over conventional stains: they make the AFB easier to see, and they allow slides to be examined much more quickly.

Because AFB are not always tubercle bacilli, patients who have positive smears do not necessarily have TB. Furthermore, patients who have negative smears may have TB because negative smears do not rule out the possibility of TB. A culture result that is positive for M. *tuberculosis* is the only definitive proof of TB disease. Nevertheless, TB treatment should be started if the smear is tound to be positive before the culture results are known. Drug susceptibility testing is recommended for the first *M. tuberculosis* isolate for all patients, and it should be performed on additional isolates if culture results remain positive after the patient has received 3 months of therapy or if the patient does not seem to respond to therapy. Drug susceptibility results should be promptly reported to the hcalth care provider and the health department.

## Contact Investigation

Contact investigation, one of the best ways to find persons who require treatment or preventive therapy for TB disease or infection, should begin as soon as a person is suspected of having TB. All new TB cases and suspected cases should be promptly reported to the health department by the health care provider. Early reporting is essential for the prompt evaluation of contacts of persons who have infectious TB. If a person's medical history and clinical findings suggest TB, health care workers should not wait for culture results before starting a contact investigation. Contact investigations are usually pertormed by the staff of health department TB control programmes, although hospital infection control officers and the staff of correctional and long-tenn care facilities may also conduct them.

Evaluations should be convenient for the contact. This may require that tuberculin testing and sputum collection be done in the field and that transportation to facilities be provided for radiographic and other examinations. The evaluation should proceed in an orderly manner, starting with persons who are most likely to have been infected, such as members of the patient's immediate family or others who have recently shared the same indoor environment with the source patient for prolonged periods. The highest priority should be given to rapidly examining close contacts who are children and persons who are HIV-infected because they are at high risk far active disease if infected with TB. For example, life-threatening TB meningitis or miliary TB can develop in newly infected children within weeks of infection unless preventive therapy is administered.

Close contacts of highly infectious persons, especially high-risk contacts (such as children and immunosuppressed persons), should be considered for preventive therapy even if their initial tuberculin skin test result is negative (less than S millimeters). A second skin test should be given 12 weeks after contact with the infectious person ended; if this result is also negative, preventive therapy may be stopped.

The HIV infection status of contacts alters the approach to both the investigation and the use of preventive therapy. Appropriate counseling and HIV testing for contacts whose HIV status is unknown is advisable. HIV-infected contacts should be considered fo preventive therapy, regardless of their tuberculin skin test results.

## HIV Counseling and Testing

Counseling is an integral part of HIV antibody testing programmes. The primary purposes of counseling and testing are to help uninfected individuals initiate and sustain behavioural changes that reduce their risk of becoming infected and to help infected individuals avoid infecting others. Pre- and post-test HIV counseling are available from specially trained health care workers in some TB control programmes or from facilities that provide these services, e.g., HIV testing and counseling centers, sexually transmitted disease (STD) clinics, and some primary care clinics. HIV counseling must be client-centered—that is, tailored to the behaviours, circumstances, and special needs of the person being served.

All persons suspected of having active TB or persons with a confirmed diagnosis of active TB should be asked about behaviours that increase the risk for HIV infection. Knowing the HIV antibody status of these persons is essential because TB skin test interpretation, preventive therapy, and treatment regimens for HIV-seropositive patients are different from those for HIV-seronegative patients. Because not all persons who engage in behaviours that put them at high risk for HIV infection will admit to these behaviours during an interview, all TB patients should be urged to have an HIV antibody test.

The HIV antibody test is not a test for AIDS; rather, it is a blood test that detects antibodies made by the body in response to infection with HIV. Persons who have a positive HIV antibody test result are infected with HIV, and they can infect others. Persons who have a negative test result probably are not infected with the virus. However, there is a slight chance that an HIV-infected person can test negative for antibodies because antibodies usually do not develop until 6 to 12 weeks after infection. Persons who test negative for HIV can become infected in the tuture if they engage in any high-risk behaviours. Informed consent should be obtained from all persons tested.

Some states mandate the reporting of all persons infected with HIV. Health care workers who perform HIV testing should learn about the laws and reporting procedures in their areas. Centers for Disease Control and Prevention (CDC) guidelines for HIV counseling and testing have been published and are available through the CDC National AIDS Clearinghouse ( 1 -800-458-5231).[6,7]

## Treatment of TB Disease

TB is usually curable if it is diagnosed early and if effective treatment is instituted without delay. TB must be treated for a long

TABLE -32.2
REGIMEN OPTIONS FOR THE TREATMENT OF TB IN CHILDREN AND ADULTS

| TB Without HIV Infection | | | TB With HIV Infection |
|---|---|---|---|
| Option 1 | Option 2 | Option 3 | |
| Administer daily INH, RIF, and PZA for 8 weeks followed by 16 weeks of INH and RIF daily or 2-3 times/week*. In areas where the INH resistance rate is not documented to <4%, EMB or SM should be added to the initial regimen until susceptibility to INH and RIF Is demonstrated. Continue treatment for at least 6 months and 3 months beyond culture conversion. Consult a TB medical expert if the patient is symptomatic or smear or culture positive after 3 months. | Administer daily INH, RIF, PZA, and SM or EMB for 2 weeks followed by 2 times/ week* administration of the same drugs for 6 weeks (by DoT§), and subsequently, 2 times/week administration of INH and RIF for 16 weeks (by DOT). Consult a TB medical expert if the patient is symptomatic or smear or culture positive after 3 months. | Treat by DOT, 3 times/week* with INH, RIF, PZA, and EMB or SM for 6 months.† Consult a TB medical expert if the patient is symptomatic or smear or culture positive after 3 months. | Options 1, 2, or 3 can be used, but treatment regimens should continue for a total of 9 months and at least 6 months beyond culture conversion. |

* All regimens administered 2 times/week or 3 times/week should be monitored by DOT for the duration of therapy.

† The strongest evidence from clinical trials is the effectiveness of all four drugs administered for the full 6 months. There is weaker evidence that SM can be discontinued after 4 months if the isolate is susceptible to all drugs. The evidence for stopping PZA before the end of 6 months is equivocal for the 3 times/week regimen, and there is no evidence on the effectiveness of this regimen with EMB for less than the full 6 months.

§ DOT—Directly observed therapy.

TABLE -32.3
Dosage Recommendations for the Treatment of TB in Children* and Adults
Dosage

| | Daily Dose | | Twice-Weekly Dose | | Thrice-Weekly Dose | |
|---|---|---|---|---|---|---|
| Drugs | Children | Adults | Children | Adults | Children | Adults |
| Isoniazid | 10-20mg/kg<br>Max. 300mg | 5 mg/kg<br>Max.300mg | 20-40mg/kg<br>Max. 900mg | 15 mg/kg<br>Max. 900mg | 20-40mg/kg<br>Max. 900mg | 15 mg/kg<br>Max. 900 mg |
| Rifampin | 10-20 mg/ kg<br>Max. 600 mg | 10 mg/kg<br>Max. 600 mg | 10-20 mg/kg<br>Max. 600 mg | 10 mg/kg<br>Max. 600 mg | 10-20 mg/kg<br>Max. 600 mg | 10 mg/kg<br>Max. 600 mg |
| Pyrazinamide | 15-30 mg/kg<br>Max. 2gm | 15-30 mg/kg<br>Max.2gm | 50-70 mg/kg | 50-70 mg/kg | 50-70 mg/kg | 50-70mg/kg |
| Ethambutol† | 15-25 mg/kg<br>Max. 2.5 gm | 15-25 mg/kg<br>Max. 2.5 gm | 50 mg/kg | 50 mg/kg | 25-30 mg/kg | 25-30 mg/kg |
| Streptomycin | 20-40 mg/kg<br>Max. 1gm | 15 mg/kg<br>Max. 1 gm | 25-30 mg/kg | 25-30 mg/kg | 25-30 mg/kg | 25-30 mg/kg |

* Children ⩽12 years of age.

† Ethambutol is generally not recommended for children whose visual acuity cannot be monitored (children <6 years of age). However, ethambutol should be considered for all children with organisms resistant to other drugs, if susceptibility to ethambutol has been demonstrated or susceptibility is likely.

time compared with most other infectious diseases. If treatment does not continue for a sufficient length of time (at least 6 months), enough tubercle bacilli may survive to make the patient ill and infectious again; also, ineffective treatment may foster the development of drug-resistant mycobacteria.

Because of the increase in drug-resistant TB, all TB patients should be given a fourdrug regimen of INH, rifampin (RIF), pyrazinamide (PZA), and ethambutol (EMB) or streptomycin (SM) until the drug susceptibility results are known. If the susceptibility results show no drug resistance, EMB or SM can be discontinued and the other drugs continued until PZA has been given for 2 months (initial phase). For HIV-negative persons, INH and RIF should then be continued for another 4 months (continuation phase), including at least 3 months of therapy after the culture results become negative. For HIV-positive persons, the continuation phase is 7 months; therapy should last a total of 9 months, including at least 6 months of therapy after the culture results become negative. In general, persons coinfected with TB and HIV respond well to TB treatment. Intermittent treatment regimens should be considered when giving daily therapy is impractical. Guidelines for the initial therapy of TB were updated and published in 1993.[8] Tables 32.2 and 32.3 (see pages 10 and 11) list regimen options and recommended dosages for the treatment of TB in adults and children.

Directly observed therapy (DOT) should be considered for all patients because of the difficulty in predicting which patients will adhere to a prescribed treatment regimen. DOT is the observation by a health care worker or other designated person of patients as they ingest anti-TB medications. The patient and provider should agree on an effective DOT routine that maintains the patient's Confidentiality and takes into account each patient's needs, living and employment conditions. and preferences. DOT can be arranged and administered in a variety of settings or locations, including TB clinics, community health centers, migrant clinics, homeless shelters, prisons or jails, nursing homes, schools, drug treatment centers, hospitals, HIV/AIDS clinics or living facilities, or occupational health clinics.

A variety of persons may administer DOT: physicians, nurses, health department personnel, health care aides, nursing home staff, correctional facility personnel, staff of community-based organizations, school nurses or teachers, staff of drug treatment centers, volunteers, social and welfare caseworkers, clergy, or other community leaders. Persons giving DOT who are not physicians or nurses should be supervised by a physician or a nurse. DOT can be given daily or intermittently (i.e., two or three times a week). Intermittent regimens are easier to implement than daily regimens, and they cost less. The use of incentives or enablers (such as transportation or car/bus fare to the DOT sites) may promote patient adherence to a DOT programme. When patients not receiving DOT demonstrate nonadherent behaviours (such as refusing pills or missing clinic appointments), the situation should be brought to the attention of the appropriate public health officials. These patients should be given DOT. Inadequate therapy is a major cause of multidrug-resistant TB.

Patients should be evaluated for and questioned about symptoms of drug toxicity at least once a month during therapy, even if no problems are apparent. Patients should be instructed to look for adverse reactions to the medications they are receiving. If symptoms suggestive of drug toxicity occur, appropriate laboratory testing and medical evaluation should be performed immediately. For patients treated with RIF who are also taking methadone, an increased methadone dosage may be necessary to avoid withdrawal symptoms caused by the interaction between the two drugs.[9]

The effectiveness of treatment can be evaluated by monitoring patients' sputum smear results. Also, sputum cultures should be obtained at least monthly until the results are negative. Appropriate consultation should be sought for patients whose smear or cut results do not convert to negative within 3 months. A positive sputum culture is the only definitive sign of treatment failure, and the persistence or reappearance of organisms in the smear should create a high index of suspicion.

As a general rule, regimens that are adequate for treating pulmonary TB in adults children are also effective for treating extrapulmonary disease. However, some experts recommend 9 months of therapy for patients with disseminated disease, miliary disease disease involving the bones or joints, or tuberculous lymphadenitis. Adjunctive therapies such as surgery and corticosteroids, may be used in some circumstances.

## MULTIDRUG-RESISTANT TB

An extremely serious aspect of the TB problem in the United States is the recent increase in multidrug-resistant TB (MDR TB). From 1990 through late 1992, CDC investigated eight outbreaks of MDR TB in hospitals and correctional facilities in New York Florida and New Jersey. These outbreaks have included almost 300 cases virtually all due to organisms resistant to both INH and RIF Some cases were due to organisms resistant to at least seven antituberculosis drugs. Most of the patients in these outbreaks were infected with HIV. Mortality among patients with MDR TB in these outbreaks ranged from 72 per cent to 89 per cent and the median intervals between TB diagnosis and death ranged from 4 to 16 weeks. The transmission ol MDR TB to health care workers and prison guards was documented in these outbreaks.

Some persons are at high risk for drug-resistant TB: persons who have been recently exposed to drug-resistant TB especially it they are immunocompromised; TB patients who failed to take medications as prescribed; TB patients who were prescribed an ineffective treatment regimen; and persons previously treated for TB. Clinicians who are not familiar with the management of patients who have MDR TB or patients who have been exposed to MDR TB should seek expert consultation.

## PREVENTION AND TREATMENT OF TB IN HEALTH CARE WORKERS

Health care facilities that provide care for patients at risk for TB should maintain active surveillance for TB among HCWs. All HCWs, including those with a history of BCG vaccination, should be given a Mantoux tuberculin skin test upon employment. For the initial tuberculin skin test, a two-step testing procedure is recommended. Two-step testing reduces the likelihood that a boosted skin test reaction will be interpreted as representing recent infection. If the reaction to the first tuberculin skin test is negative, a second test should be given 1 to 3 weeks later. If the reaction to this second test is positive, it probably represents a boosted reaction. Based on the second test result, the person should be classified as being TB infected or not and managed accordingly. HCWs known to have previous positive tuberculin test results or known to have completed adequate treatment or preventive therapy should be exempt from further screening unless they show symptoms suggestive of TB. HCWs should be educated about the signs and symptoms of TB and told to seek medical assistance promptly if these symptoms develop.

HCWs who have negative skin test results should be retested periodically to screen for new infection and disease. HCWs who may be exposed to patients with TB or who are involved in high-risk procedures (such as bronchoscopy) should be retested at least every 6 months. HCWs in other areas should be retested annually. Data on skin test conversions should be reviewed periodically to estimate the risk of acquiring new infection for each area of the facility. The frequency of retesting may be altered according to this analysis.

In addition to being screened periodically, HCWs should be evaluated for TB disease or infection if they have been exposed to a potentially infectious TB patient with whom recommended infection control procedures have not been taken. CDC has published guidelines for preventing the transmission of TB in health care settings.[10] HCWs who have been exposed to TB should be given a Mantoux tuberculin skin test as soon as possible after exposure. These HCWs should be managed in the same way as other contacts. If the initial skin test result is negative, the test should be repeated 12 weeks after the exposure ended. Exposed persons who have skin test reactions of 5 millimeters or greater or who have symptoms suggestive of TB should be evaluated with a chest radiograph. HIV infected HCWs may have a negative skin test result because of anergy. These persons should be given preventive therapy if they are likely to have been infected with TB after exposure. Persons known to have previous positive skin test reactions who have been exposed to an infectious patient do not require a repeat skin test or a chest radiograph unless they have symptoms suggestive of TB.

HCWs who have positive skin test results but who do not have active TB should be evaluated for their risk of HIV infection and considered for preventive therapy. If HIV infection is considered a possibility, counseling and HIV antibody testing should be strongly encouraged.

HCWs with pulmonary or laryngeal TB pose a risk to patients and to other employees while they are infectious. Therefore, they should be restricted from work until they begin receiving adequate treatment, they are no longer coughing, and they have three consecutive negative sputum smears. HCWs who are receiving preventive therapy for TB infection do not pose a risk to others, and they should be allowed to continue their usual work activities.

*Remember! The key to preventing TB infection, disability from TB disease, and death is to consider the diagnosis of TB in high-risk groups, make the diagnosis as quickly as possible, and initiate effective, directly observed therapy for persons found to have TB.*

## References

1. Centers for Disease Control and Prevention. 1993 revised classification system for HIV infection and expanded surveillance case definition for AIDS among adolescents and adults. *MMWR.* 1992;41 (No.RR-17): 1-19.
2. Centers for Disease Control. Purified protein derivative (PPD)-tuberculin anergy and HIV infection: guidelines for anergy testing and management of anergic persons at risk of tuberculosis. *MMWR.* 1991 ;40() (No. RR-5): 1-5.
3. Curran JW, Chamberland M. Epidemiology and prevention of AIDS and HIV infection. In: Mandell GL Douglas RG, Bennett JE. eds. *Principles and Practice of Infections Diseases* 3rd ed. New York, NY: Churchill Livingston; 1990:1029-1046.
4. Hutton MD, Stead WW, Cauthen GM, Bloch AB, Ewing WM. Nosocomial

transmission of tuberculosis associated with a draining abscess. *J Infest Dis.* 1990; 161:286-295.

5. Frampton MW. An outbreak of tuberculosis among hospital personnel caring for a patient with a skin ulcer. *Ann Intern Med.* 1992;117:312-313.
6. Centers for Disease Control and Prevention. Technical guidance on HIV counseling. *MMWR.* 1993;42(No. RR-2):8-17.
7. Centers for Disease Control. Public Health Service guidelines for counseling and antibody testing to prevent HIV infection and AIDS. *MMWR.* 1987;36(No. 31):509-515.
8. Centers for Disease Control and Prevention. Initial therapy for tuberculosis in the era of multidrug resistance: recommendations of the Advisory Council for the Elimination of Tuberculosis. *MMWR* 1993;42(No. RR-7):1-8.
9. Kreek MJ. Garfield JW, Gutjahr CL. Ginsti LM. Rif, ampin-induced methadone withdrawal. Engl. J Med 1976;294: 1104-6.
10. Centers for Disease Control. Guidelines for preventing the transmission of tuberculosis in health care settings, with special focus on HIV-related issues. *MMWR.* 1990;39(No. RR-17): 1-29.

33

# HIV Testing Policies and Guidelines

WHO-Regional Office for South-East Asia
New Delhi, India

## INTRODUCTION

The Acquired Immune Deficiency Syndrome (AIDS) was first recognized in the United States in 1981. The etiological agent, Human Immunodeficiency Virus (HIV), was isolated in 1984 and a laboratory test for HIV became commercially available the following year. This enabled health care workers to diagnose HIV infection, individuals to know whether or not they were HIV infected, and most importantly, medical science to understand HIV/AIDS better. The availability of these tests has also led to misconceptions regarding the role of HIV testing. These misconceptions were particularly witnessed worldwide during the early stages of the epidemic, and not unexpectedly are presently being noted in a number of countries in Asia. Many individuals, particularly health care workers, seem to believe that the spread of HIV can be controlled by identifying people with HIV infection, and testing of hospital patients or groups of people practising high risk behaviour are often advocated. This paper discusses some issues related to the use and appropriateness of HIV testing in the overall context of national AIDS control programmes.

## PURPOSE OF HIV TESTING

Compared to any other type of disease, the issues related to the diagnosis of HIV infection are far more complex AIDS is invariably fatal and infection is lifelong. No drugs are available to cure AIDS or to render an HIV-infected person non-infectious. Since HIV is spread mainly through sexual contact, individuals known to be infected with HIV are unfortunately often stigmatized and discriminated against. Such a situation results from the lack of proper understanding regarding the mode of transmission, particularly the fact that HIV infection cannot be transmitted by casual social contact or through the respiratory route . Unlike other diseases, identification of people with HIV infection or AIDS, therefore, is neither rational nor appropriate.

HIV testing is recommended by the World Health Organization (WHO) only for selected purposes.[1] These include (1) screening of blood including blood products, and organs and tissues for transplantation; (2) epidemiological surveillance, particularly HIV sentinel surveillance using unlinked anonymous HIV testing methodology where all personal details of the person being tested are removed from the blood samples so that the results of HIV testing cannot be linked with the identity of the person—the specific purposes of testing in these situations are to ensure blood safety or to conduct epidemiological surveillance respectively; (3) diagnosis of symptomatic infection among those clinically suspected of having AIDS; and finally (4) early diagnosis of HIV infection among asymptomatic persons who would like to know their HIV status. In the latter two situations HIV testing is carried out with informed consent and with strict maintenance of confidentiality. No situation other than the four listed above warrant HIV testing, and there is no place in national AIDS prevention and control programmes for testing without informed consent. Experience shows that any kind of HIV testing without the full and informed consent of the person concerned is counter-productive as well as wasteful of resources.

## PUBLIC HEALTH RATIONALE AGAINST MANDATORY TESTING

Public health rationale should always be kept in mind when testing of any population group including foreigners, refugees, hospital patients or individuals engaged in high risk behaviour is contemplated. The 45th World Health Assembly, to which all countries were signatory, noted that "there is no public health rationale for any measures that limit the rights of the individual, notably measures establishing mandatory screening".[2] Studies and public health experience have also shown that HIV testing carried out on a voluntary basis and with appropriate counselling is more likely to promote behaviour change than mandatory testing.[3] Furthermore, mandatory testing measures can be counter-productive because they tend to drive those at high risk of HIV infection "Underground, as a result of which such persons do not have access to education and counselling programmes". Such initiatives not only damage the credibility of the health services, but also create a false sense of security among the general public that all HIV-infected persons are known and that there is no need to take necessary precautions. From the cost point of view, testing is an expensive business, not only to National AIDS Programmes because of the high cost of HIV kits but also to individuals from the psychological point of view when the results of HIV testing are inadvertently disclosed and confidentiality is not always maintained. Additional details addressesing the question "Can mandatory HIV testing stop the AIDS epidemic?".

## HIV TESTING IN HEALTH CARE SETTINGS

Many health care workers, however, seem to mistakenly believe in programmes of mandatory HIV testing or of testing without consent because of the fear of contracting HIV in the health care setting. Although there is a risk of HIV being transmitted in these settings, this risk is very small. For example, in the United States, more than 250,000 patients have so far been diagnosed as having AIDS, including 8,467 cases among health care workers of which only six (0.07 per cent) were due to occupational transmission[4]. While thousands of needle stick injuries occur every year, only 33 documented HIV infections have so far resulted from occupational injuries in the health care setting. In studies of health care workers who were exposed to HIV through needle stick injuries, the risk has been shown to be less than 0.4 per cent.[4,5] The risk of HIV transmission following mucous membrane or skin exposure to HIV infected blood, body fluids or tissues is even lower. Based on such data, testing of ambulatory or hospitalized patients for HIV on a routine basis for HIV has not been adopted as a general policy in the United States or other countries with prolonged experience of HIV/AIDS, and is not recommended by WHO. Rather, the application of universal precautions in infection control procedures is recommended as the best way to minimize HIV transmission in the health care setting.

In spite of this, there have been a number of situations where patients attending health facilities have been or are being tested for HIV. For example, many advocate testing in antenatal clinics on the notion that women may want to know whether they are infected in order to make a decision regarding having a baby. It has, however, been seen that such women, after having been provided counselling, are likely to participate in testing voluntarily. Moreover, routine testing of pregnant women may discourage many women from attending antenatal clinics because of the fear of being tested without their knowledge. Experience in other countries shows that relatively few women elect to have an abortion when they are properly informed and counselled (Kervin O'Reilly, personat Communication). Similarly, testing of patients attending hospital, particularly for surgery, cannot be justified.

Should patients with STDs be tested for HIV routinely? This issue has been much debated because of the close association between STD and AIDS. The consensus among the international scientific community is that all STD patients should be offered appropriate counselling and STD care without having to resort to mandatory HIV testing. If HIV testing is at all required and/or asked for, this can be provided through voluntary testing with appropriate pre- and post-test counselling. From the economics point of view, any requirements for HIV testing are likely to constitute additional burdens to STD control programmes as the cost of HIV tests would add to the already high costs of STD drugs.

Regarding the testing of blood donors, WHO advocates the concept of screening of donated blood rather than the testing of donors.[6] This in essence means that blood samples are subjected to antibody testing and those found positive are discarded without relating the test to the individual. However, if blood donors are to be tested for HIV and if they are to be notified of the results, they must know in advance that the blood is to be tested for HIV and they should give their informed consent to testing. This also entails provision of pre- and post-test counselling. There is, however, a danger that if blood banks offer facilities for HIV testing, many people, including those with high risk behaviour, may use these services to determine their HIV status thus compromising/endangering the safety of blood. In summary, the only roles that HIV testing can play in the health care setting are to assist in the diagnosis of HIV infection in patients with clinical signs compatible with AIDS and to offer voluntary testing services to people who wish to know their HIV status. In both the situations, the testing should be voluntary with provision of adequate pre- as well as post-test counselling.

## VOLUNTARY TESTING AND COUNSELLING

Voluntary HIV testing always in conjunction with counselling has a place in national AIDS control programmes within the comprehensive range of measures for HIV/AIDS prevention, care and supports[7]. HIV testing, to be beneficial, should however be entirely voluntary and anonymous, with no possibility of breech of confidentiality. Voluntary HIV testing should be part of a comprehensive counselling programme which provides support services such as condoms and treatment for STDs. It should however be noted that counselling on its own is a valuable intervention even if HIV testing is not available or if the person decides not to be tested.

The current availability in the Asian region of HIV/AIDS counselling, of voluntary HIV testing and of HIV counselling and voluntary testing is limited, with the exception of Thailand. In countries where these services are not yet widely available, their introduction should proceed cautiously in order to ensure that confidentiality or anonymity is guaranteed and that the services are delivered in a manner most likely to result in benefits to the individual and to public health.

In conclusion, HIV testing has an important role to play in national AIDS control programmes. However, it should be carried out in a rational manner and without resort to coercive approaches. Mandatory testing or testing without informed consent is not only counter productive but also wasteful of scarce resources. The spread of HIV cannot be controlled by mandatory testing of hospital patients or high risk groups in the population; such efforts have failed everywhere they have been tried. HiV testing should be carried out only for those purposes which are specific objectives of National AIDS Control Programmes.

## SOME QUESTIONS AND ANSWERS ON HIV TESTING POLICIES AND GUIDELINES

### Can Mandatory HIV Testing Stop the AIDS Epidemic?

Forcing someone to undergo medical testing of any kind is an invasion of privacy and a violation of human rights. This is a fundamental reason why WHO and its member countries have taken a strong position against forced testing for HIV. But what about protecting the health of the public? The following Questions & Answers explain why compulsory HIV testing, far from protecting the public health, can actually endanger it. They have been contributed as the first of an occasional series by Suzanne Cherney, GPA's communications scientist, who encourages readers to suggest topics for exploration in future issues of Global AIDS news.

Q. **Some people say that the reason AIDS continues to spread is that we aren't aggressive enough about finding out who is infected with the human immunodeficiency virus (HIV). Shouldn't we be testing everyone for HIV—if necessary, against their will?**

A. If a person tests positive for HIV, it means that he or she has HIV infection and, scientists believe, will ultimately develop AIDS—a fatal disease for which there is at present no cure. But this can take 10 or even 15 years, and some people would prefer to live those healthy years without knowing their diagnosis. In addition, people with HIV infection or AIDS can suffer exclusion, discrimination and even persecution. *So testing for HIV is a very serious matter.*

**People who are counselled about the personal and social implications of taking an HIV test can of course decide to be tested voluntarily. But forcing someone to undergo HIV testing is a highly coercive, intrusive measure.**

**Q. But why worry only about the infected people? Surely compulsory testing is justified in the case of a fatal epidemic disease?**

A. There are a number of reasons why compulsory testing for HIV makes no sense. To begin with, *testing someone for HIV just gives you a diagnosis, and a diagnosis alone never stopped an epidemic.* Testing only helps if there are ways of breaking the chain of transmission. For example, when you test donated blood prior to transfusion and discard the infected blood, you are helping to prevent the spread of the virus. The testing of blood for transfusion, and of tissues or organs for transplantation, is the only area where testing needs to be compulsory.

**Q. Testing has helped contain other infections diseases. Why not AIDS?**

A. Because HIV is different. There is no drug available that can cure the infection or make the person uninfectious—that is, incapable of transmitting the virus to another person. And once a person is infected with HIV, it's for life. A person who tests positive for syphilis can be cured with a short course of antibiotics. A person diagnosed with tuberculosis can be made uninfectious with antibiotics. When someone tests positive for meningitis, the individuals in close contact with him or her can be treated and/or vaccinated. With HIV, there is no medical way to "test and treat" or "test and vaccinate" so as to break the chain of transmission.

**Q. Yes, but people with HIV are nevertheless a danger to others. They could be isolated.**

A. They don't need to be, because HIV infection is not "contagious" in the usual sense. Unlike tuberculosis, it doesn't spread through coughing. Unlike typhoid, it can't be transmitted through food or water. You can't catch HIV from swimming with an infected person, or sharing an office or home, or drinking from the same cup. So locking up infected people is not justified or practical. It's not even necessary isolate HIV-infected people when they're hospitalized.

We all have a responsibility to look after ourselves. And the fact that HIV spreads mainly through sexual intercourse means that uninfected people are not defenseless against the virus. They have ways of protecting themselves from HIV without locking up the infected individuals. They can abstain from sex, stay faithful to an uninfected partner, engage in sex without penetration, or else use a condom every time for sexual intercourse.

Q. **Still, if we could screen the whole population through compulsory testing and then isolate the infected people for life, it might stop the epidemic.**

A. Mass HIV testing sounds straightforward.. In practice, it's extremely costly, logistically unwieldy, incapable of identifying everyone who is infected, and fraught with problems that could be avoided by offering voluntary tests and guaranteeing the confidentiality of the test results.

Logistically, it's impossible to take blood samples from everyone, test them, and give everyone their results on the same day. So, even if the authorities managed to trace all infected people (clearly, many won't turn up voluntarily to find out their test results) and isolate them, this wouldn't prevent sexual contact between the uninfected and those who have yet to be tested.

And even if these logistic obstacles could somehow be eliminated, no mandatory testing programme can expect to identify all HIV-infected people. Individuals who think they might be infected can go to extremes to avoid testing and follow-up, given the serious consequences of a positive HIV test—especially when there is a threat of isolation.

Not all HIV-infected people will be identified even if they are tested. Most commercially available HIV tests work by detecting not the virus itself but antibodies to the virus which the person's immune system produces following infection with HIV. But it takes up to 12 weeks, or sometimes more, for those HIV antibodies to be produced and become detectable in a blood sample. This is the "window period" during which the infected person continues to test negative.

At best, an HIV test result is a "snapshot" of someone's infection status today. It's no guarantee that he or she won't become infected tomorrow, or next week or month —and how often can people be tested?

In any case, periodic testing of the entire population is prohibitively expensive in terms of staff time, transport of blood samples, and so on. (The actual HIV test kits account for only a fraction of the total costs). in many developing countries, testing the whole population just once would cost more than the government is able to spend on all health care in a year.

Q. **Surely some countries have attempted to test everyone?**

A. No. The financial and logistic impossibility of testing the whole population periodically has been recognized even by the few countries that have devoted most of their AIDS budget to testing. And most of these now realize that instead of mandatory testing—which failed to stop the epidemic—they should use their resources for preventive measures of proven effectiveness, such as informing the general public about HIV transmission, making condoms cheap and accessible, providing school-based education for young people, and ensuring blood safety.

Q. **Even if you can't identify and trace all infected people, you could at least isolate the ones you find.**

A. Apart from being a serious violation of human rights, lifetime isolation would be an unnecessary economic burden on the individuals' families and on society. In many places in Africa, and increasingly in Asia, 10 per cent or more of all young adults are infected. Isolation means forfeiting their economic productivity during the decade or so of good health that these young adults can expect. It means depriving their families of breadwinners and care-givers. And it means keeping thousands or even millions of fit individuals fed, clothed and looked after for years on end—at government expense.

Q. **I am still concerned about all the healthy people walking around with HIV who don't even know they have the virus. Granted that isolation makes no sense and that there is no medical way of curing them or making them uninfectious. Compulsory testing would at least force them to find out their diagnosis and take precautions against transmitting the virus to others.**

A. In other words, won't people who learn they are HIV-infected through compulsory testing simply avoid unsafe sex from then on? To begin with, not even voluntary counselling and testing achieves a uniformity "preventive" effect. When testing is purely voluntary, and people are presumably well motivated to protect themselves and their loved ones, the evidence shows that some infected people manage to change their sexual behaviour, others do not.*

* *(For example, helpful behaviour change (increased condom use) in couples who seek voluntary testing together and find out that just one of them is HIV infected).*

Is compulsory testing likely to be more effective than this in achieving behaviour change? On the contrary. First of all, someone who is forced to and out he or she is infected may have less interest in protecting others—or even in self-protection (safer sex protects both partners). But the main point is that a permanent, lifelong change in sexual behaviour isn't achieved automatically or quickly. The consistent use of condoms, for example, takes continuing motivation, will power, personal commitment. It takes the availability of inexpensive and readily accessible condoms. And for someone in a long-term relationship, it takes the full co-operation of the other partner. *The bottom line is that HIV prevention rests on the individual's willingness to avoid unsafe behaviour. Will power and motivation can't be coerced.* You don't gain people's voluntary co-operation by forcing them to be tested.

Q. **True, but even if the infected person doesn't voluntarily adopt safer behaviour, at least other people can be warned...**

A. Who? Medical test results are supposed to remain confidential. Imagine how suspicious we would be of doctors if they turned into law enforcement officers ! We'd stop seeking medical help for a whole range of problems if we thought our diagnoses would be handed out.

This doesn't mean that voluntary contact tracing is useless, though with HIV it's far less useful than for syphilis or gonorrhoea, where the sexual contact can be tested, treated and cured. But it's obvious that people infected with HIV will be less likely to volunteer information about their sex partners if they suspect that those individuals in turn may be forced into testing. Once again, making the test mandatory instead of voluntary makes it less rather than more effective.

Suppose an infected man refuses to use condoms or tell his wife about the infection. What will happen if the health care provider doesn't keep the diagnosis confidential but goes ahead and informs her? The wife might decide to leave the relationship, assuming she is economically able to do so. But while that might help her (if she is still uninfected), there are two reasons why it might endanger the public health. First, her rejected husband may well and new sex partners—and the epidemic will continue to spread. Or, if she is infected but doesn't know it, she might infect her new partners. Secondly, there is ample evidence that in places where test results aren't kept strictly confidential, people simply avoid HIV testing and continue to behaves though they were not infected. Helpful behaviour change that might have occurred as a result of voluntary counselling and testing is thus forfeited.

Q. **In some places, couples have to get tested for syphilis before marrying. Why not for HIV?**

A. Even with syphilis, a curable disease, experience from around the world shows that mandatory premarital screening has little or no impact on the public health. For HIV, mandatory testing makes even less sense. First, fear of a compulsory test will dissuade many couples from marrying where such a requirement exists—a disadvantage that voluntary test doesn't entail. Second, why pick the time of marriage? People often begin their sexual experimentation well before that. (indeed, if premarital sex were rate, testing before marriage would turn up virtually no positive HIV results!). And, most important sex with other partners can and does take place after marriage. For the many people whose mason risk of HIV is their partner's extramarital activity, a negative premarital test offers no protection—just an illusion of safety.

Q. **But HIV can be transmitted from an infected woman to her fetus or newborn. Wouldn't it be helpful at least to insist on testing all pregnant women?**

A. Once a woman is pregnant the fetus may well be infected already although there is no way to know this. At this stage the only possibilities for prevention are abortion, a decision not to breast-feed (although in many settings bottle-feeding may be more risky for the baby, or perhaps treatment with an antiviral drug around the time of delivery (this is still experimental). All these are major decision which cannot be forced on any woman but which she must take, if at all, voluntarily. Therefore, voluntary counselling and testing is what should be offered. Forced testing may also dissuade pregnant women from seeking medical care.

In any case, the best time for prevention is prior to pregnancy. Married or unmarried people need to be aware of all the implications of HIV infection before they decide whether to have children.

Q. **Some employers test job applicants before hiring them. Does that make sense?**

A. No. It won't protect the general public. And it won't protect the firm's employees because HIV infection is not "contagious" and doesn't spread at the workplace. The emphasis in any form should be on preventing infections among the existing workforce, which is always far larger than the number of new staff recruited each year. Some employers provide their workers with AIDS education, encouragement for condom use, and care for sexually transmitted diseases (STDs) such as syphilis and chancroid, which if left untreated greatly increase a person's susceptibility to HIV infection. They report a decrease in STD rates among their employees, which is good news on two counts. It means employees are less likely to get HIV and, for companies that offer or reimburse STD care, it means a decrease in company expenditure.

**Q. I can see why forcing ordinary people to be tested is useless. What about restricting compulsory testing to high-risk groups?**

A. At first sight this seems more practical than compulsory testing of the general population testing of the general population, but in fact it's got even more problems. To begin with, many such groups are hard to define, and even harder to locate. For example, men who have unprotected sex with prostitutes are clearly at high risk - but how do you identify them? And where do you draw the line? At those who seek out a sex worker twice a year? Or those who do so every payday? And what about their wives - are they a high-risk group to be tested? In many places, after all, most women with HIV have been infected by their one partner—their husband.

**Q. One well defined group, at least, is drug users who inject their drugs. Isn't it true that they are at high risk of acquiring HIV?**

A. Yes. If they don't use new or freshly sterilized equipment every time they inject, they can easily become infected—and pass the virus on to their sex partners. So the most urgent need is to reach them to clean their equipment carefully each time, never share it with anyone, or exchange their used syringes for sterile ones—and to encourage them to use condoms for sex. (Over the longer term, they need encouragement to switch from drug injecting to safer forms of drug use, or no drug use at all). These socalled "harm reduction" measures are clearly vital for the public health as well as for the users themselves.

The biggest hurdle for harm-reduction programmes is that drug users live on the margins of society. Almost everywhere, drug use is secretive or frankly illegal, and users are mistrustful of authorities. In many places, health workers have to persuade the local police not to arrest drug users who come in for education, new syringes, bleach or condoms. Any threat of mandatory HIV testing would scare them away even more, doom the harm-reduction programmes to failure, and endanger the public health.

Q. **Shouldn't we at least insist that sex workers be HIV-negative?**

A. This is yet another idea that sounds fine in theory but works poorly in practice. Compulsory testing is as counterproductive for prostitutes as it is for drug users. Authorities need to work with prostitutes, not against them. They need to strengthen their ability to demand condom use by clients. (This is the standard harm-reduction measure for commercial sex work). if prostitutes are harassed an driven away by the threat of mandatory testing, they will be out of reach of effective harm-reduction programmes.

Prostitutes who can't escape testing and turn out to be HIV-positive may be fired (if they work in a brothel) or lose their registration. But this doesn't protect the public health. Infected individuals will simply move on to another place. Where there is a system of registration, the infected sex workers will join the ranks of unofficial prostitutes, who generally have even less power to negotiate safer sex. Testing doesn't even protect the local clients. No matter how many "condom only" signs are posted, any brothel owner (or government official) who insists on testing sex workers - and lets the clients know that they are HIV-negative—is sending a clear message that if a client doesn't want to use a condom, he'll still be safe. Of course, the client may well be infected himself and infect the prostitute, who will then infect others who decide not to use a condom, and so on. Testing sex workers even as often as every 3 months still means that, because of the "window period", they can have HIV for nearly half a year—and infect many clients—before their infection is diagnosed.

Q. **You may well ask, why test the prostitutes and not their clients?**

A. From the standpoint of common decency, it's just as important to safeguard sex workers as sex work clients. From the standpoint of public health, protecting the prostitutes is even more important. Besides, there's something illogical about putting the responsibility for HIV prevention and safe sex on the sex worker. After all, in almost all cases, whether the prostitute is male or female, it's the client who has to wear the condom!

If condom use by men is the key, why not try to test STD patients systematically for HIV? After all, they're mostly men. And by coming down with a disease like syphilis or chancroid, they have proven that they are engaging in unsafe sex and are at risk of HIV.

There's no doubt that men (and women) with an STD are a very important "audience" indeed when it comes to HIV prevention. Attendance at a clinic or doctor's office provides the ideal opportunity for educating them about AIDS and condom promotion — just at the time they are confronted with evidence of their vulnerability to all STDs. But people with an STD need encouragement to seek care at the earliest possible sign of disease. Any threat of mandatory testing would frighten them away.

Q. **So compulsory testing can't even help with people who engage in high-risk behaviour?**

A. No. When it comes to drug injectors, sex workers and STD patients, mandatory HIV testing has nothing to recommend it—and multiple disadvantages as compared with voluntary testing. First, people are hard to track down for compulsory testing, and expensive to trace for follow-up. Then, what do you achieve? When you and infected individuals, you can't isolate them for life or enforce behaviour change. Indeed, voluntary testing is more likely to result in the adoption of safe behaviour.

Not only are the "benefits" of compulsory testing illusory, but the side effects are a positive danger to the public health. The main ones are driving vulnerable people away from harm-reduction and other prevention programmes, and encouraging a false sense of HIV-free security in the general population. Voluntary testing hasn't got these disadvantages. Hence, there's nothing to be gained for the public health, and much to be lost, by making HIV tests compulsory instead of voluntary and confidential .

Q. **Aren't coercive measures ever necessary?**

A. Yes. It is occasionally necessary to override people's individual rights in the interests of public health. For example, WHO recommended obligatory vaccination against smallpox until it was eradicated, and still endorses the need for mandatory vaccination against yellow fever for people travelling from zones where this disease is endemic. If one day a medicine is found that can make HIV-infected people noninfectious to others, WHO will re-examine its policy on HIV testing. For the moment, AIDS happens to be a disease for which coercive testing is not only pointless but harmful to the public health.

In the AIDS era, there is no way to sideline the infected people so that everyone else can go on living as before. Today, everyone has a responsibility to avoid unsafe behaviour.

## References


1. WHO Global Programme on AIDS. Recommendations for the selection and use of HIV antibody tests, Weekly Epidemiological Record No. 20, 1992, p.145-149.
2. World Health Assembly Resolution 45.35, 14 May 1992
3. WHO Global Programme on AIDS. Global strategy for the prevention and control of AIDS, 1992 update. AIDS Series No.12.
4. Ciesielski C. et al. Occupationally acquired HIV infection - United States. 9th International Conference on AIDS, Berlin, 1993 (Abstract WS-c12-1).
5. Report of a WHO Consultation on the Prevention of Human immunodeficiency Virus and Hepatitis B virus transmission in the Health Care Setting, Geneva, 11-12 April 1991.
6. Gobal Blood Safety initiative. Consensus statement on screening of blood donations for infectious agents transmissible through blood transfusion, Geneva, 30 Jan.-1 Feb..1990. WHO/LBS/91.1.
7. WHO Global Programme on AIDS. Statement from the consultation on Testing and Counselling for HIV infection, Geneva, 16-18 November 1992. WHO/GPA/INF/93.2.

# 34

# Universal Precautions for Prevention of Transmission of Human Immunodeficiency Virus, Hepatitis B Virus, and Other Bloodborne Pathogens in Health-Care Settings

## INTRODUCTION

The purpose of this report is to clarify and supplement the CDC publication entitled "Recommendations for Prevention of HIV Transmission in Health-Care Settings"[1].

In 1983, CDC published a document entitled "Guideline for Isolation Precautions in Hospitals"[2] that contained a section entitled "Blood and Body Fluid Precautions." The recommendations in this section called for blood and body fluid precautions when a patient was known or suspected to be infected with bloodborne pathogens. In August 1987, CDC published a document entitled "Recommendations for Prevention of HIV Transmission in Health-Care Settings"[1]. In contrast to the 1983 document, the 1987 document recommended that blood and body fluid precautions be consistently used for all patients regardless of their bloodborne infection status. This extension of blood and body fluid precautions to *all* patients is referred to as "Universal Blood and Body Fluid Precautions" or "Universal Precautions." Under universal precautions, blood and certain body fluids of all patients are considered potentially infectious for human immunodeficiency virus (HIV), hepatitis B virus (HBV), and other bloodborne pathogens.

Universal precautions are intended to prevent parenteral, mucous membrane, and nonintact skin exposures of health-care workers to bloodborne pathogens. In addition, immunization with HBV vaccine is recommended as an important adjunct to universal precautions for health-care workers who have exposures to blood [3,4].

Since the recommendations for universal precautions were published in August 1987, CDC and the Food and Drug Administration (FDA) have received requests for clarification of the following issues: (1) body fluids to which universal precautions apply, (2) use of protective barriers, (3) use of gloves for phlebotomy, (4) selection of gloves for use while observing universal precautions, and (5) need for making changes in waste management programmes as a result of adopting universal precautions.

## Body Fluids to Which Universal Precautions Apply

Universal precautions apply to blood and to other body fluids containing visible blood. Occupational transmission of HIV and HBV to health-care workers by blood is documented [4,5]. Blood is the single most important source of HIV, HBV, and other bloodborne pathogens in the occupational setting. Infection control efforts for HIV, HBV, and other bloodborne pathogens must focus on preventing exposures to blood as well as on delivery of HBV immunization.

Universal precautions also apply to semen and vaginal secretions. Although both of these fluids have been implicated in the sexual transmission of HIV and HBV, they have not been implicated in occupational transmission from patient to health-care worker. This observation is not unexpected, since exposure to semen in the usual health-care setting is limited, and the routine practice of wearing gloves for performing vaginal examinations protects health-care workers from exposure to potentially infectious vaginal secretions.

Universal precautions also apply to tissues and to the following fluids: cerebrospinal fluid (CSF), synovial fluid, pleural fluid, peritoneal fluid, pericardial fluid, and amniotic fluid. The risk of transmission of HIV and HBV from these fluids is unknown; epidemiologic studies in the health-care and community setting are currently inadequate to assess the potential risk to health-care workers from occupational exposures to them. However, HIV has been isolated from CSF, synovial, and amniotic fluid [6-8], and HBsAg has been detected in synovial fluid, amniotic fluid, and peritoneal fluid.[9-11] One case of HIV transmission was reported after a percutaneous exposure to bloody pleural fluid obtained by needle aspiration.[12] Whereas aseptic procedures used to obtain these fluids for diagnostic or therapeutic purposes protect health-care workers from skin exposures, they cannot prevent penetrating injuries due to contaminated needles or other sharp instruments.

## Body Fluids to Which Universal Precautions Do Not Apply

Universal precautions do not apply to feces, nasal secretions, sputum, sweat, tears, urine, and vomitus unless they contain visible blood. The risk of transmission of HIV and HBV from these fluids and materials is extremely low or nonexistent. HIV has been isolated and HBsAg has been demonstrated in some of these fluids; however, epidemiologic studies in the health-care and community setting have not implicated these fluids or materials in the transmission of HIV and HBV infections.[13,14] Some of the above fluids and excretions represent a potential source for nosocomial and community-acquired infections with other pathogens, and recommendations for preventing the transmission of nonbloodborne pathogens have been published. [2]

## Precautions for Other Body Fluids in Special Settings

Human breast milk has been implicated in perinatal transmission of HIV, and HBsAg has been found in the milk of mothers infected with HBV.[10,13] However, occupational exposure to human breast milk has not been implicated in the transmission of HIV nor HBV infection to health-care workers. Moreover, the health-care worker will not have the same type of intensive exposure to breast milk as the nursing neonate. Whereas universal precautions do not apply to human breast milk, gloves may be worn by health-care workers in situations where exposures to breast milk might be frequent, for example, in breast milk banking.

Saliva of some persons infected with HBV has been shown to contain HBV-DNA at concentrations 1/1,000 to 1/10,000 of that found in the infected person's serum.[15] HBsAg-positive saliva has been shown to be infectious when injected into experimental animals and in human bite exposures.[16,18] However, HBs Ag-positive saliva has not been shown to be infectious when applied to oral mucous membranes in experimental primate studies[18] or through contamination of musical instruments or cardiopulmonary resuscitation dummies used by HBV carriers [19.20]. Epidemiologic studies of nonsexual household contacts of HIV-infected patients, including several small series in which HIV transmission failed to occur after bites or after percutaneous inoculation or contamination of cuts and open wounds with saliva from HIV-infected patients, suggest that the potential for salivary transmission of HIV is remote. [5,13,14,21,22] One case report from Germany has suggested the possibility of transmission of HIV in a household setting from an infected child to a sibling through a human bite [23]. The bite did not break the skin or result in bleeding. Since the date of seroconversion to HIV was not known for either child in this case, evidence for the role of saliva in the transmission of virus is unclear. [23] Another case report suggested the possibility of transmission of HIV from husband to wife by contact with saliva during kissing. [24] However, follow-up studies did not confirm HIV infection in the wife [21].

Universal precautions do not apply to saliva. General infection control practices already in existence—including the use of gloves for digital examination of mucous membranes and endotracheal suctioning, and handwashing after exposure to saliva —should further minimize the minute risk, if any, for salivary transmission of HIV and HBV[1,25]. Gloves need not be worn when feeding patients and when wiping saliva from skin.

Special precautions, however, are recommended for dentistry[1]. Occupationally acquired infection with HBV in dental workers has been documented[4], and two possible cases of occupationally acquired HIV infection involving dentists have been reported [5,26]. During dental procedures, contamination of saliva with blood is predictable, trauma to health-care workers' hands is common, and blood spattering may occur. Infection control precautions for dentistry minimize the potential for nonintact skin and mucous membrane contact of dental health-care workers to blood-contaminated saliva of patients. In addition, the use of gloves for oral examinations and treatment in the dental setting may also protect the patient's oral mucous membranes from exposures to blood, which may occur from breaks in the skin of dental workers' hands.

## Use of Protective Barriers

Protective barriers reduce the risk of exposure of the health-care worker's skin or mucous membranes to potentially infective materials. For universal precautions, protective barriers reduce the risk of exposure to blood, body fluids containing visible blood, and other fluids to which universal precautions apply. Examples of protective barriers include gloves, gowns, masks, and protective eyewear. Gloves should reduce the incidence of contamination of hands, but they cannot prevent penetrating injuries due to needles or other sharp instruments. Masks and protective eyewear or face shields should reduce the incidence of contamination of mucous membranes of the mouth, nose, and eyes.

Universal precautions are intended to supplement rather than replace recommendations for routine infection controt such as handwashing and using gloves to prevent gross microbial contamination of hands. [27] Because specifying the types of barriers needed for every possible clinical situation is impractical, some judgment mum be exercised.

The risk of nosocomial transmission of HIV, HBV, and other

bloodborne pathogens can be minimized if health-care workers use the following general guidelines:*

1 Take care to prevent injuries when using needles, scalpels, and other sharp instruments or devices when handling sharp instruments aher procedures; when deaning used instruments; and when disposing of used needles Do not recap used needles by hand; do not remove used needles from disposable syringes by hand; and do not bend, break, or otherwise manipulate used needles by hand Place used deposable syringes and needles, scalpel blades, and other sharp items in puncture-resistant containers for disposal Locate the puncture-resistant containers as close to the use area as is practical.
2 Use protective barriers to prevent exposure to blood, body fluids containing visible blood, and other fluids to which universal precautions apply. The type of protective barder(s) should be appropriate for the procedure being performed and the type of exposure anticipated.
3 Immediately and thoroughly wash hands and other skin surfaces that are contaminated with blood, body fluids containing visible blood, or other body fluids to which universal precautions apply.

## Glove Use for Phlebotomy

Gloves should reduce the incidence of blood contamination of hands during phlebotomy (drawing blood samplesh, but they cannot prevent penetrating injuries caused by needles or other sharp instruments. The likelihood of hand contamination wdh blood containing HIV, HBV, or other bloodborne pathogens during phlebotomy depends on several factors: (1) the skill and technique of the health-care worker, (2) the frequency with which the health-care worker performs the procedure (other factors being equat the cumulative risk of blood exposure is higher for a health-care worker who performs more procedures (3) whether the procedure occursin a routine or emergency situation (where blood contact may be more likely and (4) the prevalence of infection with bloodborne pathogens in the patient population. The likelihood of infection after skin exposure to blood containing HIV or HBV will depend on the concentration of virus (viral concentration is much higher for hepatitis B than for HIV), the duration of contact the presence of skin lesions on the hands of the health-care worke and— for HBV—the immune status of the health-care worker. Although not accurately

† The August 1987 publication should be consulted for general information and specific recommendations not addressed in this update.

quantified, the risk of HIV infection following intact skin contact with infective blood is certainly much less than the 0.5 per cent risk following percutaneous needles tick exposures.[5] In universal precautions, all blood is assumed to be potentially infective for bloodborne pathogens, but in certain settings (e. g., volunteer blood-donation centers) the prevalence of infection with some bloodborne pathogens (e.g., HIV, HBV) is known to be very low Some institutions have relaxed recommendations for using gloves for phlebotomy procedures by skilled phlebotomists in settings where the prevalence of bloodborne pathogens is known to be very low.

Institutions that judge that routine gloving for all phlebotomies is not necessary should periodically reevaluate their policy. Gloves should always be available to health-care workers who wish to use them for phlebotomy. In addition, the following general guidelines apply:

1. Use gloves for performing phlebotomy when the health-care worker has cuts, scratches, or other breaks in his/her skin.
2. Use gloves in situations where the health-care worker judges that hand contamination with blood may occur for example, then performing phlebotomy on an uncooperative patient.
3. Use gloves for performing finger and/or heel sticks on infants and children.
4. Use gloves when persons are receiving training in phlebotomy.

## Selection of Gloves

The Center for Devices and Radiological Health, FDA, has responsibility for regulating the medical glove industry. Medical gloves include those marketed as sterile surgical or nonsterile examination gloves made of vinyl or latex. General purpose utility ("rubber") gloves are also used in the health-care sewing, but they are not regulated by FDA since they are not promoted for medical use. There are no reported differences in barrier effectiveness between intact latex and intact vinyl used to manufacture gloves. Thus, the type of gloves selected should be appropriate for the task being performed.

The following general guidelines are recommended:

1. Use sterile gloves for procedures involving contact with normally sterile areas of the body.
2. Use examination gloves for procedures involving contact with mucous membranes, unless otherwise indicated, and for other patient care or diagnostic procedures that

do not require the use of sterile gloves.

3. Change gloves between patient contacts.
4. Do not wash or disinfect surgical or examination gloves for reuse. Washing with surfactant may cause "wicking" i.e., the enhanced penetration of squids through undetected holes in the glove. Disinfecting agents may cause deterioration.
5. Use general purpose untility gloves (e.g., rubber household gloves) for housekeeping chores involving potential blood contact and for instrument cleaning and decontamination procedures. Utility gloves may be decontaminated and reused but should be discarded if they are peeling, cracked, or discolored, or if they have punctures, tears, or other evidence of deterioration.

## Waste Management

Universal precautions are not intended to change waste management programmes previously recommended by CDC for health-care settings.[1] Policies for defining, collecting, storing, decontaminating, and disposing of infective waste are generaly determined by institutions in accordance with state and local regulations. Information regarding waste management regulations in heakh-care settings may be obtained from state or local heath departments or agencies responsible for waste management.

*Reported by*: Center for Devices and Radiological Health, Food and Drug Administration, Hospital Infections Programme, AIDS Programme, and Hepatitis Br, Div of Viral Diseases, Center for Infectious Diseases, National Institute for Occupational Safety and Health, CDC.

Editorial Note: Implementation of universal precautions does not eliminate the need for other category- or disease-specific isolation precautions, such as enteric precautions for infectious diarrhea or isolation for pulmonary tuberculosis.[1,2] In addition to universal precautions, detailed precautions have been developed for the following procedures and/or settings in which prolonged or intensive exposures to blood occur: invasive procedures, dentistry, autopsies or morticians' services, dialysis, and the clinical laboratory. These detailed precautions are found in the August 21, 1987, "Recommendations for Prevention of HIV Transmission in Health-Care Settings".[1] In addition, specific precautions have been developed for research laboratories. [28]

## References

1. Centers for Disease Control. Recommendations for prevention of HIV transmission in health-care settings. MMWR 1987;36(suppl no. 2S).
2. Garner JS, Simmons BP. Guideline for isolation precautions in hospitals. Infect Control 1983:4:245-325.
3. Immunization Practices Advisory Committee. Recommendations for protection against viral hepatitis. MMWR 1985;34:313-24,329—35.
4. Department of Labour, Department of Health and Human Services. Joint advisory notice: protection against occupational exposure to hepatitis B virus (HBV) and human immunodeficiency virus (HIV). Washington, DC:US Department of Labour, US Department of Health and Human Services, 1987.
5. Centers for Disease Control. Update: Acquired immunodeficiency syndrome and human immunodeficiency virus infection among health-care workers. MMWR 1988;37:229—34,239.
6. Hollander H. Levy JA. Neurologic abnormalities and recovery of human immunodeficiency virus from cerebrospinal fluid. Ann Intern Med 1987;106:692—5.
7. Wirthrington RH, Cornes P. Harris JRW, et al. Isolation of human immunodeficiency virus from synovial fluid of a patient with reactive arthritis. Br Med J 1987;294:484.
8. Mundy DC. Schinazi RF, Gerber AR, Nahmias AJ, Randall HW. Human immunodeficiency virus isolated from amniotic fluid. Lancet 1987;2:459-60.
9. Onion DK, Crumpacker CS, Gilliland BC. Arthritis of hepatitis associated with Australia antigen. Ann Intern Med 1971;75:29-33.
10. Lee AKY, Ip HMH, Wong VCW. Mechanisms of maternal-fetal transmission of hepatitis B virus. J Infect Dis 1978;138:668-71.
11. Bond WW, Petersen NJ, Gravelle CR, Favero MS. Hepatitis B virus in peritoneal dialysis fluid: A potential hazard. Dialysis and Transplantation 1982;11:592-600.
12. Oskenhendler E, Harzic M, Le Roux J-M, Rabian C, Clauvel JP. HIV infection with seroconversion after a superficiai needlestick injury to the finger [Letter]. N Engl J Med 1986;315:582.
13. Lifson AR. Do alternate modes for transmission of human immunodeficiency virus exist? A review. JAMA 1988;259:1353-6.
14. Friedland GH, Saltzman BR, Rogers MF, et al. Lack of transmission of HTLV-III/LAV infection to household contacts of patients with AIDS or AIDS-related complex with oral candidiasis. N Engl J Med 1986;314:344-9.
15. Jenison SA, Lemon SM. Baker LN, Newbold JE. Quantitative analysis of hepatitis B virus DNA in saliva and semen of chronically infected homosexual men. J Infect Dis 1987; 156: 299-306.
16. Cancio-Bello TP, de Medina M, Shorey J. Valledor MD, Schiff ER. An institutional outbreak of hepatitis B related to a human biting carrier. J Infect Dis 1982;146:652-6.
17. MacQuarrie MB, Forghani B. Wolochow DA. Hepatitis B transmitted by a human bite. JAMA 1974;230:723-4.

18. Scott RM, Snitbhan R. Bancroft WH, Alter HJ, Tingpalapong M. Experimental transmission of hepatitis B virus by semen and saliva. J Infect Dis 1980;142:67-71.
19. Glaser JB, Nadler JP. Hepatitis B virus in a cardiopulmonary resuscitation training course. Risk of transmission from a surface antigen-positive participant. Arch Intern Med 1985;145:1653—5.
20. Osterholm MT, Bravo ER, Crosson JT, et al. Lack of transmission of viral hepatitis type B after oral exposure to HBsAg-positive saliva. Br Med J 1979;2:1263-4.
21. Curran JW, Jaffe HW, Hardy AM, et al. Epidemiology of HIV infection and AIDS in the United States. Science 1988;239:610-6.
22. Jason JM, McDougal JS, Dixon G. et al. HTLV-III/LAV antibody and immune status of household contacts and sexual partners of persons with hemophilia. JAMA 1986;255:212-5.
23. Wahn V, Kramer HH, Voit T. Broster HT, Scrampical B. Scheid A. Horizontal transmission of HIV infection between two siblings [Letter]. Lancet 1986;2:694.
24. Salahuddin SZ, Groopman JE, Markham PD, et al. HTLV-III in symptom-free seronegative persons. Lancet 1984;2:1418-20.
25. Simmons BP, Wong ES. Guideline for prevention of nosocomial pneumonia. Atlanta: US Department of Health and Human Services, Public Health Service, Centers for Disease Control, 1982.
26. Klein RS, Phelan JA, Freeman K, et al. Low occupational risk of human immunodeficiency virus infection among dental professionals. N Engl J Med 1988;318:86-90.
27. Garner JS, Favero MS. Guideline for handwashing and hospital environmental control, 1985. Atlanta: US Department of Health and Human Services, Public Health Service, Centers for Disease Control, 1985; HHS publication no. 99-1117.
28. Centers for Disease Control. 1988 Agent summary statement for human immunodeficiency virus and report on laboratory-acquired infection with human immunodeficiency virus. MMWR 1988;37(suppl no. S4:1S-22S).

# 35

# Preventing Transmission of Human Immunodeficiency Virus and Hepatitis B Virus to Patients During Exposure Prone Invasive Procedures

This document has been developed by the Centers for Disease Control (CDC) to update recommendations for prevention of transmission of human immunodeficiency virus (HIV) and hepatitis B virus (HBV) in the health-care setting. Current data suggest that the risk for such transmission from a health-care worker (HCW) to a patient during an invasive procedure is small; a precise assessment of the risk is not yet available. This document contains recommendations to provide guidance for prevention of HIV and HBV transmission during those invasive procedures that are considered exposure-prone.

## INTRODUCTION

Recommendations have been made by the Centers for Disease Control (CDC) for the prevention of transmission of the human immunodeficiency virus (HIV) and the hepatitis B virus (HBV) in health-care settings.[1-6] These recommendations emphasize adherence to universal precautions that require that blood and other specified body fluids of all patients be handled as if they contain blood-borne pathogens.[1,2]

Previous guidelines contained precautions to be used during invasive procedures and recommendations for the management of HIV- and HBV-infected health-care workers (HCWs).[1] These guidelines did not include specific recommendations on testing HCWs for HIV or HBV infection, and they did not provide guidance on which invasive procedures may represent increased risk to the patient.

The recommendations outlined in this document are based on the following considerations:

# Infected HCWs who adhere to universal precautions and who do not perform invasive procedures pose no risk for transmitting HIV or HBV to patients.
# Infected HCWs who adhere to universal precautions and who perform certain exposure-prone procedures pose a small risk for transmitting HBV to patients.
# HIV is transmitted much less readily than HBV.

In the interim, until further data are available, additional precautions are prudent to prevent HIV and HBV transmission during procedures that have been linked to HCW-to-patient HBV transmission or that are considered exposure-prone.

## BACKGROUND

### Infection-Control Practices

Previous recommendations have specified that infection-control programmes should incorporate principles of universal precautions (i.e., appropriate use of hand washing, protective barriers, and care in the use and disposal of needles and other sharp instruments) and should maintain these precautions rigorously in all health-care settings.[1,2,5] Proper application of these principles will assist in minimizing the risk of transmission of HIV or HBV from patient to HCW, HCW to patient, or patient to patient.

As part of standard infection-control practice, instruments and other reusable equipment used in performing invasive procedures should be appropriately disinfected and sterilized as follows:[7]

# Equipment and devices that enter the patient's vascular system or other normally sterile areas of the body should be sterilized before being used for each patient.
# Equipment and devices that touch intact mucous membranes but do not penetrate the patient's body surfaces should be sterilized when possible or undergo high-level disinfection if they cannot be sterilized before being used for each patient.
# Equipment and devices that do not touch the patient or that only touch intact skin of the patient need only be cleaned with a detergent or as indicated by the manufacturer.

Compliance with universal precautions and recommendations for disinfection and sterilization of medical devices should be scrupulously monitored in all health-care settings.[1,7,8] Training of

HCWs in proper infection-control technique should begin in professional and vocational schools and continue as an ongoing process. Institutions should provide all HCWs with appropriate inservice education regarding infection control and safety and should establish procedures for monitoring compliance with infection-control policies.

All HCWs who might be exposed to blood in an occupational setting should receive hepatitis B vaccine, preferably during their period of professional training and before any occupational exposures could occur.[8,9]

## Transmission of HBV During Invasive Procedures

Since the introduction of serologic testing for HBV infection in the early 1970s, there have been published reports of 20 clusters in which a total of over 300 patients were infected with HBV in association with treatment by an HBV-infected HCW. In 12 of these clusters, the implicated HCW did not routinely wear gloves; several HCWs also had skin lesions that may have facilitated HBV transmission.[10-22] These 12 clusters included nine linked to dentists or oral surgeons and one cluster each linked to a general practitioner, an inhalation therapist, and a cardiopulmonarybypass-pump technician. The clusters associated with the inhalation therapist and the cardiopulmonary-bypass-pump technician—and some of the other 10 clusters—could possibly have been prevented if current recommendations on universal precautions, including glove use, had been in effect. In the remaining eight clusters, transmission occurred despite glove use by the HCWs; five clusters were linked to obstetricians or gynecologists, and three were linked to cardiovascular surgeons.[6, 22-28] In addition, recent unpublished reports strongly suggest HBV transmission from three surgeons to patients in 1989 and 1990 during colorectal (CDC, unpublished data), abdominal, and cardiothoracic surgery.[29]

Seven of the HCWs who were linked to published clusters in the United States were allowed to perform invasive procedures following modification of invasive techniques (e.g., double gloving and restriction of certain high-risk procedures).[6,11-13,15,16,24] For five HCWs, no further transmission to patients was observed. In two instances involving an obstetrician/gynecologist and an oral surgeon, HBV was transmitted to patients after techniques were modified.[6,12]

Review of the 20 published studies indicates that a combination of risk factors accounted for transmission of HBV from HCWs to patients. Of the HCWs whose hepatitis B e antigen (HBeAg) status was determined (17 of 20), all were HBeAg positive. The presence of HBeAg in serum is associated with higher levels of circulating virus and therefore with greater infectivity of hepatitis-B-surface-antigen (HBsAg)-positive individuals; the risk of HBV transmission to an HCW after a percutaneous exposure to HBeAg-positive blood is approximately 30 per cent.[30-32] In addition, each report indicated that the potential existed for contamination of surgical wounds or traumatized tissue, either from a major break in standard infection-control practices (e.g., not wearing gloves during invasive procedures) or from unintentional injury to the infected HCW during invasive procedures (e.g., needle sticks incurred while manipulating needles without being able to see them during suturing.

Most reported clusters in the United States occurred before awareness increased of the risks of transmission of blood-borne pathogens in health-care settings and before emphasis was placed on the use of universal precautions and hepatitis B vaccine among HCWs. The limited number of reports of HBV transmission from HCWs to patients in recent years may reflect the adoption of universal precautions and increased use of HBV vaccine. However, the limited number of recent reports does not preclude the occurrence of undetected or unreported small clusters or individual instances of transmission; routine use of gloves does not prevent most injuries caused by sharp instruments and does not eliminate the potential for exposure of a patient to an HCW's blood and transmission of HBV.[6, 22-29]

## Transmission of HIV During Invasive Procedures

The risk of HIV transmission to an HCW after percutaneous exposure to HIV-infected blood is considerably lower than the risk of HBV transmission after percutaneous exposure to HBeAg-positive blood (0.3 per cent versus approximately 30 per cent).[33-35] Thus, the risk of transmission of HIV from an infected HCW to a patient during an invasive procedure is likely to.be proportionately lower than the risk of HBV transmission from an HBeAg-positive HCW to a patient during the same procedure. As with HBV, the relative infectivity of HIV probably varies among individuals and over time for a single individual. Unlike HBV infection, however, there is currently no readily available laboratory test for increased HIV infectivity.

Investigation of a cluster of HIV infections among patients in the practice of one dentist with acquired immunodeficiency syndrome (AIDS) strongly suggested that HIV was transmitted to five of the approximately 850 patients evaluated through June 1991.[38] The investigation indicates that HIV transmission occurred during dental care, although the precise mechanisms of transmission have not been determined. In two other studies, when patients cared for by a general surgeon and a surgical resident who had AIDS were tested, all patients tested, 75 and 62, respectively, were negative for HIV infection. [39,40]. In a fourth study, 143 patients who had been treated by a dental student with HIV infection and were later tested were all negative for HIV infection.[41] In another investigation, HIV antibody testing was offered to all patients whose surgical procedures had been performed by a general surgeon within 7 years before the surgeon's diagnosis of AIDS; the date at which the surgeon became infected with HIV is unknown.[42] Of 1,340 surgical patients contacted, 616 (46 per cent) were tested for HIV. One patient, a known intravenous drug user, was HIV positive when tested but may already have been infected at the time of surgery. HIV test results for the 615 other surgical patients were negative (95 per cent confidence interval for risk of transmission per operation =0.0 per cent-0.5 per cent).

The limited number of participants and the differences in procedures associated with these five investigations limit the ability to generalize from them and to define precisely the risk of HIV transmission from HIV-infected HCWs to patients. A precise estimate of the risk of HIV transmission from infected HCWs to patients can be determined only after careful evaluation of a substantially larger number of patients whose exposure-prone procedures have been performed by HIV-infected HCWs.

## Exposure-Prone Procedures

Despite adherence to the principles of universal precautions, certain invasive surgical and dental procedures have been implicated in the transmission of HBV from infected HCWs to patients, and should be considered exposure-prone. Reported examples include certain oral, cardiothoracic, colorectal (CDC, unpublished data), and obstetric/gynecologic procedures.[6, 12, 22-29]

Certain other invasive procedures should also be considered exposure-prone. In a prospective study CDC conducted in tour hospitals, one or more percutaneous injuries occurred among surgical personnel during 96 (6.9 per cent) of 1,382 operative procedures on the general surgery, gynecology, orthopedic, cardiac, and trauma services. [43] Percutaneous exposure of the patient to the HCW's blood may have occurred when the sharp object causing the injury recontacted the patient's open wound in 28 (32 per cent) of the 88 observed injuries to surgeons (range among surgical specialties=8 per cent=57 per cent; range among hospitals=24 per cent-42 per cent).

*Characteristics of exposure-prone procedures include digital palpation of a needle tip in a body cavity or the simultaneous presence of the HCW's fingers and a needle or other sharp instrument or object in a poorly visualized or highly confined anatomic site. Performance of exposure-prone procedures presents a recognized risk of percutaneous injury to the HCW, and—if such an injury occurs—the HCW's blood is likely to contact the patient's body cavity, subcutaneous tissues, and/or mucous membranes.*

Experience with HBV indicates that invasive procedures that do not have the above characteristics would be expected to pose substantially lower risk, if any, of transmission of HIV and other blood-borne pathogens from an infected HCW to patients.

## RECOMMENDATIONS

Investigations of HIV and HBV transmission from HCWs to patients indicate that, when HCWs adhere to recommended infection-control procedures, the risk of transmitting HBV from an infected HCW to a patient is small, and the risk of transmitting HIV is likely to be even smaller. However, the likelihood of exposure of the patient to an HCW's blood is greater for certain procedures designated as exposure-prone. To minimize the risk of HIV or HBV transmission, the following measures are recommended:

# All HCWs should adhere to universal precautions, including the appropriate use of hand washing, protective barriers, and care in the use and disposal of needles and other sharp instruments. HCWs who have exudative lesions or weeping dermatitis should refrain from all direct patient care and from handling patient-care equipment and devices used in performing invasive procedures until the condition resolves. HCWs should also comply with current guidelines for disinfection and sterilization of reusable devices used in invasive procedures.

# Currently available data provide no basis for recommendations to restrict the practice of HCWs infected with HIV or HBV who perform invasive procedures not identified as exposure-prone, provided the infected HCWs practice recommended surgical or dental technique and comply with universal precautions and current recommendations for sterilization/disinfection.

# Exposure-prone procedures should be identified by medical/surgical/dental organizations and institutions at which the procedures are performed.

# HCWs who perform exposure-prone procedures should know their HIV antibody status. HCWs who perform exposure-prone procedures and who do not have serologic evidence of immunity to HBV from vaccination or from previous infection should know their HBsAg status

and, if that is positive, should also know their HBeAg status.

# HCWs who are infected with HIV or HBV (and are HBeAg positive) should not perform exposure-prone procedures unless they have sought counsel from an expert review panel and been advised under what circumstances, if any, they may continue to perform these procedures.* Such circumstances would include notifying prospective patients of the HCW's seropositivity before they undergo exposure-prone invasive procedures.

# Mandatory testing of HCWs for HIV antibody, HBsAg, or HBeAg is not recommended. The current assessment of the risk that infected HCWs will transmit HIV or HBV to patients during exposure-prone procedures does not support the diversion of resources that would be required to implement mandatory testing programmes. Compliance by HCWs with recommendations can be increased through education, training, and appropriate confidentiality safeguards.

## HCWS WHOSE PRACTICES ARE MODIFIED BECAUSE OF HIV OR HBV STATUS

HCWs whose practices are modified because of their HIV or HBV infection status should, whenever possible, be provided opportunities to continue appropriate patient-care activities. Career counseling and job retraining should be encouraged to promote the continued use of the HCW's talents, knowledge, and skills. HCWs whose practices are modified because of HBV infection should be reevaluated periodically to determine whether their HBeAg status changes due to resolution of infection or as a result of treatment.[44]

## NOTIFICATION OF PATIENTS AND F LOW-UP STUDIES

The public health benefit of nofficafon of pafents who have

---

*The review panel should include experts who represent a balanced perspective. Such experts might include all of the following: a) the HCW's personal physician(s), (b) an infectious disease specialist with expertise in the epidemiology of HIV and HBV transmission, (c) a health professional with expertise in the procedures performed by the HCW, and d) state or local public health official(s). if the HCW's practice is institutionally based, the expert review panel might also include a member of the infection-control committee, preferably a hospital epidemiologist. HCWs who perform exposure-prone procedures outside the hospital/institutional setting should seek advice from appropriate state and local public health officials regarding the review process. Panels must recognize the importance of confidentiality and the privacy rights of infected HCWs.

had exposure-prone procedures performed by HCWs infected with HIV or positive for HBeAg should be considered on a case-by-case basis taking into consideration an assessment of specfic risk, confidentialy issues, and available resources. Carefully designed and implemented follow-up studies are necessary to determine more precisely the risk of transmission during such procedures. Decisions regarding notification and follow-up studies should be made in consultation with state and local public health officials.

## ADDITIONAL NEEDS

# Clearer definition of the nature, frequency, and circumstances of blood contact between parents and HCWs during invasive procedures.

# Development and evaluation of new devices, protective barriers, and techniques that may prevent such blood contact without adversely affecting the quality of parent care.

# More information on the potential for HIV and HBV transmission through contaminated instruments.

# Improvements in sterilization and disinfection techniques for certain reusable equipment and devices.

# Identification of factors that may influence the likelihood of HIV or HBV transmission after exposure to HIV- or HBV-infected blood.

## References

1. CDC. Recommendations for prevention of HIV transmission in health-care settings MMWR 1987; 36 (suppl.. no 25) 1-185
2. CDC . Update Universal precautions for prevention of transmission of human immunodeficiency virus, hepatitis B virus and other blood borne pathogens in health-care setlings. MMWR 1988;37 377-82,387-8
3. CDC. Heptitis Surveillance Report No. 48. Atlanta: U.S. Department of Health and Human Services, Public Health Service, 1982: 2-3.
4. CDC. CDC Guideline for Infection Control in Hospital Personnel Atlanta, Georgia: Public Health Service, 1983 24 pages (GPO# 6AR031 488305)
5. CDC. Guidelines for prevention of transmission of human immunodeficiency virus and hepatitis B virus to health-care and public-safety workers. MMWR 1989;38; (suppl. no. S-6): 1-37.
6. Lettau LA, Smith JD, Williams D, et al. Transmission of hepatise B with resultant restriction of surgical practice. Jama 1986; 255: 934-7.
7 CDC. Guidelines for the prevention and control of nosocomial infections guideline for handwashing and hospital environmental control Atlanta, Georgia Public Health Service, 1985: 20 pages (GPO# 544-436/24441).
8 Department of Labour, Occupational Safety and Health Administration.

Occupational exposure to bloodborne pathogens: proposed rule and notice of hearing Federal Register 1989;54. 23042-139
9 CDC.Protection against viral hepatitis: recommendations of the immunization practices advisory committee (ACIP) MMWR 1990 39:(no RR-2L)
10 Levin ML. Maddre; WC, Wands JR, Mendeloff Al. Hepatitis B transmission by dentists. JAMA 1974; 228 1139-40.
11 Rimland D, Parkin WE, Miller GB, Schrack WD. Hepatitis B outbreak traced to an oral surgeon. N Engl J Med 1977; 296: 953-8.
12. Goodwin D, Fannin SL, McCracken BB An oral-surgeon related hepatitis-B outbreak California Morbidity 1976 14.
13. Hadler SC Sorley DL, Acree KH, et al. An outbreak of hepatitis B in a dental practice. Ann Intern Med 1981 1981;95:133-8.
14. Reingold AL, Kane MA, Murphy BL, Checko P,. Francis DP, Maynard JE Transmission of hepatitis B by an oral surgeon J Infect Dis 1982;145:262-8.
15 Goodman RA, Ahtons JL, Finton RJ Hepaftis B transmission from dental personnel to patients unfinished business [Editorial. Ann Intern Med 1982;96:119.
16. Ahtons J. Goodman RA. Hepatitis B and dental personnel: transmission to patients and prevention issues J Am Dent Assoc 1983;106:219-22.
17. Shaw FE Jr, Barrett CL, Hamm R. et al. Lethal outbreak of hepatitis B in a dental practice JAMA 1986,255 3260-4.
18. CDC. Outbreak of hepatitis B associated with an oral surgeon, New Hampshire MMWR 1987;36:132-3.
19 Grob PJ, Moeschlin P. Risk to contacts of a medical practitioner carrying HBsAg [Letter] N Engl J Med 1975 293:197.
20 Grob PJ Bischof B. Naeff F. Cluster of hepatitis B transmitted by a physician Lancet 1981;2:1218-20.
21 Snydman DR, Hindman SH, Wineland MD, Bryan JA, Maynard JE Nosocomial viral hepatitis B. A cluster among staff with subsequent transmission to patients. Ann Intern Med 1976;85:573-7.
22. Coutinho RA, Albrecht-van Lent P. Stoutjesdijk L, et al Hepatitis B from doctors [Letter] Lancet 1982;1:345-6.
23. Anonymous Acuts hepatitis B associated with gynaecological surgery Lancet 1980;1:1-6.
24. Carl M, Blakey DL, Francis DP, Maynard JE. Interruption of hepatitis B transmission by modification of a gynaecologist's surgical technique. Lancet 1982;1:731-3.
25. Anonymous. Acute hepatitis B following gynaecological surgery. J Hosp Infect 1987;9:34-8.
26. Welch J. Webster M, Tilzey AJ, Noah ND, Banatvala JE. Hepatitis B infections after gynaecological surgery. Lancet 1989; 1 :205-7.
27. Haeram JW, Siebke JC, Ulstrup J. Geiram D, Helle I. HBsAg transmission from a cardiac surgeon incubating hepatitis B resulting in chronic antigenemia in four patients. Acta Med Scand 1981;210:389-92.
28. Flower AJE, Prentice M, Morgan G. et al. Hepatitis B infection following cardiothoracic surgery [Abstract].1990 International Symposium on Viral Hepatitis and Liver Diseases, Houston. 190;94.

29. Heptonstall J. Outbreaks of hepatitis B virus infection associated with infected surgical staff in the United Kingdom. Communicable Disease Reports 1991 (in press).
30. Alter HJ, Seef LB, Kaplan PM, et al. Type B hepatitis: the infectivity of blood positive for e antigen and DNA polymerase after accidental needlestick exposure. N Engl J Med 1976;295:909-13.
31. Seeff LB, Wright EC, Zimmerman HJ, et al. Type B hepatitis after needlestick exposure: prevention with hepatitis B immunoglobulin: final report of the Veterans Administration Co-operative Study. Ann Intern Med 1978;88:285-93.
32. Grady GF, Lee VA, Prince AM, et ai. Hepatitis B immune globulin for accidental exposures among medical personnel: final report of a multicenter controlled trial. J Infect Dis 1978;138:625-38.
33. Henderson DK, Fahey BJ, Willy M, et al. Risk for occupational transmission of human immunodeficiency virus type 1 (HIV-1) associated with ciinical exposures: a prospective evaluation. Ann Intern Med 1990;113:740-6.
34. Marcus R. CDC Co-operative Needlestick Study Group. Surveillance of health-care workers exposed to blood from patients infected with the human immunodeficiency virus. N Engl J Med 1988;319:1118-23.
35. Gerberding JL, Bryant-LeBlanc CE, Nelson K, et al. Risk of transmitting the human immunodeficiency virus, cytomegalovirus, and hepatitis B virus to health-care workers exposed to patients with AIDS and AIDS-related conditions. J Infect Dis 1987; 156:1 -8.
36. CDC. Possible transmission of human immunodeficiency virus to a patient during an invasive dental procedure. MMWR 1990;39:489-93.
37. CDC. Update: transmission of HIV infection during an invasive dental procedure - Florida. MMWR 1991; 40:21 -27,33.
38. CDC. Update: transmission of HIV infection during invasive dental procedures - Florida. MMWR 1991; 40: 377-81.
39. Porter JD, Cruikshank JG, Gentle PH, Robinson RG, Gill ON. Management of patients treated by a surgeon with HIV infection. [Letter] Lancet 1990;335:113-4.
40. Armstrong FP, Miner JC, Wolfe WH. Investigation of a health-care worker with symptomatic human immunodeficiency virus infection: an epidemiologic approach. Milit Med 1987;152:414-8.
41. Comer RW, Myers DR, Steadman CD, Carter MJ, Rissing JP, Tedesco FJ. Management considerations for an HIV positive dental student. J Dent Educ 1991;55:187-91.
42. Mishu B. Schaffner W. Horan JM, Wood LH, Hutcheson R. McNabb P. A surgeon with AIDS: lack of evidence of transmission to patients. JAMA 1990;264:467-70.
43. Tokars J. Bell D, Marcus R. et al. Percutaneous injuries during surgical procedures [Abstract]. Vll International Conference on AIDS. Vol 2. Florence, Italy, June 16-21, 1991:83.
44. Perrillo RP, Schiff ER, Davis GL, et al. A randomized, controlled trial of interferon alfa-2b alone and after prednisone withdrawal for the treatment of chronic hepatitis B. N Engl J Med 1990;323:295-301.

# 36

# Prevention of HIV Transmission in Health-Care Settings

## INTRODUCTION

Human immunodeficiency virus (HIV), the virus that causes acquired immunodeficiency syndrome (AIDS), is transmitted through sexual contact and exposure to infected blood or blood components and perinatally from mother to neonate. HIV has been isolated from blood, semen, vaginal secretions, saliva, tears, breast milk, cerebrospinal fluid, amniotic fluid, and urine and is likely to be isolated from other body fluids, secretions, and excretions. However, epidemiologic evidence has implicated only blood, semen, vaginal secretions, and possibly breast milk in transmission.

The increasing prevalence of HIV increases the risk that health-care workers will be exposed to blood from patients infected with HIV, especially when blood and bodyfluid precautions are not followed for all patients. Thus, this document emphasizes the need for health-care workers to consider all patients as potentially infected with HIV and/or other blood-borne pathogens and to adhere rigorously to infection-control precautions for minimizing the risk of exposure to blood and body fluids of all patients.

The recommendations contained in this document consolidate and update CDC recommendations published earlier for preventing HIV transmission in health-care settings: precautions for clinical and laboratory staffs [1] and precautions for health-care workers and allied professionals [2]; recommendations for preventing HIV transmission in the workplace [3] and during invasive procedures;[4] recommendations for preventing possible transmission of HIV from tears [5]; and recommendations for providing dialysis treatment for HIV-infected patients.[6] These recommendations also update portions of the "Guideline for Isolation Precautions in Hospitals" [7] and reemphasize some of the recommendations contained in

"Infection Control Practices for Dentistry". [8] The recommendations contained in this document have been developed for use in health-care settings and emphasize the need to treat blood and other body fluids from all patients as potentially infective. These same prudent precautions also should be taken in other settings in which persons may be exposed to blood or other body fluids.

## DEFINITION OF HEALTH-CARE WORKERS

Health-care workers are defined as persons, including students and trainees, whose activities involve contact with patients or with blood or other body fluids from patients in a health-care setting.

## HEALTH-CARE WORKERS WITH AIDS

As of July 10,1987, a total of 1,875 (5.8 per cent) of 32,395 adults with AIDS, who had been reported to the CDC national surveillance system and for whom occupational information was available, reported being employed in a health-care or clinical laboratory setting. In comparison, 6.8 million persons—representing 5.6 per cent of the U.S. labour force—were employed in health services. Of the health-care workers with AIDS, 95 per cent have been reported to exhibit high-risk behaviour; for the remaining 5 per cent, the means of HIV acquisition was undetermined. Health-care workers with AIDS were significantly more likely than other workers to have an undetermined risk (5 per cent versus 3 per cent, respectively). For both health-care workers and non-health-care workers with AIDS, the proportion with an undetermined risk has not increased since 1982.

AIDS patients initially reported as not belonging to recognized risk groups are investigated by state and local health departments to determine whether possible risk factors exist. Of all health-care workers with AIDS reported to CDC who were initially characterized as not having an identified risk and for whom follow-up information was available, 66 per cent have been reclassified because risk factors were identified or because the patient was found not to meet the surveillance case definition for AIDS. Of the 87 health-care workers currently categorized as having no identifiable risk, information is incomplete on 16 (18 per cent) because of death or refusal to be interviewed; 38 (44 per cent) are still being investigated. The remaining 33 (38 per cent) health-care workers were interviewed or had other follow-up information available. The occupations of these 33 were as follows: five physicians (15 per cent), three of whom were surgeons; one dentist (3 per cent); three nurses (9 per cent); nine nursing assistants (27 per cent);

seven housekeeping or maintenance workers (21 per cent); three clinical laboratory technicians (9 per cent); one therapist (3 per cent); and four others who did not have contact with patients (12 per cent). Although 15 of these 33 health-care workers reported parenteral and/or other non-needlestick exposure to blood or body fluids from patients in the 10 years preceding their diagnosis of AIDS, none of these exposures involved a patient with AIDS or known HIV infection.

## RISK TO HEALTH-CARE WORKERS OF ACQUIRING HIV IN HEALTH-CARE SETTINGS

Health-care workers with documented percutaneous or mucous-membrane exposures to blood or body fluids of HIV-infected patients have been prospectively evaluated to determine the risk of infection after such exposures. As of June 30,1987, 883 health-care workers have been tested for antibody to HIV in an ongoing surveillance project conducted by CDC.[9] of these, 708 (80 per cent) had percutaneous exposures to blood, and 175 (20 per cent) had a mucous membrane or an open wound contaminated by blood or body fluid. Of 396 health-care workers, each of whom had only a convalescent-phase serum sample obtained and tested ≥90 days post-exposure, one—for whom heterosexual transmission could not be ruled out—was seropositive for HIV antibody. For 425 additional health-care workers, both acute- and convalescent-phase serum samples were obtained and tested; none of 74 health-care workers with nonpercutaneous exposures seroconverted, and three (0.9 per cent) of 351 with percutaneous exposures seroconverted. None of these three health-care workers had other documented risk factors for infection.

Two other prospective studies to assess the risk of nosocomial acquisition of HIV infection for health-care workers are ongoing in the United States. As of April 30, 1987, 332 health-care workers with a total of 453 needlestick or mucous-membrane exposures to the blood or other body fluids of HIV-infected patients were tested for HIV antibody at the National Institutes of Health.[10] These exposed workers included 103 with needlestick injuries and 229 with mucous-membrane exposures; none had seroconverted. A similar study at the University of California of 129 health-care workers with documented needlestick injuries or mucous-membrane exposures to blood or other body fluids from patients with HIV infection has not identified any seroconversions.[11] Results of a prospective study in the United Kingdom identified no evidence of transmission among 150 health-care workers with parenteral or mucous-membrane exposures to blood or other body fluids, secretions, or excretions from patients with HIV infection.[12]

In addition to health-care workers enrolled in prospective studies, eight persons who provided care to infected patients and denied other risk factors have been reported to have acquired HIV infection. Three of these health-care workers had needlestick exposures to blood from infected patients.[13,15] Two were persons who provided nursing care to infected persons; although neither sustained a needlestick, both had extensive contact with blood or other body fluids, and neither observed recommended barrier precautions.[16,17] The other three were healthcare workers with non-needlestick exposures to blood from infected patients.[18] Although the exact route of transmission for these last three infections is not known, all three persons had direct contact of their skin with blood from infected patients, all had skin lesions that may have been contaminated by blood, and one also had a mucous-membrane exposure.

A total of 1,231 dentists and hygienists, many of whom practiced in areas with many AIDS cases, participated in a study to determine the prevalence of antibody to HIV; one dentist (0.1 per cent) had HIV antibody. Although no exposure to a known HIV-infected person could be documented, epidemiologic investigation did not identify any other risk factor for infection. The infected dentist, who also had a history of sustaining needlestick injuries and trauma to his hands, did not routinely wear gloves when providing dental care.[19]

## PRECAUTIONS TO PREVENT TRANSMISSION OF HIV

### Universal Precautions

Since medical history and examination cannot reliably identify all patients infected with HIV or other blood-borne pathogens, blood and body-fluid precautions should be consistently used for all patients. This approach, previously recommended by CDC [3,4], and referred to as "universal blood and body-fluid precautions" or "universal precautions," should be used in the care of all patients, especially including those in emergency-care settings in which the risk of blood exposure is increased and the infection status of the patient is usually unknown.[20]

1. All health-care workers should routinely use appropriate barrier precautions to prevent skin and mucous-membrane exposure when contact with blood or other body fluids of any patient is anticipated. Gloves should be worn for touching blood and body fluids, mucous membranes, or non-intact skin of all patients, for handling items or surfaces soiled with blood or body fluids, and for performing venipuncture and other vascular access

procedures. Gloves should be changed after contact with each patient. Masks and protective eyewear or face shields should be worn during procedures that are likely to generate droplets of blood or other body fluids to prevent exposure of mucous membranes of the mouth, nose, and eyes. Gowns or aprons should be worn during procedures that are likely to generate splashes of blood or other body fluids.

2. Hands and other skin surfaces should be washed immediately and thoroughly if contaminated with blood or other body fluids. Hands should be washed immediately after gloves are removed.
3. All health-care workers should take precautions to prevent injuries caused by needles, scalpels, and other sharp instruments or devices during procedures; when cleaning used instruments; during disposal of used needles; and when handling sharp instruments after procedures. To prevent needlestick injuries, needles should not be recapped, purposely bent or broken by hand, removed from disposable syringes, or otherwise manipulated by hand. After they are used, disposable syringes and needles, scalpel blades, and other sharp items should be placed in puncture-resistant containers for disposal; the punctureresistant containers should be located as close as practical to the use area. Large-bore reusable needles should be placed in a puncture-resistant container for transport to the reprocessing area.
4. Although saliva has not been implicated in HIV transmission, to minimize the need for emergency mouth-to-mouth resuscitation, mouthpieces, resuscitation bags, or other ventilation devices should be available for use in areas in which the need for resuscitation is predictable.
5. Health-care workers who have exudative lesions or weeping dermatitis should refrain from all direct patient care and from handling patient-care equipment until the condition resolves.
6. Pregnant health-care workers are not known to be at greater risk of contracting HIV infection than health-care workers who are not pregnant; however, if a health-care worker develops HIV infection during pregnancy, the infant is at risk of infection resulting from perinatal transmission. Because of this risk, pregnant health-care workers should be especially familiar with and strictly adhere to precautions to minimize the risk of HIV transmission.

Implementation of universal blood and body-fluid precautions for all patients eliminates the need for use of the isolation category of "Blood and Body Fluid Precautions" previously recommended by CDC [7] for patients known or suspected to be infected with blood-borne pathogens. Isolation precautions (e.g., enteric, "AFB" [7]) should be used as necessary if associated conditions, such as infectious diarrhea or tuberculosis, are diagnosed or suspected.

## Precautions for Invasive Procedures

In this document, an invasive procedure is defined as surgical entry into tissues, cavities, or organs or repair of major traumatic injuries (1) in an operating or delivery room, emergency department, or outpatient setting, including both physicians' and dentists' offices; (2) cardiac catheterization and angiographic procedures; (3) a vaginal or cesarean delivery or other invasive obstetric procedure during which bleeding may occur; or (4) the manipulation, cutting, or removal of any oral or perioral tissues, including tooth structure, during which bleeding occurs or the potential for bleeding exists. The universal blood and body-fluid precautions listed above, combined with the precautions listed below, should be the minimum precautions for all such invasive procedures.

1. All health-care workers who participate in invasive procedures must routinely use appropriate barrier precautions to prevent skin and mucous-membrane contact with blood and other body fluids of all patients. Gloves and surgical masks must be worn for all invasive procedures. Protective eyewear or face shields should be worn for procedures that commonly result in the generation of droplets, smashing of blood or other body fluids, or the generation of bone chips. Gowns or aprons made of materials that provide an effective barrier should be worn during invasive procedures that are likely to result in the splashing of blood or other body fluids. All health-care workers who perform or assist in vaginal or cesarean deliveries should wear gloves and gowns when handling the placenta or the infant until blood and amniotic fluid have been removed from the infant's skin and should wear gloves during post-delivery care of the umbilical cord.
2. If a glove is torn or a needlestick or other injury occurs, the glove should be removed and a new glove used as promptly as patient safety permits; the needle or instrument involved in the incident should also be removed from the sterile field.

## Precautions for Dentistry*

Blood, saliva, and gingival fluid from all dental patients should be considered infective. Special emphasis should be placed on the following precautions for preventing transmission of blood-borne pathogens in dental practice in both institutional and non-institutional settings.

1. In addition to wearing gloves for contact with oral mucous membranes of all patients, all dental workers should wear surgical masks and protective eyewear or chin-length plastic face shields during dental procedures in which splashing or spattering of blood, saliva, or gingival fluids is likely. Rubber dams, highspeed evacuation, and proper patient positioning, when appropriate, should be utilized to minimize generation of droplets and spatter.
2. Handpieces should be sterilized after use with each patient, since blood, saliva, or gingival fluid of patients may be aspirated into the handpiece or waterline. Handpieces that cannot be sterilized should at least be flushed, the outside surface cleaned and wiped with a suitable chemical germicide, and then rinsed. Handpieces should be flushed at the beginning of the day and after use with each patient. Manufacturers' recommendations should be followed for use and maintenance of waterlines and check valves and for flushing of handpieces. The same precautions should be used for ultrasonic scalers and air/water syringes.
3. Blood and saliva should be thoroughly and carefully cleaned from material that has been used in the mouth (e.g., impression materials, bite registration), especially before polishing and grinding intra-oral devices. Contaminated materials, impressions, and intra-oral devices should also be cleaned and disinfected before being handled in the dental laboratory and before they are placed in the patient's mouth. Because of the increasing variety of dental materials used intra-orally, dental workers should consult with manufacturers as to the stability of specific materials when using disinfection procedures.
4. Dental equipment and surfaces that are difficult to disinfect (e.g., light handles or X-ray-unit heads) and that may become contaminated should be wrapped with impervious-backed paper, aluminum foil, or clear plastic wrap. The coverings should be removed and discarded, and clean coverings should be put in place after use with each patient.

* General infection-control precautions are more specifically addressed in previous recommendations for infection-control practices for dentistry.[8]

## Precautions for Autopsies or Morticians' Services

In addition to the universal blood and body-fluid precautions listed above, the following precautions should be used by persons performing postmortem procedures:

1. All persons performing or assisting in postmortem procedures should wear gloves, masks, protective eyewear, gowns, and waterproof aprons.
2. Instruments and surfaces contaminated during postmortem procedures should be decontaminated with an appropriate chemical germicide.

## Precautions for Dialysis

Patients with end-stage renal disease who are undergoing maintenance dialysis and who have HIV infection can be dialyzed in hospital-based or free-standing dialysis units using conventional infection-control precautions.[21] Universal blood and body-fluid precautions should be used when dialyzing all patients.

Strategies for disinfecting the dialysis fluid pathways of the hemodialysis machine are targeted to control bacterial contamination and generally consist of using 500-750 parts per million (ppm) of sodium hypochlorite (household bleach) for 30-40 minutes or 1.5 per cent-2.0 per cent formaldehyde overnight. In addition, several chemical germicides formulated to disinfect dialysis machines are commercially available. None of these protocols or procedures need to be changed for dialyzing patients infected with HIV.

Patients infected with HIV can be dialyzed by either hemodialysis or peritoneal dialysis and do not need to be isolated from other patients. The type of dialysis treatment (i.e., hemodialysis or peritoneal dialysis) should be based on the needs of the patient. The dialyzer may be discarded after each use. Alternatively, centers that reuse dialyzers—i.e., a specific single-use dialyzer is issued to a specific patient, removed, cleaned, disinfected, and reused several times on the same patient only— may include HIV-infected patients in the dialyzer-reuse programme. An individual dialyzer must never be used on more than one patient.

## Precautions for Laboratories †

Blood and other body fluids from all patients should be considered infective. To supplement the universal blood and body-fluid precautions listed above, the following precautions are recommended for health-care workers in clinical laboratories.

---

† Additional precautions for research and industrial laboratories are addressed elsewhere.[22,23]

1. All specimens of blood and body fluids should be put in a well-constructed container with a secure lid to prevent leaking during transport. Care should be taken when collecting each specimen to avoid contaminating the outside of the container and of the laboratory form accompanying the specimen.
2. All persons processing blood and body-fluid specimens (e.g., removing tops from vacuum tubes) should wear gloves. Masks and protective eyewear should be worn if mucous-membrane contact with blood or body fluids is anticipated. Gloves should be changed and hands washed after completion of specimen processing.
3. For routine procedures, such as histologic and pathologic studies or microbiologic culturing, a biological safety cabinet is not necessary. However, biological safety cabinets (Class I or II) should be used whenever procedures are conducted that have a high potential for generating droplets. These include activities such as blending, sonicating, and vigorous mixing.
4. Mechanical pipetting devices should be used for manipulating all liquids in the laboratory. Mouth pipetting must not be done.
5. Use of needles and syringes should be limited to situations in which there is no alternative, and the recommendations for preventing injuries with needles outlined under universal precautions should be followed.
6. Laboratory work surfaces should be decontaminated with an appropriate chemical germicide after a spill of blood or other body fluids and when work activities are completed.
7. Contaminated materials used in laboratory tests should be decontaminated before reprocessing or be placed in bags and disposed of in accordance with institutional policies for disposal of infective waste.[24]
8. Scientific equipment that has been contaminated with blood or other body fluids should be decontaminated and cleaned before being repaired in the laboratory or transported to the manufacturer.
9. All persons should wash their hands after completing laboratory activities and should remove protective clothing before leaving the laboratory.

Implementation of universal blood and body-fluid precautions for all patients eliminates the need for warning labels on specimens since blood and other body fluids from all patients should be considered infective.

## ENVIRONMENTAL CONSIDERATIONS FOR HIV TRANSMISSION

No environmentally mediated mode of HIV transmission has been documented. Nevertheless, the precautions described below should be taken routinely in the care of all patients.

### Sterilization and Disinfection

Standard sterilization and disinfection procedures for patient-care equipment currently recommended for use [25,26] in a variety of health-care settings—including hospitals, medical and dental clinics and offices, hemodialysis centers, emergency care facilities, and long-term nursing-care facilities—are adequate to sterilize or disinfect instruments, devices, or other items contaminated with blood or other body fluids from persons infected with bloodborne pathogens including HIV. [21,23]

Instruments or devices that enter sterile tissue or the vascular system of any patient or through which blood flows should be sterilized before reuse. Devices or items that contact intact mucous membranes should be sterilized or receive highlevel disinfection, a procedure that kills vegetative organisms and viruses but not necessarily large numbers of bacterial spores. Chemical germicides that are registered with the U.S. Environmental Protection Agency (EPA) as "sterilants" may be used either for sterilization or for high-level disinfection depending on contact rims.

Contact lenses used in trial fittings should be disinfected after each fitting by using a hydrogen peroxide contact lens disinfecting system or, if compatible, with heat (78 C-80 C [172.4 F-176.0 F] for 10 minutes.

Medical devices or instruments that require sterilization or disinfection should be thoroughly cleaned before being exposed to the germicide, and the manufacturers instructions for the use of the germicide should be followed. Further it is important that the manufacturer's specifications for compatibility of the medical device with chemical germicides be closely followed. Information on specific label claims of commercial germicides can be obtained by writing to the Disinfectants Branch, Office of Pesticides, Environmental Protection Agency, 401 M Street, SW, Washington, D.C. 20460.

Studies have shown that HIV is inactivated rapidly after being exposed to commonly used chemical germicides at concentrations that are much lower than used in practice.[27-30] Embalming fluids are similar to the types of chemical germicides that have been tested and found to completely inactivate HIV. In addition to commercially available chemical germicides, a solution of sodium hypochlorite (household bleach) prepared daily is an inexpensive and effective germicide. Concentrations ranging from approximately 500 ppm (1:100 dilution of household bleach) sodium hypochlorite to 5,000 ppm (1:10 dilution of household bleach) are effective depending on the amount of organic material (e.g., blood, mucus present on the surface to be cleaned and disinfected.. Commercially available chemical germicides may be more compatible with certain medical devices that might be corroded by repeated exposure to sodium hypochlorite, especially to the 1:10 dilution

## Survival of HIV in the Environment

The most extensive study on the survival of HIV after drying involved greatly concentrated HIV samples, i.e., 10 million tissue-culture infectious doses per milliliter. This concentration is at least 100,000 times greater than that typically found in the blood or serum of patients with HIV infection. HIV was detectable by tissue-culture techniques 1-3 days after drying, but the rate of inactivation was rapid. Studies performed at CDC have also shown that drying HIV causes a rapid (within several hours) 1-2 log (90 per cent-99 per cent) reduction in HIV concentration. In tissue-culture fluid, cell-free HIV could be detected up to 15 days at room temperature, up to 11 days at 37 C (98.6 F), and up to 1 day if the HIV was cell-associated.

When considered in the context of environmental conditions in health-care faculties, these results do not require any changes in currency recommended sterilization, disinfection, or housekeeping strategies. When medical devices are contaminated with blood or other body fluids, existing recommendations include the cleaning of these instruments, followed by disinfection or sterilization, depending on the type of medical device. These protocols assume "worstcase" conditions of extreme virologic and micrological contamination, and whether viruses have been inactivated after drying plays no role in formulating these strategies. Consequently, no changes in published procedures for cleaning, disinfecting, or sterilizing need to be made.

## Housekeeping

Environmental surfaces such as walls, floors, and other surfaces are not associated with transmission of infections to patients or health-care workers. Therefore, extraordinary attempts to disinfect or sterilize these environmental surfaces are not necessary. However, cleaning and removal of soil should be done routinely.

Cleaning schedules and methods vary according to the area of the hospital or institution, type of surface to be cleaned, and the amount and type of soil present. Horizontal surfaces (e.g., bedside tables and hard-surfaced flooring) in patient-care areas are usually cleaned on a regular basis, when soiling or spills occur, and when a patient is discharged. Cleaning of walls, blinds, and curtains is recommended only if they are visibly soiled. Disinfectant fogging is an unsatisfactory method of decontaminating air and surfaces and is not recommended.

Disinfectant-detergent formulations registered by EPA can be used for cleaning environmental surfaces, but the actual physical removal of micro-organisms by scrubbing is probably at least as important as any antimicrobial effect of the cleaning agent used. Therefore, cost, safely, and acceptability by housekeepers can be the main criteria for selecting any such registered agent. The manufacturers' instructions for appropriate use should be followed.

## Cleaning and Decontaminating Spills of Blood or Other Body Fluids

Chemical germicides that are approved for use as "hospital disinfectants" and are tuberculocidal when used at recommended dilutions can be used to decontaminate spills of blood and other body fluids. Strategies for decontaminating spills of blood and other body fluids in a patient-care setting are different than for spills of cultures or other materials in clinical, public health, or research laboratories. In patient-care areas, visible material should first be removed and then the area should be decontaminated. With large spills of cultured or concentrated infectious agents in the laboratory, the contaminated areas should be flooded with a germicide before cleaning, then decontaminated with fresh germicidal chemical. In both settings, gloves should be worn during the cleaning and decontaminating procedures.

## Laundry

Although soiled linen has been identified as a source of large numbers of certain pathogenic micro-organisms, the risk of actual disease transmission is negligible. Rather than rigid procedures and specifications, hygienic and common-sense storage and processing of clean and soiled linen are recommended .[26] Soiled linen should be handled as little as possible and with minimum agitation to prevent gross microbial contamination of the air and of persons handling the linen. All soiled linen should be bagged at the location where it was used; it should not be sorted or rinsed in patient-care areas. Linen soiled with blood or body fluids should be placed and transported in bags that prevent leakage. If hot water is used, linen should be washed with detergent in water at least 71 C

(160 F.) for 25 minutes. If low-temperature ($\leqslant$ 70 C [158 F.]) laundry cycles are used, chemicals suitable for low-temperature washing at proper use concentration should be used.

## Infective Waste

There is no epidemiologic evidence to suggest that most hospital waste is any more infective than residential waste. Moreover, there is no epidemiologic evidence that hospital waste has caused disease in the community as a result of improper disposal. Therefore, identifying wastes for which special precautions are indicated is largely a matter of judgment about the relative risk of disease transmission. The most practical approach to the management of infective waste is to identify those wastes with the potential for causing infection during handling and disposal and for which some special precautions appear prudent. Hospital wastes for which special precautions appear prudent include microbiology laboratory waste, pathology waste, and blood specimens or blood products. While any item that has had contact with blood, exudates, or secretions may be potentially infective, it is not usually considered practical or necessary to treat all such waste as infective.[23,26] Infective waste, in general, should either be incinerated or should be autoclaved before disposal in a sanitary landfill. Bulk blood, suctioned fluids, excretions, and secretions may be carefully poured down a drain connected to a sanitary sewer. Sanitary sewers may also be used to dispose of other infectious wastes capable of being ground and flushed into the sewer.

## Implementation of Recommended Precautions

Employers of health-care workers should ensure that policies exist for:

1. Initial orientation and continuing education and training of all health-care workers—including students and trainees—on the epidemiology, modes of transmission, and prevention of HIV and other blood-borne infections and the need for routine use of universal blood and body-fluid precautions for all patients.
2. Provision of equipment and supplies necessary to minimize the risk of infection with HIV and other blood-borne pathogens.
3. Monitoring adherence to recommended protective measures. When monitoring reveals a failure to follow recommended precautions, counseling, education, and/or re-training should be provided, and, if necessary, appropriate disciplinary action should be considered.

Professional associations and labour organizations, through continuing education efforts, should emphasize the need for health-care workers to follow recommended precautions.

## Serologic Testing for HIV Infection

*Background*

A person is identified as infected with HIV when a sequence of tests, starting with repeated enzyme immunoassays (EIA) and including a Western blot or similar, more specific assay, are repeatedly reactive. Persons infected with HIV usually develop antibody against the virus within 6-12 weeks after infection.

The sensitivity of the currently licensed EIA tests is at least 99 per cent when they are performed under optimal laboratory conditions on serum specimens from persons infected for ⩾ 12 weeks. Optimal laboratory conditions include the use of reliable reagents, provision of continuing education of personnel, quality control of procedures, and participation in performance-evaluation programmes. Given this performance, the probability of a false-negative test is remote except during the first several weeks after infection, before detectable antibody is present. The proportion of infected persons with a false-negative test attributed to absence of antibody in the early stages of infection is dependent on both the incidence and prevalence of HIV infection in a population (Table 36.1).

The specificity of the currently licensed EIA tests is approximately 99 per cent when repeatedly reactive tests are considered. Repeat testing of initially reactive specimens by EIA is required to reduce the likelihood of laboratory error. To increase further the specificity of serologic tests, laboratories must use a supplemental test, most often the Western blot, to validate repeatedly reactive EIA results. Under optimal laboratory conditions, the sensitivity of the Western blot test is comparable to or greater than that of a repeatedly reactive EIA, and the Western blot is highly specific when strict criteria are used to interpret the test results. The testing sequence of a repeatedly reactive EIA and a positive Western blot test is highly predictive of HIV infection, even in a population with a low prevalence of infection (Table 36.2). If the Western blot test result is indeterminant, the testina sequence is considered equivocal for HIV infection.

When this occurs, the Western blot test should be repeated on the same serum sample, and, if still indeterminant, the testing sequence should be repeated on a sample collected 3-6 months later. Use of other supplemental tests may aid in interpreting of results on samples that are persistently indeterminant by Western blot.

TABLE -36.1.

**Estimated Annual Number of Patients Infected with HIV not Detected by HIV-Antibody Testing in a Hypothetical Hospital with 10,000 Admissions/year***

| Beginning pre valence of HIV Infection | Annual incidence of HIV Infection | Approximate number of HIV-infected patients | Approximate number of HIV-infected patients not detected |
|---|---|---|---|
| 5.0% | 1.0% | 550 | 17-18 |
| 5.0% | 0.5% | 525 | 11-12 |
| 1.0% | 0.2% | 110 | 3 4 |
| 1.0% | 0.1% | 105 | 2-3 |
| 0.1% | 0.02% | 11 | 0-1 |
| 0.1% | 0.01% | 11 | 0-1 |

* The estimates are based on the following assumptions: (1) the sensitivity of the screening test is 99 per cent (i.e., 99 per cent of HIV-infected persons with antibody will be detected), (2) persons infected with HIV will not develop detectable antibody (seroconvert) until 6 weeks (1.5 months) after infection; (3) new infections occur at an equal rate throughout the year; (4) calculations of the number of HIV-infected persons in the patient population are based on the mid-year prevalence, which is the beginning prevalence plus half the annual incidence of infections.

TABLE -36.2.

**Predictive Value of Positive HIV-Antibody Tests in Hypothetical Populations with Different Prevalences of Infection**

| | Prevalence of infection | Predictive value of positive test |
|---|---|---|
| Repeatedly reactive enzyme immunoassay (EIA)† | 0.2% | 28.41% |
| | 2.0% | 80.16% |
| | 20.0% | 98.02% |
| Repeatedly reactive EIA followed by positive Western blot (WB)§ | 0.2% | 99.75% |
| | 2.0% | 99.97% |
| | 20.0% | 99.99% |

* Proportion of persons with positive test results who are actually infected with HIV.

† Assumes EIA sensitivity of 99.0% and specificity of 99.5%.

§ Assumes WB sensitivity of 99.0% and specificity of 99.9%.

## Testing of Patients

Previous CDC recommendations have emphasized the value of HIV serologic testing of patients for: (1) management of parenteral or mucous-membrane exposures of health-care workers, (2) patient diagnosis and management, and (3) counseling and serologic testing to prevent and control HIV transmission in the community. In addition, more recent recommendations have stated that hospitals, in conjunction with state and local health departments, should periodically determine the prevalence of HIV infection among patients from age groups at highest risk of infection.[32]

Adherence to universal blood and body-fluid precautions recommended for the care of all patients will minimize the risk of transmission of HIV and other blood-borne pathogens from patients to health-care workers. The utility of routine HIV serologic testing of patients as an adjunct to universal precautions is unknown. Results of such testing may not be available in emergency or outpatient settings. In addition, some recently infected patients will not have detectable antibody to HIV (Table 36.1).

Personnel in some hospitals have advocated serologic testing of patients in settings in which exposure of health-care workers to large amounts of patients' blood may be anticipated. Specific patients for whom serologic testing has been advocated include those undergoing major operative procedures and those undergoing treatment in critical-care units, especially if they have conditions involving uncontrolled bleeding. Decisions regarding the need to establish testing programmes for patients should be made by physicians or individual institutions. In addition, when deemed appropriate, testing of individual patients may be performed on agreement between the patient and the physician providing care.

In addition to the universal precautions recommended for all patients, certain additional precautions for the care of HIV-infected patients undergoing major surgical operations have been proposed by personnel in some hospitals. For example, surgical procedures on an HIV-infected patient might be altered so that hand-to-hand passing of sharp instruments would be eliminated; stapling instruments rather than hand-suturing equipment might be used to perform tissue approximation; electrocautery devices rather than scalpels might be used as cutting instruments; and, even though uncomfortable, gowns that totally prevent seepage of blood onto the skin of members of the operative team might be worn. While such modifications might further minimize the risk of HIV infection for members of the operative team, some of these techniques could result in prolongation of operative time and could potentially have an adverse effect on the patient.

Testing programmes, if developed, should include the following principles:

- # Obtaining consent for testing.
- # Informing patients of test results, and providing counseling for seropositive patients by properly trained persons.

# Assuring that confidentiality safeguards are in place to limit knowledge of test results to those directly involved in the care of infected patients or as required by law.

# Assuring that identification of infected patients will not result in denial of needed care or provision of suboptimal care.

# Evaluating prospectively, (1) the efficacy of the programme in reducing the incidence of parenteral, mucous-membrane, or significant cutaneous exposures of health-care workers to the blood or other body fluids of HIV-infected patients and (2) the effect of modified procedures on patients.

## Testing of Health-Care Workers

Although transmission of HIV from infected health-care workers to patients has not been reported, transmission during invasive procedures remains a possibility. Transmission of hepatitis B virus (HBV)—a blood-borne agent with a considerably greater potential for nosocomial spread—from health-care workers to patients has been documented. Such transmission has occurred in situations (e.g., oral and gynecologic surgery) in which health-care workers, when tested, had very high concentrations of HBV in their blood (at least 100 million infectious virus particles per milliliter, a concentration much higher than occurs with HIV infection), and the health-care workers sustained a puncture wound while performing invasive procedures or had exudative or weeping lesions or microlacerations that allowed virus to contaminate instruments or open wounds of patients.[33,34]

The hepatitis B experience indicates that only those health-care workers who perform certain types of invasive procedures have transmitted HBV to patients. Adherence to recommendations in this document will minimize the risk of transmission of HIV and other blood-borne pathogens from health-care workers to patients during invasive procedures. Since transmission of HIV from infected health-care workers performing invasive procedures to their patients has not been reported and would be expected to occur only very rarely, if at all, the utility of routine testing of such health-care workers to prevent transmission of HIV cannot be assessed. If consideration is given to developing a serologic testing programme for health-care workers who perform invasive procedures, the frequency of testing, as well as the issues of consent, confidentiality, and consequences of test results—as previously outlined for testing programmes for patients—must be addressed.

## Management of Infected Health-Care Workers

Health-care workers with impaired immune systems resulting from HIV infection or other causes are at increased risk of acquiring or experiencing serious complications of infectious disease. Of particular concern is the risk of severe infection following exposure to patients with infectious diseases that are easily transmitted if appropriate precautions are not taken (e.g., measles, varicella). Any health-care worker with an impaired immune system should be counseled about the potential risk associated with taking care of patients with any transmissible infection and should continue to follow existing recommendations for infection control to minimize risk of exposure to other infectious agents.[7,35] Recommendations of the Immunization Practices Advisory Committee (ACIP) and institutional policies concerning requirements for vaccinating health-care workers with live-virus vaccines (e.g., measles, rubella) should also be considered.

The question of whether workers infected with HIV—especially those who perform invasive procedures—can adequately and safely be allowed to perform patient-care duties or whether their work assignments should be changed must be determined on an individual basis. These decisions should be made by the health-care worker's personal physician(s) in conjunction with the medical directors and personnel health service staff of the employing institution or hospital.

## Management of Exposures

If a health-care worker has a parenteral (e.g., needlestick or cut) or mucousmembrane (e.g., splash to the eye or mouth) exposure to blood or other body fluids or has a cutaneous exposure involving large amounts of blood or prolonged contact with blood—especially when the exposed skin is chapped, abraded, or afflicted with dermatitis—the source patient should be informed of the incident and tested for serologic evidence of HIV infection after consent is obtained. Policies should be developed for testing source patients in situations in which consent cannot be obtained (e.g., an unconscious patient).

If the source patient has AIDS, is positive for HIV antibody, or refuses the test, the health-care worker should be counseled regarding the risk of infection and evaluated clinically and serologically for evidence of HIV infection as soon as possible after the exposure. The health-care worker should be advised to report and seek medical evaluation for any acute febrile illness that occurs within 12 weeks after the exposure. Such an illness—particularly one characterized by fever, rash, or lymphadenopathy— may be indicative of recent HIV infection. Seronegative health-care workers should be retested 6 weeks post-exposure and on a periodic basis thereafter (e.g., 12 weeks and 6 months after exposure) to determine whether transmission has occurred. During this follow-up period—especially the first 6-12 weeks after exposure, when most infected persons are expected to seroconvert—exposed health-care workers should follow U.S. Public Health Service (PHS) recommendations for preventing transmission of HIV.[36,37]

No further follow-up of a health-care worker exposed to infection as described above is necessary if the source patient is seronegative unless the source patient is at high risk of HIV infection. In the latter case, a subsequent specimen (e.g., 12 weeks following exposure) may be obtained from the health-care worker for antibody testing. If the source patient cannot be identified, decisions regarding appropriate follow-up should be individualized. Serologic testing should be available to a health-care workers who are concerned that they may have been infected with HIV.

If a patient has a parenteral or mucous-membrane exposure to blood or other body fluid of a health-care worker, the patient should be informed of the incident, and the same procedure outlined above for management of exposures should be followed for both the source health-care worker and the exposed patient.

## References

1. CDC. Acquired immunodeficiency syndrome (AIDS): Precautions for clinical and laboratory staffs. MMWR 1982;31:577-80.
2. CDC. Acquired immunodeficiency syndrome (Aids) Precautions for health-care workers and allied professionals. MMWA 1983;32:450-1.
3. CDC. Recommendations for preventing transmission of infection with human T-lymphotropic virus type III,/ lymphadenopathy-associated virus in the workplace. MMWA 1985;34:681-6, 691-5.
4. CDC. Recommendations for preventing transmission of infection with human T-lymphotropic virus type III/ lymphadenopathy-associated virus during Invasive procedures. MMWR 1986;35:221-3.
5. CDC. Recommendations for preventing possible transmission of human T-lymphotropic virus type III, /lymphadenopathy-associated virus from tears. MMWR 1985;34:533-4.
6. CDC. Recommendations for providing dialysis treatment to patients infected with human T-lymphotropic virus type III/lymphadenopathy-associated virus infection. MMWR 1986;35:376-8, 383.
7. Garner JS, Simmons BP. Guideline for isolation precautions in hospitals. Infect Control 1983;4 (suppl) :245-325.
8. CDC. Recommended infection control practices for dentists MMWR 1986;35:237-42.
9. McCray E, The Co-operative Needlestick Surveillance Group. Occupational risk of the acquired immunodeficiency syndrome among health care workers. N Engl J Med 1986;314:1127-32.

10. Henderson DK, Saah AJ, Zak BJ, at al Risk of nosocomial infection with human T-cell Iymphotropic virus type III/ymphadenopathy-associated virus in a large cohort of intensively exposed health care workers. Ann Intern Med 1986; 104:W-7.
11. Gerberding JL, Bryant--LeBlanc CE, Nelson K, et al Risk of transmitting the human immunodeficiency virus, cytomegalovirus, and hepatitis B virus to health care workers exposed to patients with AIDS and AIDS-related conditions. J Infect Dis 1987;156:1-8.
12. McEvoy M, Poner K, Mortimer P. Simmons N. Shanson D. Prospective study of clinical, laboratory, and concillory staff with accidental exposures to blood or other body fiuids from patients infected with HIV. Bo Med J 1987;29:1595-7.
13. Anonymous. Needlestick transmission of HTLV-III from a patient infected in Africa. Lancet 1984;2:1376-7.
14. Oksenhendler E, Haizic M, he, Le Roux JM, Rabian C, Clauvel JP. HIV infection with seroconversion after a superficial needlesfick injury to the finger. N Engl. J Med 1986;315:582.
15. Neisson-Vernant C, Arfi S., Mathez D, Leibowdch J. Monplaisir N. Needlestick HIV seroconversion in a nurse. Lancet 1986;2:814.
16. Grint P. McEvoy M. Two associated cases of the acquired immune deficiency syndrome (AIDS). PHLS Commun Dis Rep 1985;42:4.
17. CDC. Apparent transmission of human T-lymphotropic virus type III/lymphadenopathy associated virus from a child to a mother providing health care. MMWR 1986;35:76-9.
18. CDC. Update: Human immunodeficiency virus infections in health-care workers exposed to blood of infected patients. MMWR 1987;36:285-9.
19. Kline RS, Phelan J. Friedland GH, et al Low occupational risk for HIV infection for dental professionals [Abstracts] fin: Abstracts from the III International Conference on AIDS, 1-5 June 1985. Washington, DC: 155.
20. Baker JL, Kelen GD, Sivenson KT, Quinn TC. Unsuspected human immunodeficiency virus in critically ill emergency patients. JAMA 1987;257:Z609-11.
21. Favero My. Dialysis-associated diseases and their control in: Bennett JV, Brachman PS, eds. Hospital infections. Boston: Little, Brown and Company, 1985:Z 67-84.
22. Richardson JH, Barkley WE, eds. Biosafety in microbiological and biomedical laboratories, 1984. Washington, DC: US Department of Health and Human Services, Public Health Service. HHS publication no. (CDC) 84-8395.
23. CDC. Human T-lymphotropic virus type III/lymphadenopathy-associated virus: Agent summary statement. MMWR 1986,35:540-2, 547-9.
24. Environmental Protection Agency. EPA guide for infectious waste management. Washington, DC : U.S. Environmental Protection Agency, May 1986 (Publication no. EPA/530-SW-86-014).
25. Favero MS. Sterilization, disinfection, arid antisepsis in the hospital. In: Manual of clinical microbiology. 4th ed. Washington, DC: American Society for Microbiology, 1985:129-37.

26. Garner JS, Favero MS. Guideline for handwashing and hospital environmental control, 1985. Atlanta: Public Health Service, Centers for Disease Control, 1985. HHS publication no. 99-1117.
27. Spire B. Montagnier L, Barre-Sinoussi F. Chermann JC. Inactivation of lymphadenopathy associated virus by chemical disinfectants. Lancet 1984;2:899-901.
28. Martin LS, McDougal JS, Loskoski SL. Disinfection and inactivation of the human T lymphotropic virus type III/lymphadenopathy-associated virus. J Infect Dis 1985; 152:400-3.
29. McDougal JS, Martin LS, Cort SP, et al. Thermal inactivation of the acquired immunodeficiency syndrome virus-III/lymphadenopathy-associated virus, with special reference to antihemophilic factor. J Clin Invest 1985;76:875-7.
30. Spire B. Barre-Sinoussi,,F, Doront D, Montagnier L, Chermann JC. Inactivation of lymphadenopathy-associated virus by heat, gamma rays, and ultraviolet light. Lancet 1985;1:188-9.
31. Resnik L, Veren K, Salahuddin SZ, Tondreau S. Markham PD. Stability and inactivation of HTLV-III/LAV under clinical and laboratory environments. JAMA 1986;255:1887-91.
32. CDC. Public Health Service (PHS) guidelines for counseling and antibody testing to prevent HIV infection and AIDS. MMWR 1987,3:509-15..
33. Kane MA, Lenau LA. Transmission of HBV from dental personnel to patients. J Am Dent Assoc 1985;110:634-6.
34. Lettau LA, Smith JD, Williams D, et. al. Transmission of hepatitis B with resultant restriction of surgical practice. JAMA 1986;255:934-7.
35. Williams WW. Guideline for infection control in hospital personnel. Infect Control 1983,4 (supply) :326-49.
36. CDC. Prevention of acquired immune deficiency syndrome (AIDS): Report of inter-agency recommendations. MMWR 1983;32:101-3.
37. CDC. Provisional Public Health Service inter-agency recommendations for screening donated blood and plasma for antibody to the virus causing acquired immunodeficiency syndrome. MMWR 1985;34:1-5.

# 37

# HIV in the Workplace: Dealing with the Issues

Joyce Leyones and
Jenny Huddart
UNDP, New York

## INTRODUCTION

*Vinod, a skilled mechanic, has recently disclosed he is infected with HIV to his fellow worker and good friend Jyoti. He now sits isolated in the cafeteria.*

*Teresita, a beloved teacher in a rural community, has been dismissed from her job because of her HIV positive status.*

What is obvious in these scenarios is that education about, and an understanding of, HIV has not taken place. Discrimination and dismissal will not remove the threat of HIV infection nor help to create a congenial workplace environment. The only protection we have against the spread of HIV is education. Clear, concise and medically correct facts help to reduce the fear and anxiety commonly associated with HIV and to prevent any loss in worker productivity which may result from these far too common responses.

### Why is an Understanding of the Implications of HIV Important to the Workplace?

"Today there are 2.3 billion economically active people in the world. The workplace environment plays a central role in the lives of people everywhere. A consideration of HIV/ AIDS and the workplace will strengthen the capacity to deal effectively with the problem of HIV/AIDS at the local, national and international levels." (Statement from the Consultation on AIDS and the Workplace, WHO/ILO Geneva, June 1988).

HIV is a nondiscriminatory virus, affecting people of all cultures, religions and races. The most common route of transmission is unprotected sexual activity. This fact makes men and women in their most productive and sexually active years, those between 18-45 years of age, the most vulnerable group for becoming infected. The largest organized target audience of the vulnerable age group is found in the workplace where employers have a lot to lose if employees become infected with the virus.

Because of its infection pattern, unlike other epidemics, HIV directly affects the social and economic environment of the workplace. Due to the fear and stigma currently surrounding the virus, HIV can cause interpersonal, social and discriminatory problems within the workplace.

It can also affect the company's productivity when in later stages of the infection, increased absenteeism, loss of skilled labour, and costs of retraining or hiring new workers begin to take their toll.

One vital factor which distinguishes HIV from other diseases is that it can remain dormant in an individual for many years before the onset of illness. During this time, the individual can lead a healthy and productive life; this has psychological and economic implications for the worker as well as for the employer. Each can continue to receive the full benefits of the working relationship.

Another significant point about this virus, unlike other viruses, is that infection can be prevented by changes in personal behaviour. To lessen the impact of HIV on the workplace, it is important to develop a comprehensive HIV/ AIDS programme which includes workplace policies to ensure humane treatment of those who are HIV positive, prepares managers to answer questions and confrontations related to HIV, and teaches workers how the infection is transmitted and what they can do to prevent it. All employees should be supplied with the facts and support needed to practice the preventive behaviour which will reduce their vulnerability to infection and their fear of those infected. Some employers will also want to consider offering additional health services.

## The Purpose of the Role Plays

Statistics have shown us that information alone is important but not enough to make people adopt the changes in behaviour necessary to protect themselves from HIV infection. This should not come as a surprise, for example, advertising campaigns against smoking do not stop smokers. Often a more personal experience is necessary to convince people to change their behaviour. The media have been successful in using well known characters to tell stories about living with HIV; community members with HIV have been able to convey the message. To reach a large audience, videos, films and slide shows have also been effective.

Another technique, which has great value in helping individuals to personalize issues, is to give them an opportunity to explore the predicament by involving them as participants in a simulation experience. Keeping this in mind, these role plays, based on reports of actual situations, have been developed to help managers confront and discuss the issues related to HIV in the workplace.

The role plays assist participants to:

1. Explore the issues surrounding HIV/AIDS in the workplace;
2. Identify the potential contributions of NGOs in assisting the business sector to address the issues of HIV/AIDS in the workplace;
3. Practice skills in developing co-operative strategies for dealing with HIV/AIDS in the workplace.

Before implementing these role plays, a basic understanding of HIV and AIDS is needed, including how the infection is (and is not) transmitted and its progression from infection to AIDS-related symptoms.

## BACKGROUND

### Basic Facts

*What is AIDS?*

Acquired Immunodeficiency Syndrome, AIDS is the result of infection with the Human Immunodeficiency Virus (HIV). The virus is transmitted primarily through sexual intercourse, although infection can also occur through the transmission of infected blood and blood products. Slowly, the virus disables the immune system which is the body's primary line of defense against disease. As the body's immune system breaks down, it becomes more vulnerable to a host of opportunistic infections which leave a person susceptible to pneumonia, tuberculosis, oral lesions and occasionally rare forms of cancer—diseases which rarely affect healthy immune systems. The symptoms and signs of HIV related illnesses are complex, vary greatly and can include persistent diarrhea, weight loss, oral and skin lesions, and loss of appetite. It is impossible to tell from looking at a person or by hearing his symptoms whether or not he is infected with the virus. It is important to note that these symptoms are commonly associated with many other diseases. Diagnosis of HIV infection can only be made through a blood test .

We know a great deal more about HIV now than we did when it was first identified in 1985. We know how it is transmitted, how the body reacts to it and most importantly, we know how to protect ourselves. We still do not know how to cure it and there is no definitive answer as to the origin of the virus. This gap in our knowledge has no bearing on the development of a workplace programme to control its transmission. The knowledge we do have clearly shows that casual contact, such as in the workplace setting, does not put a person at risk of infection.

## HOW IS HIV TRANSMITTED?

There are only three ways the virus can be transmitted.

1. By having unprotected sexual intercourse with a person who has the virus. This accounts for approximately 80 per cent of the worldwide transmission of the virus; the percentage in developing countries is even greater.
2. By being injected with contaminated blood, blood products or unsterile equipment; 35 per cent of the worldwide transmissions occur in this manner. Five to ten per cent of global infections are due to the reuse of contaminated needles by intravenous drug users.
3. By an infected mother passing the virus onto her child through pregnancy or breastfeeding; this comprises 5-10 per cent of the entire transmission figure.

### HOW IS HIV NOT TRANSMITTED?

The virus cannot be transmitted:

1. Through the air, by sneezing, coughing, or breathing
2. Through casual physical contact, such as touching, hugging or kissing
3. Through water, as in swimming pools
4. Through sharing utensils or food or the same telephone
5. Through toilets
6. Through mosquitoes

### HOW CAN HIV TRANSMISSION BE PREVENTED?

1. By practicing safer sex: keeping to one partner whose sexual history is known to you; practicing non-penetrative sex or using a high quality latex condom for every act of sexual intercourse.
2. By always using clean, sterilized needles and avoiding unnecessary skin piercing.
3. By never sharing injecting drug equipment.
4. By receiving blood transfusions only when necessary and only with properly screened blood.

## ISSUES

### What are the Issues that HIV Brings into the Workplace?

As HIV enters the workplace, government agencies, companies and labour unions are all struggling to develop strategies to respond to the issues it raises. What follows is a discussion of these issues; relevant policy statements of the United Nations are included as a guide to help others determine their own response. (The complete UN HIV/AIDS Personnel Policy can be found in the p. No. 483).

1. DENIAL: A common misconception is that HIV is someone else's problem. It is a disease of selected groups commonly referred to as "high risk" groups, i.e., promiscuous people, intravenous drug users, foreigners.

This ignores the evidence that the greatest single mode of transmission of HIV is unprotected heterosexual intercourse. The virus does not put groups at risk. People practicing unsafe behaviour put themselves at risk.

Statistics demonstrate that the virus is already spreading at an alarming rate in Asia. By the year 2000, the number of the new cases in Asia is expected to surpass that of Africa, the overwhelming majority of them, men and women in their most economically productive years.

Continued beliefs that HIV only affects a selected population is a dangerous practice, allowing large sectors of society to feel protected from the epidemic thus blocking the understanding of the necessity to develop effective intervention strategies.

2. FEAR: Ten years into the epidemic and still the most common response to the subject of AIDS is fear Misinformation, misconceptions and dread of the unknown heighten the anxiety felt by those who have their first encounter with a person with AIDS, or someone known to have HIV.

   Fear is best handled by allowing people to express openly their concerns. Acknowledgment of their feelings and discussion about them helps to dissipate the fear.

3. DISCRIMINATION: Fear often leads to discrimination against people who have HIV Loss of jobs, friends, homes are not uncommon occurrences. Mistaken beliefs that casual contacts can spread the virus have led to the isolation and loss of dignity and respect to which people infected with the virus often become subject.

Presenting medically correct facts and discussing the

misconceptions that cause fear will reduce the discrimination that results from it.

4. CONFIDENTIALITY: A person's medical history is confidential Revelation of items such as a person's HIV status can lead to the consequences of his/her being stigmatized and subjected to discrimination.

HIV is still associated with discrimination and stigma due to misconceptions of how the virus is transmitted. Cases of people losing their jobs, homes and families have occurred after disclosure that they are infected with the HIV virus. The medical facts regarding transmission of the virus clearly prove that ordinary workplace behaviour and interaction does not lead to the spread of infection. To reduce disruption in the workplace and protect the infected individual, privacy about his/her status is required.

United Nations Policy states "Confidentiality regarding all medical information, including HIV/AIDS status, must be maintained "

5. SCREENING: To attempt to create an HIV free environment business may consider screening or pretesting potential employees to determine their HIV status as a condition of employment.

The practice of eliminating HIV positive people from the workforce has no justification as a public health measure nor is it considered fair employment practice. Furthermore due to the "window period" or amount of time it takes between becoming infected and having antibodies to the virus form in the blood, screening would not even reveal all individuals who are HIV+. Even if the employer believed that screening would reduce the number of infected people who gain entrance into the workplace, pre-employment testing certainly does not prevent an employee from practicing behaviours that will expose him or her to infection after employment.

UN Policy states: "There will be no screening of candidates for recruitment".

6. TESTING: Testing of employees has also been used as a means to eliminate workers who contract HIV while employed

Testing for HIV is not 100 per cent accurate; the "window period" makes the exact date upon which antibodies will appear in the blood undeterminable. Estimates range from 6 weeks to 6 months; however, researchers have found that some individuals take longer, sometimes years, to develop antibodies. Testing is an expensive prospect which must be repeated every 3-6 months if its objective is to identify all cases of HIV. In many countries, legal regulations limit the type of testing that can be required.

Testing should not be done unless a person is fully aware of the meaning and consequences of the test results and has provided his or her consent. An interview with a trained counsellor should give the individual interested in being tested an opportunity to express his concerns and to ask questions about the test. It is important to assure the individual that confidentiality is guaranteed. Counselling is essential both before testing and upon receipt of test results.

UN Policy states: "Voluntary testing with pre-and post-counselling and assured confidentiality should be made available to all UN staff members and their families".

7. POLICY: Issues related to sick leave, increased inability to perform the same strenuous job, health insurance needs, retirement rules, and policies on hiring and dismissal will all need to be reviewed."

Policies should reflect the medical facts, confirm basic human rights, and ensure workplace harmony. In many instances, HIV can be added to the policy in existence on serious illnesses. In all cases, the policy should be endorsed by top management and understood at all levels.

A person's job not only provides him or her with daily subsistence but helps to define a person's life. Most people who have discovered themselves to be HIV+ are fully capable of carrying out their job responsibilities and find comfort in continuing their daily employment.

Under what circumstances should an HIV+ individual be dismissed or deemed ineligible for employment? Facts show that a person infected with HIV does not present a risk of infection for others in daily casual contact. Facts also show that once a person is infected, s/he can lead a healthy, active and productive life for an average of 7-10 years. If this person is capable of performing in his or her job, there is no medical justification for dismissal.

When related illnesses cause a person with HIV to need special attention, such as longer sick leave or a less strenuous job, businesses should accommodate the situation following the same policies as are applied to other illnesses.

UN Policy states: (a) The only medical criteria for recruitment is fitness to work . (b) HIV infection or AIDS should not, of itself, be considered as a basis for termination of employment. (c) If fitness to work is impaired by HIV-related illness, reasonable alternative working arrangements should be made. (d) UN staff members should enjoy health and social protection in the same manner as other UN employees suffering from serious illness."

8. RESPONSIBILITY: Having a healthy and productive workforce is essential to the workplace. Preventive services such as condom promotion and counsellin.g referrals can be offered to ensure the personal health of workers Companies that provide health care should consider offering services for counselling and treatment of sexually transmitted diseases.

The simplest way to help employees protect themselves against infection is to provide accurate and up-to-date information. Messages on the need to have medical check ups for STD (Sexually Transmitted Disease) control are also important. The vulnerability to HIV increases when an STD is present.

After education, the best defense we have against HIV is the use of high quality condoms. Condoms act as a barrier preventing the virus from passing through, thereby reducing the risk of transmission. Having condoms available at the workplace for distribution or purchase is an innovative way of helping to ensure safer behaviour.

In the absence of a cure, counselling for individuals who have HIV or who suspect they might be infected takes on new significance. People need to express their frustration and anger. Often a linkup with a local health center or NGO can set up a referral system for pre- and post-test counselling, as well as, for illness related help.

Established links with hospitals or health care centers in which blood is known to be screened for the HIV virus can be a life saving matter.

UN Policy: (a) UN Staff and their families should be provided with sufficient, updated information to enable them to protect themselves from HIV infection and to cope with the presence of AIDS. (b) All UN staff members and their families should be made aware of where safe blood may be obtained. (c) All UN staff members and their families should have access to condoms."

## How can these Issues Best be Addressed?

The disruption in the workplace caused by the fear of HIV can be minimized by providing an HIV education and support system to all employees and by establishing HIV related personnel policies well in advance of any problems. However, only a comprehensive educational programme supported by top management will encourage employees to comply.

Successful workplace education programmes have approached executives first to help them develop an understanding of the basic facts regarding HIV. This knowledge can then be used to develop appropriate policy measures that will maintain a high level of worker productivity, ensure the rights and dignity of all, clarify legal issues, and create an atmosphere conducive to caring for and promoting the health of all workers.

Next, managers must understand and support the policy developed by their company and be knowledgeable enough about HIV/AIDS to respond to the concerns of their subordinates. They must be informed about their obligations once an employee becomes ill. They also need to know how to handle fearful workers and potential crisis situations.

Finally, a workplace education programme meeting the needs of all workers must be developed. Each programme must be tailored to the particular audience and company. Union representatives or worker spokespersons can be involved in the design of the educational programme. Logistical decisions regarding who, where, how and when this programme should be undertaken must be determined both to meet the objectives of the programme and to create the minimum disruption in the workplace.

## Methods of Addressing the Issues

The first step in addressing the issues is acknowledging the need for an HIV/AIDS education programme. This needs to be followed up by contacts with professional groups who can assist in the development of that programme. In some countries, local health departments or National AIDS Committees may have material to assist in this process. The WHO has several publications that may be relevant. In other countries, local non-government agencies may be your strongest ally.

As the epidemic spreads at an increasing rate, many NGOs have realized the importance of developing preventive programmes. Many have targeted the workplace as an appropriate setting for their efforts. Training modules, videos, peer training programmes, and written materials have been developed to assist in comprehensive workplace intervention programmes. A business/NGO collaboration is a strong deterrent to the spread of HIV.

An NGO, after providing basic education about the medical facts and societal realities of HIV, can help management prepare workplace policies that will guide the company's response to questions and concerns about HIV. An NGO can also be asked to prepare management to deal with HIV related issues that are likely to arise in the workplace. Then, in conjunction with management, it can draw up the most effective and efficient method of providing training to line workers. If necessary, the NGO can offer ongoing support in the form of pre and post-test counselling, individual sessions or training of trainers; others can offer legal guidance, support for condom distribution, family counselling or education and an opportunity to allow people openly to discuss sexuality.

## What Else can be Done?

As the worker actually begins to display signs of illness, accommodations may be worked out. Shorter work weeks, being able to work at home, more rest periods, a reduced work load, a restructuring of the job, relocation to a less demanding position have all been methods of dealing with an increased inabi'ity to perform the normal assignment.

## How Else Can Business Contribute?

To increase the understanding of HIV in society and to reach other workplaces, the following suggestions are provided:

1. Share your company's experience with other companies. Personal experience works in helping others follow the lead. Use the media, Chambers of Commerce or newsletters.
2. Produce a video on AIDS in the Workplace for your company's educational programmeme. Share it with other firms.
3. Become an advocate for AIDS in the workplace legislation.
4. Host an AIDS in the Workplace Conference.
5. Volunteer to work for AIDS organizations and encourage employees to do the same.
6. Contributions from business to the non government community can include printing of brochures, photocopying of leaflets, providing space for meetings.
7. Start a resource library of AIDS information.
8. Raise funds for research or care facilities.
9. Provide HIV/AIDS information for the worker's family. Organize a meeting for spouses. Produce simple material for presentation to their children.
10. Provide informed speakers for schools and community groups.

## *I. GLOSSARY*

AIDS.: Acquired Immune Deficiency Syndrome (AIDS) is the last stage of the virus known as HIV. The body's immune system has been seriously damaged, leaving it vulnerable to infections that can ultimately result in death.

ANTIBODY: A protein produced in the blood to fight infection.

AT RISK: Practicing behaviours which could lead to becoming infected with HIV, e.g., engaging in unprotected sex, sharing of unsterilized injecting equipment.

HIV: Human Immunodeficiency Virus (HIV) is the virus that causes AIDS.

HIV-: Having been tested for HIV antibodies in the blood and discovering that none exist.

HIV+: This signifies the status of one who has been found to have, through blood screening, antibodies to HIV in the blood. It indicates that one is infected with HIV and can infect others but it does not indicate a person has AIDS. It can also be referred to as being seropositive.

HIV TESTING: Screening the blood for HIV antibodies. The two most common tests are the ELISA and Western Blot.

NGO: Non Government Organization usually performing a service.

SAFER SEX: Engaging in sexual intercourse with the protection of a condom; having fewer sexual partners, keeping to one sexual partner whose sexual history is known to you.

SERONEGATIVE: see HIV

SEROPOSITIVE: See HIV+

STD: Sexually Transmitted Disease whose presence increases the possibility of HIV receptivity. HIV is predominately a sexually transmitted infection.

WINDOW PERIOD: The time between infection and the appearance of HIV antibodies in the blood system. This can vary greatly in length. It is also why mandatory testing is not an effective devise to determine the HIV status of individuals.

## II. *UN HIV/AIDS*

### *Personnel Policy*

### A. Information, Education and Other Preventive Health Measures

(i) UN Staff and their families should be provided with sufficient, updated information to enable them to protect themselves from HIV infection and to cope with the presence of AIDS.

To this end all UN bodies are encouraged to develop and implement an active staff education strategy for HIV/AIDS utilizing inter alia, the handbook on AIDS for UN employees and their families produced by WHO and identifying in the field local sources experienced by HIV/ AIDS counselling, to provide confidential follow up. The staff of the UN Medical Service should be fully involved in such staff education programmes. They should receive any additional professional education that they may be required; and all pertinent information material on HIV and ADDS, supplied and updated by WHO, should be available through them at all duty stations

(ii) All UN staff members and their families should be made aware of where safe blood may be obtained.

To accomplish this task, the WHO Global Blood Safety Initiative, in co-operation with the UN Medical Service, should establish and regularly update a list of reliable and operational blood transfusion centres for circulation to UN headquarters, regional offices and duty stations. The UN Medical Services should also make efforts to ensure that blood transfusions are performed only when absolutely necessary.

(iii) UN Resident Co-ordinators must exercise their responsibility to adopt measures to reduce the frequency of motor vehicle accidents, not only because of their attendant high mortality and morbidity, but because they present a particular risk for HIV infection in those localities lacking safe blood supplies.

UN Resident Co-ordinators are, therefore, encouraged to consider the following measures for reinforcement or for general adoption if not already applied; and to circulate them to all personnel at the duty station together with instructions on the use of public transport.

* the fitting of and compulsory use of seat belts in all UN vehicles;
* proper training in off-road use of 4-wheel drives;
* prohibition against the personal use of vehicles when an official driver is available;
* compulsory use of helmets for all riders of motorbikes;
* organization of first-aid training sessions; and
* equipping UN vehicles with first-aid kits containing macromolecular solutions (plasma expanders).

(iv) All UN staff members and their families should have access to disposable syringes and needles.

The UN Medical Service should provide disposable syringes and needles to staff on duty travel to areas where there is no guarantee of the proper sterilization of such materials. They should be accompanied by a certificate in all UN official languages explaining the reasons why they are being carried. Regional offices and other duty stations should stock disposable injection material for the use of UN staff and their families. This stock should be available at UN dispensaries, where such exist, or at the WHO duty station in the country.

(v) All UN staff members and their families should have access to condoms.

Condoms should be available through UNFPA and/or WHO at those duty stations where there is not a reliable and consistent supply of high quality condoms from the private sector. Access should be free, simple and discreet.

## B. Voluntary Testing, Counselling and Confidentialily

Voluntary testing with pre- and postcounselling and assured confidentiality should be made available to all UN staff members and their families.

Adequate and confidential facilities for voluntary and confirmatory testing and counselling should be made available locally to UN staff members and their families, with UN bodies acting in close collaboration with the UN Medical Service and WHO. Specific procedures must be developed by UN bodies to maintain confidentiality with respect to negative as well as positive results from an HIV test, including whether such a test has been taken. Only the person tested has the right to release information concerning his/her HIV status.

## C. Terms of Appointment and Service

Pre-recruitment and Employment Prospects

(i) The only medical criterion for recruitment is fitness to work.

(ii) HIV infection does not, in itself, constitute a lack of fitness to work.

(iii) There will be no HIV screening of candidates for recruitment.

(iv) AIDS will be treated as any other medical condition in considering medical classification.

(v) HIV testing with the specific and informed consent of the candidate may be requited if AIDS is clinically suspected.

(vi) Nothing in the pre-employment examination should be considered as obliging any candidate to declare his or her HIV status.

(vii) For any assignment in a country which requires HIV testing for residence, this requirement must appear in the vacancy notice.

### Continuity of Employment

(i) HIV infection or AIDS should not, of itself, be considered as a basis for termination of employment.

(ii) If fitness to work is impaired by HIV-related illness, reasonable alternative working arrangements should be made.

(iii) UN staff members with AIDS should enjoy health and social protection in the same manner as other UN employees suffering from serious illness.

(a) HIV/AIDS screening, whether direct (HIV testing), indirect (assessment of risk behaviours) or asking questions about tests already taken, should not be required.

(b) Confidentiality regarding all medical information, including HIV/AIDS status, must be maintained.

(c) There should be no obligation on the part of the employee to inform the employer regarding his or her HIV/AIDS status.

(d) Persons in the workplace affected by, or perceived to be affected by HIV/AIDS, must be protected from stigmatization and discrimination by co-workers, unions, employers or clients.

(e) HIV-infected employees and those with AIDS should not be discriminated against, including access to and receipt of benefits from statutory social security programmes and occupationally related schemes.

The administrative, personnel and financial implications of these principles under terms of appointment and service should be monitored and periodically reviewed.

## D. Health Insurance Benefits Programmes

(i) Health insurance coverage should be available for all UN employees regardless of HIV status.

There should be no pre- or post-employment testing for HIV infection.

(ii) Health insurance premiums for UN employees should not be affected by HIV status.

No testing for HIV infection should be permitted with respect to any health insurance scheme.

## III. RESPONDING TO AIDS: TEN PRINCIPLES FOR THE WORKPLACE

1. People with AIDS or HIV (Human Immunodeficiency Virus) infection are entitled to the same rights and opportunities as people with other serious or life threatening illnesses.
2. Employment policies must, at a minimum, comply with federal, state and local laws and regulations.
3. Employment policies should be based on the scientific and epidemiological evidence that people with AIDS or HIV infection do not pose a risk of transmission of the virus to coworkers through ordinary workplace contact.
4. The highest levels of management and union leadership should unequivocally endorse non discriminatory employment policies and education programmes about AIDS.
5. Employers and unions should communicate their support of these policies to workers in simple, clear and unambiguous terms.
6. Employers should provide employees with sensitive, accurate and up-to date education about risk reduction in their personal lives.
7. Employers have a duty to protect the confidentiality of employees' medical information.
8. To prevent work disruption and rejection by coworkers of an employee with AIDS or HIV infection, employers and unions should undertake education for all employees before such an incident occurs and as needed thereafter.
9. Employers should not require HIV screening as part of general pre-employment or workplace physical examinations.
10. In those special occupational settings where there may be a potential risk of exposure to HIV (for example, in health care, where workers may be exposed to blood or blood products), employers should provide specific, ongoing education and training, as well as the necessary equipment, to reinforce appropriate infection control procedures and ensure that they are implemented.

*CITIZENS COMMISSION ON AIDS*

February 1988

## References

AIDS Education in the Workplace, An Education Guide for Managers produced by The San Francisco AIDS Foundation, 333 Valencia Street, Fourth Floor, P. O. Box 6182, San Francisco, California 94101-6182, USA.

Statement from the Consultation on AIDS and the Workplace, World Health Organization in association with International Labour Organization, Geneva, June 1988.

38

# AIDS Prevention and Care in the Workplace:

## Enhancing the Role of the Private Sector

**Report of a Regional Work Shop, New Delhi, 12-13 January, 1995**

---

### BACKGROUND

In South-East Asia, the human immunodeficiency virus (HIV), which causes acquired immunodeficiency syndrome (AIDS), is spreading as fast as it did in Africa a decade ago. Asia with its large population may soon surpass Africa in terms of both the total numbers of people infected and the number of new infections each year. WHO estimates that while there are over 18 million adults and 1.5 million children infected with HIV, this global figure will more than double, to between 30 and 40 million infections, by the year 2000. In South-East Asia, the epidemic's spread will be even more dramatic. The 2 million HIV infections now estimated in this region are projected to increase five-fold, to over 10 million by the year 2000.

HIV infection and AIDS do not only seriously affect health and life expectancy; if left unchecked, the epidemic will also greatly undermine the social and economic development of Asian countries. The epidemic will force national resources to be diverted from economic development to the health care of people with AIDS. This set-back for the business sector will be further accentuated by the loss of productivity when workers are forced to stay home either because they are sick themselves or because they need to take care of sick relatives. With industry facing a loss of skilled workers, the indirect costs of training or retraining new workers will be high. Moreover, the epidemic may even reduce consumer markets as increasing amounts of personal income will be spent on hospital bills and treatment for AIDS-related health problems. The need to check the epidemic is, therefore, urgent.

Unfortunately, there is no cure in sight, nor is a vaccine likely to be available in the foreseeable future. Only preventive measures can check the epidemic and these must, therefore, be implemented rapidly. This demands that each sector of society understands the implications of HIV infection and AIDS and responds to the challenge. The private sector in general, and business leaders in particular, represent a crucial component in this response. Apart from the self-interest involved, this sector could also play an effective leadership role in the fight against AIDS. Provision of education and information to the labour force, condom promotion, provision of access for the treatment of sexually transmitted diseases, institution of policies to stop discrimination and stigmatization are important contributions the private sector can make to reduce both the health and socio-economic impact of AIDS in the Region.

In order to discuss the role of the private sector, the South-East Asia Regional Office of the World Health Organization (WHO/SEARO) organized a regional workshop in New Delhi in January 1995. The specific objectives of the meeting were:

(1) To review the existing role of the private sector in HIV/AIDS prevention and care world wide in general and in the South-East Asia Region in particular;

(2) To identify and recommend strategies for developing or further strengthening HIV/AIDS prevention and care in business and other private sector workplaces, in the context of national AIDS programmes, and

(3) To develop guidelines, where possible, for the implementation of such policies and programmes at country level during 1995.

The meeting was opened by Dr. Samlee Plianbangchang, Acting Regional Director of WHO's South-East Asia Region, on behalf of Dr. Uton Muchtar Rafei, Regional Director. Expressing concern at the spread of HIV/AIDS in SEAR countries, particularly among people in their most productive years of life, Dr. Samlee. urged the private sector to actively participate in the national response by developing workplace policies and services. For the technical sessions of the workshop, Mr. P.R. Dasgupta from India was nominated as chairman, Dr. Supanya Lamsam from Thailand as co-chairman and Dr. Nyoman Suesan from Indonesia as rapporteur. For the list of participants and the programme of the workshop.

## HIV AND AIDS IN SOUTH-EAST ASIA AND ITS IMPACT ON HEALTH

In the South-East Asia Region of WHO, HIV infection was first reported in 1984 from Thailand, but in most other countries in the Region the infection was not reported until 1986 and even later. However, it has now spread extremely rapidly and all the countries of the Region except DPR Korea have reported HIV infection. WHO estimates that currently there are more than two million HIV-infected people in South-East Asia (see Figure 38.1).

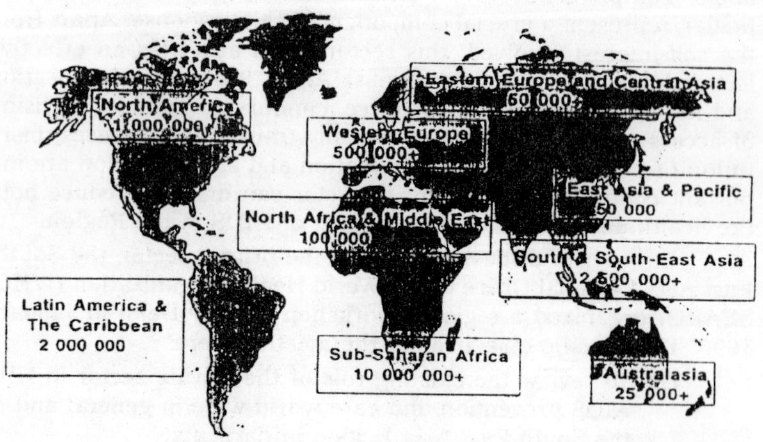


*Figure 38.1. Estimated distribution of total adult HIV infections until mid-1994*

The annual incidence of AIDS cases shows a steep rise in South-East Asia (see Figure 38.2). As of 1 October 1994, a total of 14,625 cases of AIDS have been reported in this region, Thailand and India contributing the largest numbers, viz. 13,246 and 905 respectively and thus accounting for almost 95 per cent of the total cases reported. The number reported each year is also increasing rapidly. In Thailand it increased from 82 in 1992 to 730 in 1992 and to 2092 in 1993. Of the cases reported in Thailand in 1994, nearly 80 per cent occurred in people between 20-44 years. Of these, 75 per cent occurred among 20-39-year olds, the most productive years of life. (see Figure 38.3).

Sentinel surveillance data and those from other studies indicate a rapid increase in HIV prevalence among individuals with risk-associated behaviour. For example, between 1985 and 1987, injecting drug users (IDUs) in Bangkok accounted for less than 1 per cent of the local HIV prevalence. This percentage dramatically increased to 40 by 1988 and appears to have stabilized at this level. In Manipur, India, HIV prevalence among IDUs is 54 per cent and in Myanmar a study indicates that in certain parts of the country it was as high as 71 per cent-in 1990-1991. Among female sex

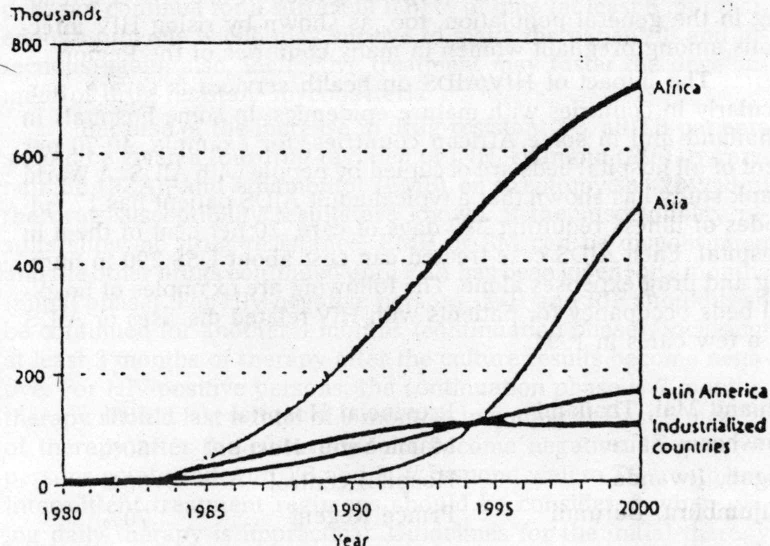


*Figure 38.2. Estimated and projected annual AIDS incidences by "macro" region- 1980-2000*

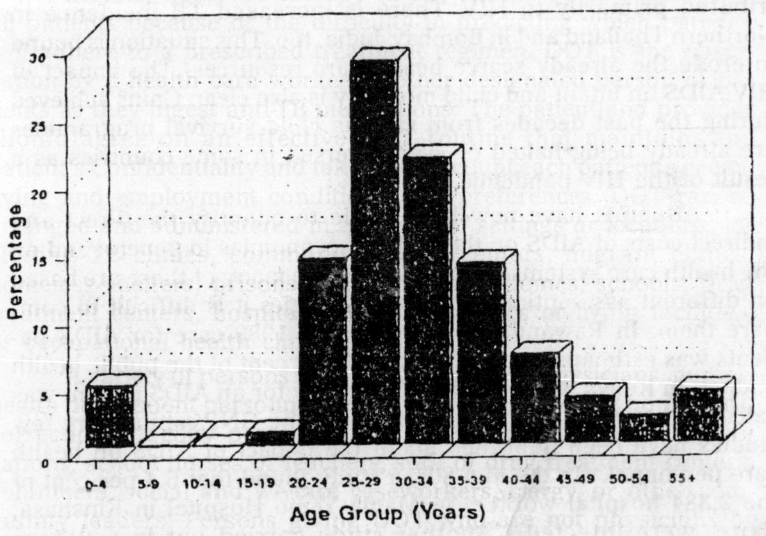


*Figure 38.3. Reported AIDS cases by age, 1994*

workers remarkable increases in HIV infection have also occurred in many parts of Thailand, India and Myanmar during the early 1990s. However, data are now beginning to show that HIV is spreading in the general population, too, as shown by rising HIV infections among pregnant women in many countries of the Region.

The impact of HIV/AIDS on health services is severe, particularly in countries with mature epidemics. In some hospitals in Thailand and in some African countries, for example, 40-70 per cent of all hospital beds are occupied by people with AIDS. A World Bank study has shown that a typical adult AIDS patient has 17 episodes of illness requiring 280 days of care, 20 per cent of them in hospital. Each AIDS case treated can cost about US$ 290 in nursing and drug expenses alone. The following are examples of hospital beds occupancy for patients with HIV-related diseases or AIDS in a few cities in 1994:

| | | |
|---|---|---|
| Chiang Mai, Thailand | Provincial Hospital | 50% |
| Kinshasa, Zaire | Mama Yemo Hospital | 50% |
| Kigali, Rwanda | Hospital central | 60% |
| Bujumbura, Burundi | Prince Regent | 70% |

There is an added burden now with the establishment of the association between HIV and tuberculosis. In many African countries, tuberculosis has shown an increase of 100-200 per cent attributed primarily to HIV. There is increased TB incidence in Northern Thailand and in Bombay, India, too. This situation is bound to erode the already scarce health care resources. The impact of HIV/AIDS on infant and child mortality is also clear. Gains achieved during the past decades from various child survival programmes are already being halted or even reversed in some countries as a result of the HIV pandemic.

Attempts have now been made to quantify the direct and indirect costs of AIDS on the national economies in general and on the health care systems in particular. Since many of these are based on different assumptions and methodologies it is difficult to compare them. In Rawanda, for example, in 1989 care for AIDS patients was estimated to absorb about 5 per cent of the public health budget. In Kenya, the cost of a 60-day stay for an AIDS patient was calculated to be three times higher than the GNP/capita. Very few studies have been published about the impact of AIDS on health care personnel. "In the mid-80s, a study found that 6.4 per cent of the 2,384 hospital workers in Mama Yemo Hospital in Kinshasa, Zaire, were infected". Another study carried out in southern Zambia found that "the mortality rate among nurses in two hospitals had risen from 0.5 in 1980 to 2.7 per cent in 1991, presumably due to AIDS". Other studies are under way in eastern and southern Africa which will help in comparing the situation in different countries. The preliminary results seem to indicate the same trend. Apart from the rising financial costs that will be incurred, the attrition rates among these highly skilled and highly technical personnel will far exceed the training capacity of the countries concerned.

## THE SOCIO-ECONOMIC IMPACT OF AIDS

Even though there is lack of well-planned social and behavioural research studies, it is clear that HIV primarily affects people during the most productive years of life, leading to premature death. Many of them are not only the mainstay of their families but that of the workforce as well. AIDS has a serious socio-economic impact. Virtually every adult who dies of AIDS leaves behind dependent family members. It is estimated that, by the year 2000 close to five million children would lose their mothers or both parents due to AIDS. Thus, in economic terms the indirect costs due to loss of productivity far exceed the health care costs. In Thailand, it is estimated that the health care cost for an AIDS patient is US$ 1500, as compared to the indirect cost to the economy of US$ 22, 000 in case of death. By the year 2000, the overall cost to Thailand and India on account of AIDS has been estimated at US$ 9 and 11 billion respectively. (see **Figure** 38.4). In addition, AIDS would have a negative impact on foreign investments and labour remittances from abroad.

Studies in Rawanda, Swaziland, Zaire and Zimbabwe point out that AIDS affects primarily people in the higher socio-economic bracket, those who represent the skilled workers, supervisors and managers of all important sectors of the economies of African countries. To replace them, a younger and less experienced labour and management workforce would have to be recruited. The consequences of this situation will vary according to the economic sector involved. In the mining industry in Zambia, for example, "the result is not necessarily a sudden collapse in output; rather there will be a steady but noticeable increase in breakdowns, accidents, delays and misjudgments, and output will suffer".

In every major company in countries with high prevalence rates of HIV and AIDS, there is anecdotal evidence to support this situation. A comment often made by company managers in Cote d'lvoire, Ghana, Kenya, Zambia and Zimbabwe is that in recent years they have noticed that death rates among staff are sometimes more than twice or three times higher than the rates observed over the previous years. These examples are drawn from sectors as diverse as the mining industry, banking, petroleum, insurance and transport, large commercial farms and agro-industries. Presumably,

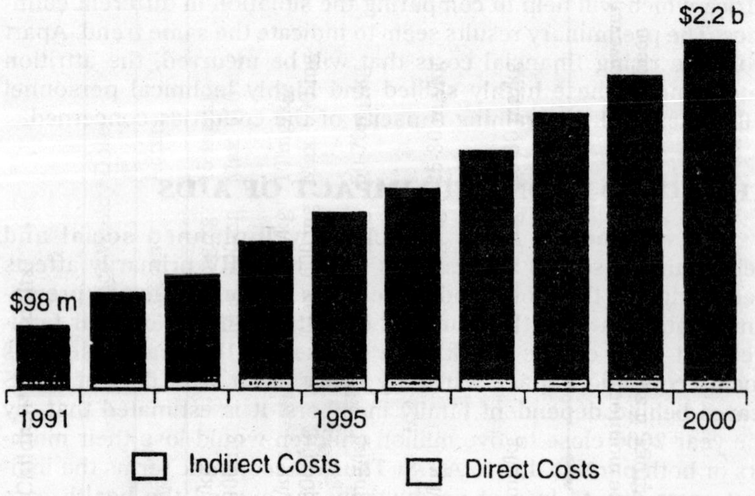


*Figure 38.4. Estimated Direct and Indirect Costs, Thailand*

the increases are related to the consequences of HIV and AIDS. One vivid example of the impact of HIV/AIDS on the private sector comes from Zambia. In 1987, of 12,204 employees in 33 businesses, 2.5 out of every 1000 employees died of AIDS. This figure increased to 18.3 in 1993—an eight-fold increase in annual employee deaths due to AIDS!

In the productive sector, an immediate consequence of HIV-related diseases and AIDS is the high level of absenteeism. A study carried out in Kenya substantiates this (see Fig. 38.5). As workers become increasingly afflicted with AIDS-related illness, their overall health conditions worsen and they take a longer time away from work to seek treatment. Even healthy workers are not spared because many, especially women, will also take time off to attend to the health needs of those family members who are infected and need care. A few companies have documented the high number of days their staff are away from work to attend funerals of family members and co-workers. As one interviewee in a study carried out in Uganda put it, death has become so common that if one wants to attend funerals one could easily end up losing a month's work

Another example of the socio-economic impact of the HIV pandemic comes from Nakambala sugar estate (NSE), Zambia. AIDS has resulted in 50 per cent of all the man-hours lost in the estate. If diarrhoeal diseases often associated with HIV are added as well, the figure rises to 60 per cent. Even when they return to work, infected workers often cannot perform their duties satisfactorily. Estimated numbers of AIDS deaths and medical releases due

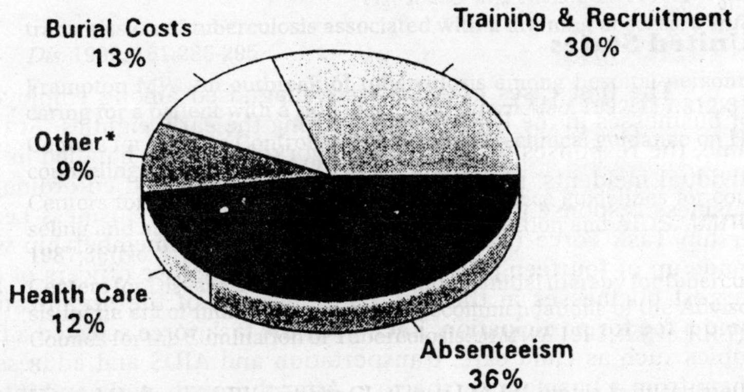


*Other includes labor turnover, funeral attendance, and productivity losses due to the inexperience of new workers

Sources: AIDS captions March 1995

*Figure 38.5: AIDS-related costs to Kanyan business*

to HIV/AIDS could well increase to 70 per cent during the year 1995/96.

As in many other African communities, healthy employees also absent themselves from work to care for sick relatives and to attend funerals. Absenteeism due to tuberculosis has also increased.

The social impact is considerable. HIV/AIDS-affected families in caring for the sick have to meet increasing medical expenses. Following death, the family loses not only the income, but also entitlement for housing 6 months after death. Those in seasonal employment are even more vulnerable because they do not get the full range of benefits. The number of orphans in the surrounding villages of Nakambala is also on the rise.

## EXAMPLES OF PRIVATE SECTOR RESPONSE AND EXPERIENCES

The contribution of the private sector and the business community as equal partners in the national, regional and global efforts is crucial for the prevention and care of HIV/AIDS. Business and government leaders need to work together to set up AIDS programmes in the workplace. These programmes include AIDS education to prevent new infections among employees and their dependents. Programmes should also ensure that people with HIV infection and AIDS are treated fairly, humanely and without discrimination. A number of countries have put in place an HIV/AIDS programme in the workplace. Some examples are as follows:

**United States**

The first cases of AIDS were diagnosed among employees of businesses in the United States during the early eighties. At that time, the responses to AIDS in the workplace were handled as individual incidents, usually in a crisis mode. The first co-ordinated business response to AIDS began in 1985 with the Business Leadership Task Force (BLTF) in San Francisco. Its membership was made up of fourteen presidents and chief executive officers of the largest businesses in the city. Each member of the organization paid a fee for participation. Each year, the task force selected a few topics such as child care, transportation and AIDS and addressed them from a business perspective. After thorough study and investigation, materials were produced and presented at a conference for effectiv involvement of the private sector in public sector issues.

The conference, "An Epidemic of Fear: AIDS In The Workplace, held in March 1986, discussed the question of how employers should deal with AIDS in the workplace in a businesslike, consistent, cost-effective and compassionate way. The conference as well as the package or materials developed by BLTF and distributed to the members was the first attempt in the United States to address the impact of AIDS on business and set an early standard for a comprehensive business response to AIDS. Since then, other regions in the United States have also developed similar collaborative programmes. An example is the New England Corporate Consortium for AIDS Education, which produces timely and useful materials on AIDS at the workplace. Many big and small business houses are members of this consortium, which also organizes an annual conference on "WORLD AIDS DAY" to encourage and help the employers in New England to address AIDS issues in responsible, ethical and cost-effective ways. In 1986, the Surgeon-General of the United States urged that worksites should have a plan in operation for education of the workforce and care for patients with AIDS even before the first such case appeared at the worksite. Employees with AIDS should be treated like any other worker with a chronic illness.

Another significant response to the AIDS epidemic from business leaders in the United States was the founding, in 1987, of the National Leadership Coalition on AIDS, a non-profit charitable organization which brings together the collective resources of the private sector. The Coalition has grown steadily and now has a membership of more than 200 business houses. In the late 1980s, the US Congress provided funding for the Center for Disease Control (CDC) Atlanta, and the American Red Cross to develop comprehensive AIDS education and prevention activities for the workplace. Programmes designed by and for business underscore the principle that AIDS should be treated like any other life-threatening illness. Their AIDS policies thus are modelled on the policies existing for other life-threatening illnesses.

Employers of workers who have a higher risk of on-the job infection (hospitals, police departments, fire departments and emergency workers) have also developed specific infection control procedures and begun to use the concept of "universal precautions" to minimize the possibility of the spread of infection on the job, for all illnesses including AIDS.

Smaller businesses and some major industries such as airlines and restaurants have, however, only now begun to address AIDS and, for the most part, did not respond well initially.

The legal framework in the United States covering people with HIV/AIDS in the workplace is found in the federal law of 1990 pertaining to disabilities. This law took effect in July 1992 and is applicable to every business enterprise having more than 25 employees. In July 1993, all businesses with more than 15 employees were included. In addition to the federal law, at least 36 of the 50 states in the US provide state protection against discrimination in the workplace to people with disabilities.

Private sector standards as expressed by ten principles for the workplace developed by the Citizens Commission on AIDS for New York City/Northern New Jersey Region are also supported by the World Health Organization, the International Labour Organisation and major multinational corporations as well as by international business groups in Europe, North America, South America and Asia.

## Africa

The business community in certain African countries, particularly those in sub-Saharan Africa which are hardest hit by the AIDS pandemic, have now begun to take an active interest in AIDS prevention and control. In a tripartite workshop on the role of the organized sector in reproductive health and AIDS prevention, held in 1994, the business community realized some important facts, viz. that AIDS leads to the loss of output and productivity, there is drain on the family income on account of caring for the sick and funerals; the cost to industry includes high cost of training, retraining and replacement of the workforce; possible increase in wage cost due to labour shortages and loss of consumer markets which will have a direct impact on several industrial sectors and an indirect impact on tourism and other service industries. Studies conducted in a bank in Zambia confirm these concerns. In June 1992, among 1800 staff, 40 deaths had already taken place and it is projected that by 1995 about 140 will die of AIDS. A snap check carried out on staff absentees on 17 July 1991 showed that 10 employees were on leave to attend funerals and 53 were on sick leave. Death claims on the state insurance corporation had increased from 200 in 1986 to nearly 800 in 1991. Many businesses have now started including AIDS in the workplace programmes. Although the involvement of the private sector in Africa is still at an early stage, it is nevertheless gathering momentum.

One example of the private sector in Africa actively engaged in AIDS prevention and control is that of the Debswana Diamond Company (Pty) Ltd., Botswana. The AIDS programme is implemented as a part of their occupational health programme, with the objective of raising the level of awareness among employees on HIV/AIDS through formal lectures, drama, distribution of literature and through briefing by people living with HIV/AIDS. The programme also aims to establish counselling and care support services through training the company hospital nurses as AIDS counsellors and using the existing professional counsellors working in the employee assistance programme.

**Nepal**

General Paper Industries, based in Kathmandu, which contributes 10 per cent of its annual export value for various community development activities, has organized camps to bring basic health services and simple AIDS awareness information to four remote mountainous villages in Nepal.

The HIV/AIDS awareness efforts received a boost in early 1993 when the company sponsored a half-page advertisement in the *Gorkhapatra* daily with the message "Use condoms to protect yourself against AIDS".

The first target population chosen for AIDS awareness were truck drivers who ply along the national transport route and are among the country's largest mobile groups. By educating drivers it was also possible to disseminate AIDS messages to distant parts of the country. Drivers are given prevention packages when they queue up to complete the required traffic registration at the Nagdhunga traffic police post. Each package contains two condoms, a simple brochure describing HIV transmission and its prevention, and a match box with the message *"Use Condoms to Protect yourself against Aids"* inscribed on it. The industry also organizes competitions among the transport workers and awards attractive prizes to the best five suggestions on how to improve the AIDS education messages.

**India**

Since 1991, many small businesses in different parts of India have got involved in creating AIDS awareness. Attempts have been made by the private sector and nongovernmental organizations to provide condoms to long distance transport workers, and collaboration between agencies involved in such programmes is being strengthened.

Numerous corporate sector organizations, such as the Confederation of Indian Industry (CII) and the West Bengal Chamber of Commerce and Industry, have begun collaborating with the National AIDS Control Organization (NACO) for the integration of HIV/AIDS/STD prevention and control activities into health care, educational and other social sector activities already being carried out under the auspices of the corporate sector. A strategic plan is currently being developed by the West Bengal Chamber of Commerce to reach all member industries. The CII has prepared a proposal for initiating AIDS activities in the workplace and many other industries have expressed interest in initiating similar activities. As stated in a folder brought out by CII recently, it is committed to programmes related to AIDS and the workplace and states that "it is essential to plan. If you wait until you have a crisis in your hands, it may be too late to take effective and appropriate action". in partnership with ILO and WHO, a pilot programme is being planned to develop approaches and materials for the industrial sector, and the Indian Tobacco Company is discussing a possible partnership with NACO and the West Bengal State AIDS Cell to provide management assistance for intervention projects in the redlight areas of Calcutta.

The Shriram Industrial Enterprises Limited (SIEL) has also been active in HIV/AIDS prevention. In 1993 an AIDS sensitization programme organized by the company was attended by the top management of industries. SIEL now plans to hold national and regional seminars and workshops on AIDS in conjunction with NACO and WHO. Activities related to AIDS prevention will be carried out along with those on STD control and drug and alcohol abuse. SIEL also holds regular "AIDS Awareness Weeks" in its factories along with workshops and discussions at different managerial levels. Posters and banners are displayed and other educational materials distributed. A major activity in AIDS awareness was carried out through the Annual Marathon which was covered well by the media. The company is now in the process of formulating a programme of AIDS education and counselling and a workplace policy in consultation with the labour unions.

Deepam Educational Society for Health (DESH) based in Madras has been able to educate more than 200,000 employees about AIDS through the involvement of management associations and trade unions. The Society has conducted interactive programmes with many agencies such as the Southern Railway, large industrial houses like Ashok Leyland Ltd., Addison & Co. Ltd., Dock Labour Board, Binny Ltd., and the Madras Port Trust in Madras, India Cements in Salem and Cuddapah, and Larsen & Toubro Ltd. and Cable Corporation in Bombay. Workshops have also been organized for the benefit of employees of the Small Industries Service Institute. Through the Central Board of Workers Education worker-teachers representing various organizations have been trained. These training sessions have been well received, with requests for repeat workshops. More importantly, the programmes seem to have brought about a positive attitudinal change. The motto of DESH is to promote the fact that "the HIV/AIDS epidemic is everyone's concem", and to develop policies which will prepare the organizations to deal with the epidemic responsibly and knowledgeably and in a businesslike way.

## Thailand

Until 1993, the response to AIDS in Thailand was mainly from the governmental and international agencies and nongovernmental organizations. There was no co-ordinated response from the private sector. A survey of the business community in 1992-93 revealed that while many were concerned about AIDS, particularly its impact on productivity, office morale and on health, few had done anything about it and many did not know where to go for education and information.

The Thai Business Coalition on AIDS (TBCA) was subsequently formed in 1993 as a non-profit organization of the private sector, for providing leadership through and beyond the AIDS epidemic. The need forAIDS education and information in the workplace and the establishment of workplace policies were supported by the Government, international agencies, universities and NGOs. The main role of TBCA is to develop leadership, promote education and information and co-ordinate the activities of the private sector. The present membership consists mostly of multinational companies and many large and medium Thai industries. Members of TBCA benefit through briefings given to key managers, in-house training and publication of a newsletter and manuals on workplace policies.

TBCA assists businesses in providing AIDS education to the workforce and in the development of a workplace policy. The Coalition expects to have 150 new corporate members by 1995-1996, and plans to provide 300 copies of workplace manuals and train about 30,000 employees and managers. The activities have so far received extensive media coverage and donations from NGOs and other agencies. Among its ten-point workplace principles are (i) combating discrimination against employees with HIV infection, (ii) maintenance of confidentiality, and (iii) providing workplace education and health care to all employees irrespective of their HIV status.

The several problems yet to be overcome include lack of adequate seed money, reluctance of local firms to join the Coalition and insufficient local training. However, given the many opportunities such as wide exposure and co-operation from the public sector, the coalition is expected to develop into a good model of the private sector's response in Asia. TBCA's future plan includes activities related to advocacy, co-ordinating training resources, undertaking community-based projects and developing regional branches.

## PRIVATE SECTOR AND AIDS: A MODEL FOR HIV/AIDS PREVENTION AND CARE

### Role of Private Sector

The impact of the AIDS epidemic is increasingly being felt by businesses across Asia. AIDS is fast becoming an obstacle to economic development, and the epidemic is forcing us to re-examine the role of the private sector in disease prevention and health promotion. The workplace is an appropriate and important setting for AIDS prevention because most people spend a significant part of their time at work. Thus, AIDS is an important private sector concern, and AIDS prevention makes good business sense.

An effective workplace AIDS prevention and care programme consists of a comprehensive and co-ordinated set of components, such as:

- # Policy development and practices that are clearly defined, understood, and consistently followed, and
- # Implementation of a workplace AIDS programme.

### Policy Development and Practice

Policy is the foundation of a workplace AIDS prevention programme. An AIDS policy defines a company's position and its practices as they relate to employees with AIDS. Policies set standards of behaviour expected of all employees as well as standards for communication about AIDS. Policies help employees to know where to go for assistance and instruct supervisors and managers on how to manage AIDS in their work groups. Businesses that have successfully addressed HIV/AIDS suggest that it is useful to have a written policy stating the company's position and procedures that tell managers and employees about what is expected of them. A policy does not provide an entire HIV/AIDS prevention programme, it is the foundation, the first step, upon which a strong prevention programme can be built.

In June 1988, a group of experts representing governments, trade unions, business, public health, medicine, the legal profession and educators agreed on a joint WHO and ILO declaration on AIDS and the workplace which incorporated the following principles:

1. HIV/AIDS screening as part of an assessment of fitness to work is unnecessary and should not be required.
2. For persons already in employment, HIV/AIDS screening, whether direct (HIV testing), indirect (assessment of risk behaviour) or asking questions about tests already taken, should not be required.
3. Confidentiality regarding all medical information including HIV/AIDS must be maintained.
4. There should be no obligation on the employee to inform the employer of his or her HIV/AIDS status.
5. Persons in the workplace infected, or perceived to be infected, by HIV/AIDS must be protected from stigmatization and discrimination by co-workers, unions, employers or clients. Information and education are essential to maintain the climate of mutual understanding necessary to ensure this protection.
6. Employees and their families should have access to information and educational programmes on HIV/AIDS as well as to relevant counselling and appropriate referral.
7. HIV-infected employees should not be discriminated against; this means that they should have unreserved access to and receipt of standard social security and occupationally related benefits.
8. HIV infection by itself is not associated with any limitation on fitness to work. If fitness to work is impaired by HIV-related illness, reasonable working arrangements should be made.
9. HIV infection is not a ground for termination of employment. As with many other illnesses, persons with HIV-related illnesses should be able to work as long as they are medically fit for available and appropriate work.
10. In any situation requiring first aid in the workplace,

precautions should be taken to reduce the risk of the transmission of blood-borne infections, including hepatitis B, and standard precautions will be equally effective against HIV transmission.

Most businesses find that developing an HIV/AIDS policy takes less time than expected and is an interesting, informative and valuable experience. They also find that management and worker responses are surprisingly favourable. The biggest benefit is the knowledge that they are prepared to deal effectively with a serious problem and reduce the health and socio-economic impact of the epidemic significantly.

Successful HIV/AIDS policies used by businesses around the world share a number of the following basic principles.

1. People with HIV/AIDS are entitled to the same rights, benefits and opportunities as people with other serious or life-threatening illnesses.
2. Employment practices must, at a minimum, comply with national, regional and local laws and regulations.
3. Employment policies should be based on the scientific and epidemiological evidence that people with HIV/AIDS do not pose a risk of transmission of the virus to co-workers through ordinary workplace contact.
4. The highest levels of management and union leadership should unequivocally endorse nondiscriminatory employment policies and educational programmes related to the prevention and care of HIV/AIDS.
5. Employers and union leaders should communicate their support of these policies to workers in simple, clear and unambiguous terms.
6. Employers should provide employees with sensitive, accurate and up-to-date education about risk reduction in their personal lives.
7. Employers have a duty to protect the confidentiality of medical information in respect of all their employees.
8. To prevent work disruption and rejection by co-workers of an HIV/AIDS employee, employers and unions should undertake education for all employees before such an incident thereafter as needed.
9. Employers should not require HIV screening as part of pre-employment or general workplace physical examinations.
10. In special occupational settings where there may be a potential risk of exposure to HIV (working with blood or blood products). employers should provide specific. on-

going education and training, as well as the necessary equipment, to reinforce appropriate infection control procedures and ensure that they are implemented.

## Implementation of Workplace AIDS Programmes

A comprehensive and on-going HIV/AIDS education and prevention programme must aim at bringing about changes in behaviour that will reduce the spread of AIDS through:

# Formal and informal education
# Condom distribution
# Diagnosis and treatment of sexually transmitted diseases (STD).
# Care, counselling and support services for workers and their families.

### *Formal and Informal Education*

HIV/AIDS education includes a variety of approaches to address a broad range of issues. No matter what forms or approaches are used, there are specific core issues that should always be included as part of the educational programme. These are:

# the company's policy or position on HIV/AIDS and procedures for handling HIV/AIDS-related problems or concerns
# How HIV/AIDS is and is not transmitted
# how to prevent the spread of HIV
# how to respond to a co-worker with HIV/AIDS
# benefits available to workers and family members with HIV/AIDS
# confidentiality and privacy requirements
# where to go for help and for additional information.

### *Use of Peers as Educators*

Peer education is universally considered the most effective way to provide workers with HIV/AIDS education to initiate prevention activities focusing on behavioural change. Peer education will, however, need specific training and support, to be able to function effectively.

Peer educator training requires between two and five days of specialized instruction to develop in the trainees the necessary skills for education and prevention activities.

Some organizations may decide that instead of peer education, individuals or a small group of people should be responsible for conducting the company's formal and informal HIV/AIDS education and prevention activities. In any case, it is essential that the people identified as HIV/AIDS educators receive adequate training—even doctors who may not be equipped to deal with issues such as those related to sex, sexuality, condom use and behavioural change.

Trade unions also have a major role to play in educating their members on AIDS prevention.

*Condom Distribution, Establishing System(s) that Maximize Condom use for AIDS Prevention*

Condom distribution is a necessary part of an effective workplace HIV/AIDS prevention programme. Workers must be educated on how to use condoms correctly and simultaneously must also have easy access to them through an effective distribution system. Condoms will also prevent other sexually transmitted diseases (STDs).

*Diagnosis and Treatment of Sexually Transmitted Diseases*

Sexually transmitted diseases (STDs) are common among workers and contribute not only to absenteeism and medica care costs but also to the increased possibility of HIV transmission during sexual intercourse. HIV/AIDS education and prevention activities must, therefore, include learning and discussions among workers about STDs and their relationship to the transmission of HIV/AIDS as well as the provision of STD diagnosis and treatment services using, where appropriate, the syndrome approach. According to some studies, the cost of diagnosis and treatment for a worker with an STD is less than one day's wages whereas the costs of absenteeism and the resulting impact on productivity, medical costs, and other expenses can be many times the cost of diagnosis and treatment. It thus makes it cost effective to provide STD diagnosis and treatment as a support service to HIV/AIDS education and prevention activities. I many situations, provision of STD treatment services may not be possible for the company. However, it is the company's responsibility to ensur that employees are informed where these services are available and how they can access them. STD diagnosis and treatment should also include counselling services for workers and their families.

*Care, Counselling and Support Services for Workers and their Families*

Care includes counselling and support services for concerned

Workers and those diagnosed with HIV (following voluntary testing and counselling services), for workers who have AIDS and for their families. Care is an important part of a comprehensive workplace AIDS programme. Counselling and support are important both for the physical and mental welfare of workers and their families. Such services also increase the probability of sustained behavioural change and will help prevent the transmission of HIV.

Provision of comprehensive care services irrespective of the HIV status makes the other prevention activities concrete and real in the lives of workers and their families, because they provide personal and individual reinforcement for behavioural change, outside of the formal and informal group activities offered at work. Without the reinforcement of these services, HIV/AIDS education and prevention activities remain merely educational exercises without real-life application and are unlikely to bring about sustained behavioural change or reduce the transmission of HIV/AIDS.

## CONCLUSIONS AND RECOMMENDATIONS

The private sector plays a significant and essential role in HIV/AIDS prevention and has the potential for impacting necessary behavioural change as no other sector in society can. Clear, straightforward, factual policies prepare businesses to deal with HIV/AIDS smoothly, responsibly and cost-effectively. HIV/AIDS education and prevention activities and services assist workers and their families to prevent the spread of HIV/AIDS and businesses derive the benefits of reduced costs, stable productivity, and a healthier workforce.

A comprehensive HIV/AIDS education and prevention programme must be developed which would include policy, education and prevention activities for workers, and accompanying support services. A responsible, assertive stand on HIV/AIDS can place a company among the ranks of business leaders in Asia, and around the world, who are collaborating successfully in confronting the HIV/AIDS epidemic.

The workshop deliberated in groups and, after discussions in the plenary, made the following recommendations·

1. In view of the fact that HIV/AIDS largely affects people in the most economically productive years of their lives, it is imperative that AIDS prevention and care activities are initiated at the workplace.
2. As the private sector has a crucial role to play in the provision of STD/HIV/AIDS education and prevention services to its employees, its resources must be harnessed to develop appropriate AIDS prevention and control

programmes in the workplace that will adequately respond to the unique national and local needs and situations prevalent in the respective countries.

3. The role of the private sector must fit into the overall national plan of action co-ordinated by the national AIDS programme of the respective countries. It is, therefore, important that the precise role the private sector can play in HIV prevention and care be defined by all parties, including the private sector itself.
4. In order to encourage and facilitate the participation of the private sector, information with respect to HIV/STD/AIDS, especially the projected national and/or sectoral impact (economic and otherwise) of the pandemic, be provided to the private sector in a business context.
5. To initiate an HIV/STD/AIDS education and prevention programme, it is necessary for the private sector to identify and involve key industrial leaders and workers' representatives in the planning, development and/or implementation of such programmes in the workplace.
6. To facilitate a partnership between the private sector and the national AIDS programme, the latter should initiate the establishment of a forum for regular exchange of information, experience and activities related to the private sector's response to HIV/STD/AIDS at regional, national and local levels.
7. Since policy is the foundation of a workplace AIDS prevention programme, a national policy for a workplace response to HIV/STD/AIDS should be developed through collaboration between the national programme and the corporate and workers' representatives as appropriate to each country.
8. In order to be cost-effective, HIV/STD/AIDS prevention and care programmes for the workplace should be developed, implemented and monitored utilizing existing structures through the development adaptation of manuals and appropriate training within existing human resources development programmes and through networking with relevant NGOs or community groups. In this process the skills, capacities and resources of the private sector should be utilized to the maximum extent.
9. In order to suport and sustain HIV/STD/AIDS prevention and care programmes in the workplace, mechanisms must be established for generating funds through the private sector.
10. To foster the private sector's response to the AIDS pan-

demic, a network should be established for the exchange of experiences between all industries and other businesses involved in HIV/STD/AIDS prevention and care activities, within and among countries.

## SUMMARY

The human immunodeficiency virus (HIV), which causes AIDS, has now spread to all continents of the world. In Asia, HIV appeared later than in other parts of the world but is now spreading at a pace reminiscent of the situation in Africa about 10 years ago. Asia last year reported the biggest increase in the number of HIV infections, the cumulative infections todate being more than 2.5 million. More and more people are expected to be infected each year and soon there will be more Asians infected with HIV annually than those in Africa. The end of the pandemic is nowhere in sight. If left unchecked, it is estimated that between 30 and 40 million people worldwide will be infected by HIV by the year 2000, and of these, 8 to 10 million will be in Asia. The AIDS pandemic has, in addition, brought with it the resurgence of tuberculosis, which already accounts for over 1.5 million deaths annually in Asia. The devastating effect of this deadly combination has already been seen in Africa, where the incidence of tuberculosis has doubled and even tripled in many countries over the last five years.

As the dimension of HIV/AIDS increases, the workplace assumes very great importance. In 1994, about 2.3 billion people in the world were associated with the workplace either in the public sector or in the private sector. When AIDS affects, it is not only the breadwinners who die, but they leave behind families, old parents, children and spouses. AIDS therefore affects not only individuals and families but also communities in which businesses are located. AIDS particularly affects the private sector or businesses in profound and costly ways—in terms of illnesses and disabilities thereby causing decrease in productivity as workers remain absent due to illnesses or are away to care for sick families. In economic terms, the indirect costs due to loss of productivity far outweigh the health care costs. In Thailand, for example, a well-documented study estimates the health care cost for an AIDS patient at US$ 1,500, as compared to the indirect cost to the economy of US$ 22,000 in case of death. By the year 2000, the overall costs to Thailand and India on account of AIDS have been estimated at US$ 9 and 11 billion respectively.

The prevention and control of HIV infections and AIDS require the broadest possible commitment to supporting community-based initiatives to encourage young people to adopt and maintain protective social norms and practices. The contribution of the private sector and the business community as equal partners in national, regional and global efforts is crucial in this regard. To effectively meet the challenge posed by AIDS, business and government leadership must work together. In all countries, governments, through their national programmes, have taken initiatives to prevent HIV infection and to provide care and social support to those affected by HIV/AIDS and their families.

Besides supporting the national AIDS programmes in their work, what can individual businesses and the private sector do to prevent the spread of HIV/AIDS? To begin with, businesses can establish and urgently begin to implement workplace policies and programmes. The two main components of such programmes are: first, to ensure that people with HIV infection and AIDS are treated fairly, humanely and without discrimination; and second, to set up AIDS education programmes in the workplace with the objective of preventing new infections among employees and their dependents. The adoption of a corporate policy on AIDS, highlighting provision of education and information to employees and their families on a regular basis irrespective of their HIV status; strengthening facilities for the treatment of sexually transmitted diseases; ensuring accessibility to condoms and promoting 'no' to pre-employment HIV screening must be the goal of each business or industry. Advocacy by the management and fellow workers is an important component of a workplace policy against HIV-related discrimination. The private sector can also play a major advocacy role in helping to shape the national response to the AIDS epidemic. For example, the Thai Business Coalition on AIDS subscribes to its famous "Ten Principles". These principles recognize the need for businesses to treat people with AIDS in the same way as people with any other serious condition; to have non-discriminatory employment practices; and to protect the confidentiality of employees' medical and insurance information. They also include a policy on AIDS prevention by stating that AIDS education is to be provided to all staff. Provision of care and support is also included in the workplace initiatives.

To enhance implementation of these policies by the private sector, much advocacy and support is needed from the government sector. Orientation of, and group educational activities for, executives and trade union leaders will go a long way in evoking an early response. While educational and information programmes at the workplace are the responsibility of the private sector, technical and material support can be obtained from the national AIDS programme. Moreover, as each private enterprise may not have facilities for treatment of STDs, the management should have information about the nearest place where such facilities are available. The same is true with respect to availability of condoms. In some situations, some seed money will have to be provided to the private sector for conducting group educational activities and promoting peer education, but ultimately contributions must come from within the private sector itself. Press coverage of the AIDS control activities of the private sector will not only strengthen such activities but will also encourage many other private enterprises to join in this effort.

In the long term, continued dialogue with the management is needed to convince them that any delay in their responding to the pandemic will have grave consequences and that investing early in AIDS prevention does indeed make sound business sense!

39

# Guidelines for Prevention of Transmission of Human Immunodeficiency Virus and Hepatitis B Virus to Health-Care and Public-Safety Workers

## I. INTRODUCTION

### A. Background

This document is a response to recently enacted legislation, Public Law 100-607, The Health Omnibus Programmes Extension Act of 1988, Title II, Programmes with Respect to Acquired Immune Deficiency Syndrome ("AIDS Amendments of 1988"). Subtitle E, General Provisions, Section 253(a) of Title II specifies that "the Secretary of Health and Human Services, acting through the Director of the Centers for Disease Control, shall develop, issue, and disseminate guidelines to all health workers, public safety workers (including emergency response employees) in the United States concerning

1. methods to reduce the risk in the workplace of becoming infected with the etiologic agent for acquired immune deficiency syndrome; and
2. circumstances under which exposure to such etiologic agent may occur."

It is further noted that "The Secretary [of Health and Human Services] shall transmit the guidelines issued under subsection (a) to the Secretary of Labour for use by the Secretary of Labour in the development of standards to be issued under the Occupational Safety and Health Act of 1970," and that "the Secretary, acting through the Director of the Centers for Disease Control, shall develop a model curriculum for emergency response employees with respect to the prevention of exposure to the etiologic agent for acquired immune deficiency syndrome during the process of responding to emergencies."

Following development of these guidelines and curriculum, "[t]he Secretary shall.

(a) transmit to State public health officers copies of the guidelines and the model curriculum developed under paragraph (1) with the request that such officers disseminate such copies as appropriate throughout the State; and

(b) make such copies available to the public."

## B. Purpose and Organization of Document

The purpose of this document is to provide an overview of the modes of transmission of human immunodeficiency virus (HIV) in the workplace, an assessment of the risk of transmission under various assumptions, principles underlying the control of risk, and specific risk-control recommendations for employers and workers. This document also includes information on medical management of persons who have sustained an exposure at the workplace to these viruses (e.g., an emergency medical technicians who incur a needle-stick injury while performing professional duties). These guidelines are intended for we by a technically informed audience. As noted above, a separate model curriculum based on the principles and practices discussed in this document is being developed for use in training workers and will contain less technical wording.

Information concerning the protection of workers against acquisition of the human immunodeficiency virus (HIV) while performing job duties, the virus that causes AIDS, is presented here. Information on hepatitis B virus ( HBV) is also presented in this document on the basis of the following assumptions:

- # the modes of transmission for hepatitis B virus (HBV) are similar to those of HIV,
- # the potential for HBV transmission in the occupational setting is greater than for HIV,
- # there is a larger body of experience relating to controlling transmission of HBV in the workplace, and
- # general practices to prevent the transmission of HBV will also minimize the risk of transmission of HIV.

Blood-borne transmission of other pathogens not specifically addressed here will be interrupted by adherence to the precautions noted below. It is important to note that the implementation of control measures for HIV and HBV does not obviate the need for continued adherence to general infection-control principles and general hygiene measures (e.g., hand washing) for preventing transmission of other infectious diseases to both worker and client. General guidelines for control of these diseases have been published.[1,2,3]

This document was developed primarily to provide guidelines for fire-service personnel, emergency medical technicians, paramedics (see section IV), and law-enforcement and correctional-facility personnel (see sectionV). Throughout the report, paramedics and emergency medical technicians are called "emergency medical workers" and fire-service, law-enforcement, and correctional-facility personnel, "public-safety workers." Previously issued guidelines address the needs of hospital-, laboratory-, and clinic-based health-care workers.[4,5] A condensation of general guidelines for protection of workers from transmission of blood-borne pathogens, derived from the Joint Advisory Notice of the Departments of Labour and Health and Human Services [6], is provided in section.[III]

## C. Modes and Risk of Virus Transmission in the Workplace

Although the potential for HBV transmission in the workplace setting is greater than for HIV, the modes of transmission for these two viruses are similar. Both have been transmitted in occupational settings only by percutaneous inoculation or contact with an open wound, nonintact (e.g., chapped, abraded, weeping, or dermatitic) skin, or mucous membranes to blood, blood-contaminated body fluids, or concentrated virus. Blood is the single most important source of HIV and HBV in the workplace setting. Protection measures against HIV and HBV for workers should focus primarily on preventing these types of exposures to blood as well as on delivery of HBV vaccination.

The risk of hepatitis B infection following a parenteral (i.e., needle stick or cut) exposure to blood is directly proportional to the probability that the blood contains hepatitis B surface antigen (HBsAg), the immunity status of the recipient, and on the efficiency of transmission[7]. The probability of the source of the blood being HBsAg positive varies from 1 to 3 per thousand in the general population to 5 per cent-15 per cent in groups at high risk for HBV infection, such as immigrants from areas of high endemicity (China and Southeast Asia, sub-Saharan Africa, most Pacific islands, and the Amazon Basin); clients in institutions for the mentally retarded; intravenous drug users; homosexually active males; and household ( sexual and non-sexual ) contacts of HBV carriers. Of persons who have not had prior hepatitis B vaccination or postexposure prophylaxis, 6 per cent-30 per cent of persons who receive a needle-stick exposure from an HBsAg-positive individual will become infected[7].

The risk of infection with HIV following one needle-stick exposure to blood from a patient known to be infected with HIV is approximately 0.5 per cent.[4,5] This rate of transmission is considerably lower than that for HBV, probably as a result of the significantly lower concentrations of virus in the blood of HIV-infected persons. Table 39.1 off presents theoretical data concerning the likelihood of infection given repeated needlestick injuries involving patients whose HIV serostatus is unknown. Though inadequately quantified, the risk from exposure of nonintact skin or mucous membranes is likely to be far less than that from percutaneous inoculation.

**Table 39.1.**
**The Risk of HIV Infection Following Needlestick Injury: Hypothetical Model**

| Prevalence of HIV Infection (A) | Probability of Infection given Needlestick Injury with Blood Containing H1V (B) | Problility of Infection given Random Needlestick (Unknown Serostatus) A * B = (C) | Probabihty of Infection Given 10 Random Needlesticks $1-(1-C)^{10}$ | Probability of Infection Given 100 Random Needlesticks $1-(1-C)^{100}$ |
|---|---|---|---|---|
| 0.0001 | 0.001 | 0.0000001 | 0.000001 | 0.00001 |
| 0.0001 | 0.005 | 0.0000005 | 0.000005 | 0.00005 |
| 0.001 | 0.001 | 0.000001 | 0.00001 | 0.0001 |
| 0.001 | 0.005 | 0.000005 | 0.00005 | 0.0005 |
| 0.01 | 0.001 | 0.00001 | 0.0001 | 0.001 |
| 0.01* | 0.005 | 0.00005 | 0.0005 | 0.005 |
| 0.05 | 0.001 | 0.00005 | 0.0005 | 0.005 |
| 0.05 | 0.005 | 0.00025 | 0.0025 | 0.025 |

* For example, if the prevalence of infection in the population is 0.01 (i.e., 1 per 100) and the risk of a seroconversion following a needlestick with blood known to contain HIV is 0.005 (i.e., 1 in 200), then the probability of HIV infection given a random needlestick is 0.00005 (i.e., 5 in 100,000). If an individual sustains 10 needlestick injuries, the probability of acquiring HIV infection is 0.0005 (i.e., 1 in 2,000); if the individual sustains 100 needlestick injuries, the probability of acquiring HIV infection is 0.005 (i.e., 1 in 200).

## D. Transmission of Hepatitis B Virus to Workers

*1. Health-care workers*

In 1987, the CDC estimated the total number of HBV infections in the United States to be 300,000 per year, with approximately 75,000 (25 per cent) of infected persons developing acute hepatitis. Of these infected individuals, 18,000-30,000 (6 per cent-10 per cent) will become HBV carriers, at risk of developing chronic liver disease (chronic active hepatitis, cirrhosis, and primary liver cancer), and infectious to others.

CDC has estimated that 12,000 health-care workers whose jobs entail exposure to blood become infected with HBV each year, that 500-600 of them are hospitalized as a result of that infection, and that 700-1,200 of those infected become HBV carriers. Of the infected workers,approximately 250 will die (12-15 from fulminant hepatitis,170-200 from cirrhosis, and 40-50 from liver cancer) . Studies indicate that 10 per cent-30 per cent of health-care or dental workers show serologic evidence of past or present HBV infection.

*2. Emergency medical and public-safety workers*

Emergency medical workers have an increased risk for hepatitis B infection.[8,9,10] The degree of risk correlates with the frequency and extent of blood exposure during the conduct of work activities. A few studies are available concerning risk of HBV infection for other groups of public-safety workers (law-enforcement personnel and correctional-facility workers ), but reports that have been published do not document any increased risk for HBV infection.[11,12,13] Nevertheless, in occupational settings in which workers may be routinely exposed to blood or other body fluids as described below, an increased risk for occupational acquisition of HBV infection must be assumed to be present.

*3. Vaccination for hepatitis B virus*

A safe and effective vaccine to prevent hepatitis B has been available since 1982. Vaccination has been recommended for health-care workers regularly exposed to blood and other body fluids potentially contaminated with HBV. [7,14,15] In 1987, the Department of Health and Human Services and the Department of Labour stated that hepatitis B vaccine should be provided to all such workers at no charge to the worker. [6]

Available vaccines stimulate active immunity against HBV infection and provide over 90 per cent protection against hepatitis B for 7 or more years following vaccination.[7] Hepatitis B vaccines also are 70-88 per cent effective when given within 1 week after

HBV exposure. Hepatitis B immune globulin (HBIG), a preparation of immunoglobulin with high levels of antibody to HBV (anti-HBs), provides temporary passive protection following exposure to HBV. Combination treatment with hepatitis B vaccine and HBIG is over 90 per cent effective in preventing hepatitis B following a documented exposure.[7]

## E. Transmission of Human Immunodeficiency Virus to Workers

### *1. Health-care workers with AIDS*

As of September 19, 1988, a total of 3,182 (5.1 per cent) of 61,929 adults with AIDS, who had been reported to the CDC national surveillance system and for whom occupational information was available, reported being employed in a health-care setting. Of the health-care workers with AIDS, 95 per cent reported high-risk behaviour; for the remaining 5 per cent (169 workers), the means of HIV acquisition was undetermined.

Of these 169 health-care workers with AIDS with undetermined risk, information is incomplete for 28 (17 per cent) because of death or refusal to be interviewed; 97 (57 per cent ) are still being investigated. The remaining 44 (26 per cent) health-care workers were interviewed directly or had other follow-up information available. The occupations of these 44 were nine nursing assistants (20 per cent); eight physicians (18 per cent), four of whom were surgeons; eight housekeeping or maintenance workers (18 per cent); six nurses (14per cent); four clinical laboratory technicians (9 per cent); two respiratory therapists (5 per cent) ; one dentist (2 per cent); one paramedic (2 per cent); one embalmer (2 per cent); and four others who did not have contact with patients (9 per cent). Eighteen of these 44 health-care workers reported parenteral and/or other non-needle-stick exposure to blood or other body fluids from patients in the 10 years preceding their diagnosis of AIDS. None of these exposures involved a patient with AIDS or known HIV infection, and HIV seroconversion of the health-care worker was not documented following a specific exposure.

### *2. Human immunodeficiency virus transmission in the workplace*

As of July 31,1988,1,201 health-care workers had been enrolled and tested for HIV antibodyinongoing CDC surveillance of health-care workers exposed vianeedle stick or splashes to skin or mucous membranes to blood from patients known to be HIV-infected.[16] Of 860 workers who had received needle-stick injuries or cuts with sharp objects (i.e., parenteral exposures) and whose serum had been tested for HIV antibody at least 180 days after exposure, 4 were positive, yielding a seroprevalence rate of 0.47 per cent. Three of these individuals experienced an acute retroviral syndrome associated with documented seroconversion. Investigation revealed no non-occupational risk factors for these three workers. Serum collected within 30 days of exposure was not available from the fourth person. This worker had an HIV-seropositive sexual partner, and heterosexual acquisition of infection cannot be excluded. None of the 103 workers who had contamination of mucous membranes or nonintact skin and whose serum had been tested at least 180 days after exposure developed serologic evidence of HIV infection.

Two other ongoing prospective studies assess the risk of nosocomial acquisition of HIV infection among health-care workers in the United States. As of April 1988, the National Institutes of Health had tested 983 health-care workers, 137 with documented needle-stick injuries and 345 health-care workers who had sustained mucousmembrane exposures to blood or other body fluids of HIV-infected patients; none had seroconverted[17] (one health-care worker who subsequently experienced an occupational HIV seroconversion has since been reported from NIH).[18] As of March 15, 1988, a similar study at the University of California of 212 health-care workers with 625 documented accidental parenteral exposures involving HIV-infected patients had identified one seroconversion following a needle stick.[19] Prospective studies in the United Kingdom and Canada show no evidence of HIV transmission among 220 health-care workers with parenteral, mucous-membrane, or cutaneous exposures.[20,21]

In addition to the health-care workers enrolled in these longitudinal surveillance studies, case histories have been published in the scientific literature for 19 HIV infected health-care workers (13 with documented seroconversion and 6 without documented sero conversion). None of these workers reported non-occupational risk factors (see Tabler 39.2).

*3. Emergency medical service and public-safety workers*

In addition to the one paramedic with undetermined risk discussed above, three public-safety workers ( law-enforcement officers) are classified in the undetermined risk group. Follow-up investigations of these workers could not determine conclusively if HIV infection was acquired during the performance of job duties.

**Table 39.2**
**HIV-Infected Health-Care Workers with no Reported Non-occupational Risk Factors and for whom Case Histories have been Published in the Scientific Literature**

Cases with Documented Seroconversion

| Case | Occupation | Country | Type of Exposure | Source |
|---|---|---|---|---|
| 1. * | NS† | United States | Needlestick | AIDS patient |
| 2. | NS | United States | Needlestick | AIDS patient |
| 3. | NS | United States | Needlestick | AIDS patient |
| 4. | NS | United States | 2 Needlesticks | AIDS patient, HIV-infected patient |
| 5. | NS | United States | Needlestick | AIDS patient |
| 6. | Nurse | England | Needlestick | AIDS patient |
| 7. | Nurse | France | Needlestick | HIV-infected patient |
| 8. | Nurse | Martinique | Needlestick | AIDS patient |
| 9. | Research lab worker | United States | Cut with sharp object | Concentrated virus |
| 10. | Home health-care worker | United States | Cutaneous# | AIDS patient |
| 11. | NS | United States | Nonintact skin | AIDS patient |
| 12. | Phlebotomist | United States | Mucous-membrane | HIV-infected patient |
| 13. | Technologist | United States | Nonintact skin | HIV-infected patient |
| 14. | NS | United States | Needlestick | AIDS patient |
| 15. | Nurse | Italy | Mucous membrane | HIV-infected patient |
| 16. | Nurse | France | Needlestick | AIDS patient |
| 17. | Navy medic | United States | Needlestick | AIDS patient |
| 18. | Clinical lab worker | United States | Cut with sharp object | AIDS patient |
| 19. | NS | United States | Puncture wound | AIDS patient |
| 20. | NS | United States | 2 Needlesticks | 2 AIDS patients |
| 21. | Research lab worker | United States | Nonintact skin | Concentrated virus |
| 22. | Home health-care provider | England | Nonintact skin | AIDS patient |
| 23. | Dentist | United States | Multiple needle-sticks | Unknown |
| 24..* | Technician | Mexico | Multiple needle-sticks and mucous-membrane | Unknown |
| 25. | Lab worker | United States | Needlestick, puncture wound | Unknown |

#AIDS case.

{Cont.}.......

† Not specified.
# Motherwho provided nursing care for her child with HIV infection; extensive contact with the child's blood and body secretion and excretions occurred; the mother did not wear gloves and often did not wash her hands immediately after exposure.

---

## II. PRINCIPLES OF INFECTION CONTROL AND THEIR APPLICATION TO EMERGENCY AND PUBLIC SAFETY WORKERS

### A. General Infection Control

Within the health-care setting, general infection control procedures have been developed to minimize the risk of patient acquisition of infection from contact with contaminated devices, objects, or surfaces or of transmission of an infectious agent from health-care workers to patients.[1,2,3] Such procedures also protect workers from the risk of becoming infected. General infection-control procedures are designed to prevent transmission of a wide range of microbiological agents and to provide a wide margin of safety in the varied situations encountered in the health-care environment.

General infection-control principles are applicable to other work environments where workers contact other individuals and where transmission of infectious agents may occur. The modes of transmission noted in the hospital and medical office environment are observed in the work situations of emergency and public-safety workers, as well. Therefore, the principles of infection control developed for hospital and other health-care settings are also applicable to these work situations. Use of general infection control measures, as adapted to the work environments of emergency and public-safety workers, is important to protect both workers and individuals with whom they work from a variety of infectious agents, not just HIV and HBV.

Because emergency and public-safety workers work in environments that provide inherently unpredictable risks of exposures, general infection-control procedures should be adapted to these work situations. Exposures are unpredictable, and protective measures may often be used in situations that do not appear to present risk. Emergency and public-safety workers perform their duties in the community under extremely variable conditions; thus, control measures that are simple and uniform across all situations have the greatest likelihood of worker compliance. Administrative procedures to ensure compliance also can be more readily developed than when procedures are complex and highly variable.

## B. Universal Blood and Body Fluid Precautions to Prevent Occupational HIV and HBV Transmission

In 1985, CDC developed the strategy of "universal blood and body fluid precautions" to address concerns regarding transmission of HIV in the health-care setting.[4] The concept, now referred to simply as universal precautions stresses that all patients should be assumed to be infectious for HIV and other blood-borne pathogens. In the hospital and other health-care setting, universal precautions" should be followed when workers are exposed to blood, certain other body fluids (amniotic fluid, pericardial fluid, peritoneal fluid, pleural fluid, synovial fluid, cerebrospinal fluid, semen, and vaginal secretions), or any body fluid visibly contaminated with blood. Since HIV and HBV transmission has not been documented from exposure to other body fluids (feces, nasal secretions, sputum, sweat, tears, urine, and vomitus), "universal precautions" do not apply to these fluids. Universal precautions also do not apply to saliva, except in the dental setting, where saliva is likely to be contaminated with blood.[7]

For the purpose of this document, human "exposure" is defined as contact with blood or other body fluids to which universal precautions apply through percutaneous inoculation or contact with an open wound, nonintact skin, or mucous membrane during the performance of normal job duties. An "exposed worker" is defined, for the purposes of this document, as an individual exposed, as described above, while performing normal job duties.

The unpredictable and emergent nature of exposures encountered by emergency and public-safety workers may make differentiation between hazardous body fluids and those which are not hazardous very difficult and often impossible. For example, poor lighting may limit the worker s ability to detect visible blood in vomitus or feces. Therefore, when emergency medical and public-safety workers encounter body fluids under uncontrolled, emergency circumstances in which differentiation between fluid types is difficulty if not impossible, they should treat all body fluids as potentially hazardous.

The application of the principles of universal precautions to the situations encountered by these workers results in the development of guidelines (listed below) for work practices, use of personal protective equipment, and other protective measures. To minimize the risks of acquiring HIV and HBV during performance of job duties, emergency and public-safety workers should be protected from exposure to blood and other body fluids as circumstances dictate. Protection can be achieved through adherence to workpractices designed to minimize or eliminate exposure and through use of personal protective equipment (i.e., gloves, masks, and protective clothing), whichprovide a barrier between the worker and the exposure source. In some situations, redesign of selected aspects of the job through equipment modifications or environmental control can further reduce risk. These approaches to primary prevention should be used together to achieve maximal reduction of the risk of exposure.

If exposure of an individual worker occurs, medical management, consisting of collection of pertinent medical and occupational history, provision of treatment, and counseling regarding future work and personal behaviours, may reduce risk of developing disease as a result of the exposure episode.[22] Following episodic (or continuous) exposure, decontamination and disinfection of the work environment, devices, equipment, and clothing or other forms of personal protective equipment can reduce subsequent risk of exposures. Proper disposal of contaminated waste has similar benefits.

## III. EMPLOYER RESPONSIBILITIES

### A. General

Detailed recommendations for employer responsibilities in protecting workers from acquisition of blood-borne diseases in the workplace have been published in the Department of Labour and Department of Health and Human Services Joint Advisory Notice and are summarized here.[6] In developing programmes to protect workers, employers should follow a series of steps: (1) classification of work activity, (2) development of standard operating procedures, (3) provision of training and education, (4) development of procedures to ensure and monitor compliance, and (5 ) workplace redesign. As a first step, every employer should classify work activities into one of three categories of potential exposure (see Table 39.3). Employers should make protective equipment available to all workers when they are engaged in Category I or II activities. Employers should ensure that the appropriate protective equipment is used by workers when they perform Category I activities.

As a second step, employers should establish a detailed work practices programme that includes standard operating procedures (SOPs) for all activities having the potential for exposure. Once these SOPs are developed, an initial and periodic worker education programme to assure familiarity with work practices should be provided to potentially exposed workers. No worker should engage in such tasks or activities before receiving training pertaining to the SOPs, work practices, and protective equipment required for that task. Examples of personal protective equipment for the pre hospital setting (defined as a setting where delivery of emergency health care takes place away from a hospital or other health-care setting) are provided in Table 39.4. (A curriculum for such training programmes is being developed in conjunction with these guidelines and should be consulted for further information concerning such training programmes.

**Table 39.3**
**Summary of Task Categorization and Implications for Personal Protective Equipment**

| Joint Advisory Notice Category[1] | Nature of Task/Activity | Personal protective equipment should be: Available? | Worn? |
|---|---|---|---|
| I. | Directcontact with blood or other body fluids to which universal precautions apply | Yes | Yes |
| II. | Activity performed without blood exposure but exposure may occur in emergency | Yes | No |
| III. | Task/activity does not entail predictable or unpredictable exposure to blood | No | No |

[1] U.S. Department of Labour, U.S. Department of Health and Human Services. Joint advisory notice: protection against occupational exposure to hepatitis B virus (HBV) and human immunodeficiency virus (HIV). Washington, DC: US Department of Labour, US Department of Health and Human Services, 1987.

To facilitate and monitor compliance with SOPs, administrative procedures should be developed and records kept as described in the Joint Advisory Notice.[6] Employers should monitor the workplace to ensure that required work practices are observed and that protective clothing and equipment are provided and properly used. The employer should maintain records documenting the administrative procedures used to classify job activities and copies of all SOPs for tasks or activities involving predictable or unpredictable exposure to blood or other body fluids to which universal precautions apply. In addition, training records, indicating the dates of training sessions, the content of those training sessions along with the names of all persons conducting the training, and the names of all those receiving training should also be maintained.

Whenever possible, the employer should identify devices and other approaches to modifying the work environment which will reduce exposure risk. Such approaches are desirable, since they don't require individual worker action or management activity. For example, jails and correctional facilities should have classification procedures that require the segregation of offenders who indicate through their actions or words that they intend to attack correctional-facility staff with the intent of transmitting HIV or HBV.

**Table 39.4**
**Examples of Recommended Personal Protective Equipment for Worker Protection Against HIV and HBV Transmission in Prehospital[1] Settings**

| Task or Activity | Disposable Gloves | Gown | Mask | Protective Eyewear |
|---|---|---|---|---|
| Bleeding control with spurting blood | Yes | Yes | Yes | Yes |
| Bleeding control with minimal bleeding | Yes | No | No | No |
| Emergency child birth | Yes | Yes | Yes if splashing is likely | Yes if splashing is likely |
| Blood drawing | At certain times[4] | No | No | No |
| Starting an intravenous (IV) line | Yes | No | No | No |
| Endotracheal intubation esophageal obturator use | Yes | No | No unless splashing is likely | No unless splashing is likely |
| Oral/nasal suctioning manually cleaning airway | Yes[5] | No | No, unless splashing is likely | No, unless splashing is likely |
| Handling and cleaning instruments with microbial contamination | Yes | No, unless soiling is likely | No | No |
| Measuring blood pressure | No | No | No | No |
| Measuring temperature | No | No | No | No |
| Giving an injection | No | No | No | No |

[1] The examples provided in this table are based on application of universal precautions Universal precautions are intended to supplement rather than replace recom

{Cont.}.........

mendations for routine infection control, such as handwashing and using gloves to prevent gross microbial contamination of hands (e g, contact with urine or feces)

[2] Defined as setting where delivery of emergency health are takes place away from a hospital or other health-care facility.

[3] Refers to protective masks to prevent exposure of mucous membranes to blood or other potentially contaminated body fluids. The use of resuscitation devices, some of which are also referred to as "masks".

[4] For clarification see A, and B.

[5] While not clearly necessary to prevent HIV or HBV transmission unless blood is present, gloves are recommended to prevent transmission of other agents (e.g., Her per simplex).

---

## B. Medical

In addition to the general responsibilities noted above, the employer has the specific responsibility to make available to the worker a programme of medical management. This programme is designed to provide for the reduction of risk of infection by HBV and for counseling workers concerning issues regarding HIV and HBV. These services should be provided by a licensed health professional. All phases of medical management and counseling should ensure that the confidentiality of the worker's and client's medical data is protected.

### *1. Hepatitis B vaccination*

All workers whose jobs involve participation in tasks or activities with exposure to blood or other body fluids to which universal precautions apply ( as defined above) should be vaccinated with hepatitis B vaccine.

### *2. Management of percutaneous exposure to blood and other infectious body fluids*

Once an exposure has occurred (as defined above a blood sample should be drawn after consent is obtained from the individual from whom exposur eoccurred and tested for hepatitis B surface antigen (HBsAg ) and antibody to human immunodeficiency virus (HIV antibody). Local laws regarding consent for testing source individuals should be followed. Policies should be available for testing source individuals in situations where consent cannot be obtained (e.g., an unconscious patient). Testing of the source individual should be done at a location where appropriate pretest counseling is available; posttest counseling and referral for treatment should be provided. It is extremely important that all individuals who seek consultation for any HIV-related concerns receive counseling as outlined in the "Public Health Service Guidelines for Counseling and Antibody Testing to Prevent HIV Infection and AIDS". [22]

(a) **Hepatitis B virus postexposure management**

For an exposure to a source individual found to be positive for HBsAg, the worker who has not previously been given hepatitis B vaccine should receive the vaccine series. A single dose of hepatitis B immune globulin (HBIG) is also recommended, if this can be given within 7 days of exposure. For exposures from an HBsAg-positive source to workers who have previously received vaccine, the exposed worker should be tested for antibody to hepatitis B surface antigen (anti-HBs), and given one dose of vaccine and one dose of HBIG if the antibody level in the worker's blood sample is inadequate (i.e.< 10 SRU by RIA, negative by EIA).[7]

If the source individual is negative for HBsAg and the worker has not been vaccinated, this opportunity should be taken to provide hepatitis B vaccination.

If the source individual refuses testing or he/she cannot be identified, the unvaccinated worker should receive the hepatitis B vaccine series. HBIG administration should be considered on an individual basis when the source individual is known or suspected to be at high risk of HBV infection. Management and treatment, if any, of previously vaccinated workers who receive an exposure from a source who refuses testing or is not identifiable should be individualized.[7]

(b) **Human immunodeficiency virus postexposure management**

For any exposure to a source individual who has AIDS, who is found to be positive for HIV infection,[4] or who refuses testing, the worker should be counseled regarding the risk of infection and evaluated clinically and serologically for evidence of HIV infection as soon as possible after the exposure. In view of the evolving nature of HIV post exposure management, the health care provider should be well informed of current PHS guidelines on this subject. The worker should be advised to report and seek medical evaluation for any acute febrile illness that occurs within 12 weeks after the exposure. Such an illness, particularly one characterized by fever, rash, or lymphadenopathy, may be indicative of recent HIV infection. Following the initial test at the time of exposure, seronegative workers shoul be retested

6 weeks, 12 weeks, and 6 months after exposure to determine whether transmission has occurred. During this follow-up period (especially the first 6-12 weeks after exposure, when most infected persons are expected to seroconvert), exposed workers should follow U.S. Public Health Service (PHS) recommendations for preventing transmission of HIV. [22] These include refraining from blood donation and using appropriate protection during sexual intercourse. [23] During all phases of follow-up, it is vital that worker confidentiality be protected.

If the source individual was tested and found to be seronegative, baseline testing of the exposed worker with follow-up testing 12 weeks later may be performed if desired by the worker or recommended by the health-care provider.

If the source individual cannot be identified, decisions regarding appropriate follow-up should be individualized. Serologic testing should be made available by the employer to ahl workers who may be concerned they have been infected with HIV through an occupational exposure as defined above.

### *3. Management of Human Bites*

On occasion, police and correctional-facility officers are intentionally bitten by suspects or prisoners. When such bites occur, routine medical and surgical therapy (including an assessment of tetanus vaccination status) should be implemented as soon as possible, since such bites frequently result in infection with organisms other than HIV and HBV. Victims of bites should be evaluated as described above exposure to blood or other infection body fluids.

Saliva of some persons infected with HBV has been shown to contain HBV-DNA at concentrations 1/1,000 to 1/10,000 of that found in the infected person's serum. [5,24] HBsAg-positive saliva has been shown to be infectious when injected into experimental animals and in human bite exposures.[25-27] However, HBsAg-positive saliva has not been shown to be infectious when applied to oral mucous membranes in experimental primate studies [27] or through contamination of musical instruments or cardiopulmonary resuscitation dummies used by HBV carriers. [28,29] Epidemiologic studies of nonsexual household contacts of HIV-infected patients, including several small series in which HIV transmission failed to occur after bites or after percutaneous inoculation or contamination of cuts and open wounds with saliva from HIV-infected patients, suggest that the potential for salivary transmission of HIV is remote.[5,30-33] One case report from Germany has suggested the possibility of transmission of HIV in a household setting from an infected child to a sibling through a human bite.[34] The bite did not break the skin or result in bleeding. Since the date of seroconversion to HIV was not known for either child in this case, evidence for the role of saliva in the transmission of virus is unclear.[34]

### *4. Documentation of Exposure and Reporting*

As part of the confidential medical record, the circumstances of exposure should be recorded. Relevant information includes the activity in which the worker was engaged at the time of exposure, the extent to which appropriate work practices and protective equipment were used, and a description of the source of exposure.

Employers have a responsibility under various federal and state laws and regulations to report occupational illnesses and injuries. Existing programmes in the National Institute for Occupational Safety and Health (NIOSH), Department of Health and Human Services; the Bureau of Labour Statistics, Department of Labour (DoL); and the Occupational safety and Health Administration (DOL) receive such information for the purposes of surveillance and other objectives. Cases of infectious disease, including AIDS and HBV infection, are reported to the Centers for Disease Control through State health departments.

### *5. Management of HBV- or HIV-infected workers*

Transmission of HBV from health-care workers to patients has been documented. Such transmission has occurred during certain types of invasive procedures (e.g., oral and gynecologic surgery) in which health-care workers, when tested, had very high concentrations of HBV in their blood (at least 100 million infectious virus particles per milliliter, a concentration much higher than occurs with HIV infection), and the health-care workers sustained a puncture wound while performing invasive procedures or had exudative or weeping lesions or microlacerations that allowed virus to contaminate instruments or open wounds of patients. [35,36] A worker who is HBsAg positive and who has transmitted hepatitis B virus to another individual during the performance of his or her job duties should be excluded from the performance of those job duties which place other individuals at risk for acquisition of hepatitis B infection.

Workers with impaired immune systems resulting from HIV infection or other causes are at increased risk of acquiring or experiencing serious complications of infectious disease. Of particular concern is the risk of severe infection following exposure to other persons with infectious diseases that are easily transmitted if appropriate precautions are not taken (e.g., measles, varicella). Any worker with an impaired immune system should be counseled about the potential risk associated with providing health care to persons with any transmissible infection and should continue to follow existing recommendations for infection control to minimize risk of exposure to other infectious agents.[2,3] Recommendations of the Immunization Practices Advisory Committee (ACIP) and institutional policies concerning requirements for vaccinating workers with live-virus vaccines (e.g., measles, rubella) should also be considered.

The question of whether workers infected with HIV can adequately and safely be allowed to perform patient-care duties or whether their work assignments should be changed must be determined on an individual basis. These decisions should be made by the worker's personal physician(s) in conjunction with the employer's medical advisors.

## C. Disinfection, Decontamination, and Disposal

As described in Section I.C. (4), the only documented occupational risks of HIV and HBV infection are associated with parenteral (including open wound) and mucous membrane exposure to blood and other potentially infectious body fluids. Nevertheless, the precautions described below should be routinely followed.

### 1. Needle and sharps disposal

All workers should take precautions to prevent injuries caused by needles, scalpel blades, andother sharp instruments or devices during procedures; when cleaning used instruments; during disposal of used needles; and when handling sharp instruments after procedures. To prevent needle-stick injuries, needles should not be recapped, purposely bent or broken by hand, removed from disposable syringes, or otherwise manipulated by hand. After they are used, disposable syringes and needles, scalpel blades, and other sharp items should be placed in puncture-resistant containers for disposal; the puncture-resistant containers should be located as close as practical to the use area (e.g., in the ambulance or, if sharps are carried to the scene of victim assistance from the ambulance, a small puncture—resistant container should be carried to the scene, as well ). Reusable needles should be left on the syringe body and should be placed in a puncture-resistant container for transport to the reprocessing area.

*2. Hand washing*

Hands and other skin surfaces should be washed immediately and thoroughly if contaminated with blood, other body fluids to which universal precautions apply, or potentially contaminated articles. Hands should always be washed after gloves are removed, even if the gloves appear to be intact. Hand washing should be completed using the appropriate facilities, such as utility or restroom sinks. Waterless antiseptic hand cleanser should be provided on responding units to use when hand-washing facilities are not available. When hand-washing facilities are available, wash hands with warm water and soap. When hand-washing facilities are not available, use a waterless antiseptic hand cleanser. The manufacturer's recommendations for the product should be followed.

*3. Cleaning, disinfecting, and sterilizing*

Table 39.5 presents the methods and applications for cleaning, disinfecting, and sterilizing equipment and surfaces in the prehospital setting. These methods also apply to housekeeping and other cleaning tasks. Previously issued guidelines for health-care workers contain more detailed descriptions.[4]

*4. Cleaning and decontaminating spills of blood*

All spills of blood and blood-contaminated fluids should be promptly cleaned up using an EPA-approved germicide or a 1:100 solution of household bleach in the following manner while wearing gloves. Visible material should first be removed with disposable towels or other appropriate means that will ensure against direct contact with blood. If splashing is anticipated, protective eyewear should be worn along with an impervious gown or apron which provides an effective barrier to splashes. The area should then be decontaminated with an appropriate germicide. Hands should be washed following removal of gloves. Soiled cleaning equipment shouldbe cleaned and decontaminated or placed in an appropriate container and disposed of according to agency policy. Plastic bags should be available for removal of contaminated items from the site of the spill.

Shoes and boots can become contaminated with blood in certain instances. Where there is massive blood contamination on floors, the use of disposable impervious shoe coverings should be considered. Protective gloves should be worn to remove contaminated shoe coverings. The coverings and gloves should be disposed of in plastic bags. A plastic bag should be included in the crime scene kit or the car which is to be used for the disposal of contaminated items. Extra plastic bags should be stored in the police cruiser or emergency vehicle.

*5. Laundry*

Although soiled linen may be contaminated with pathogenic micro organisms, the risk of actual disease transmission is negligible. Rather than rigid procedures and specifications, hygienic storage and processing of clean and soiled linen are recommended. Laundry facilities and/or services should be made routinely available by the employer. Soiled linen should be handled as little as possible and with minimum agitation to prevent gross microbial contamination of the air and of persons handling the linen. All soiled linen should be bagged at the location where it was used. Linen soiled with blood should be placed and transported in bags that prevent leakage. Normal laundry cycles should be used according to the washer and detergent manufacturers' recommendations.

*6. Decontamination and laundering of protective clothing*

Protective work clothing contaminated with blood or other body fluids to which universal precautions apply should be placed and transported in bags or containers that prevent leakage. Personnel involved in the bagging, transport, and laundering of contaminated clothing should wear gloves. Protective clothing and station and work uniforms should be washed and dried according to the manufacturer's instructions. Boots and leather goods may be brush-scrubbed with soap and hot water to remove contamination.

*7. Infective waste*

The selection of procedures for disposal of infective waste is determined by the relative risk of disease transmission and application of local regulations, which vary widely. In all cases, local regulations should be consulted prior to disposal procedures and followed. Infective waste, in general, should either be incinerated or should be decontaminated before disposal in a sanitary landfill. Bulk blood, suctioned fluids, excretions and secretiond may be carefully poured down a drain connected to a sanitary sewer, where permitted sanitary sewers may also be used to dispose of other infectious wastes capable of being ground and ushed into the sewer, where permited sharp items should be placed in puncture-proof containers and other blood-contaminated items should be placed in leak-proof plastic bags for transport to an appropriate disposal location.

Prior to the removal of protective equipment, personnel remainingon the scene after the patient has been cared for should carefully search for and remove contaminated materials Debris should be disposed of as noted above.

## IV. FIRE AND EMERGENCY MEDICAL SERVICES

The guidelines that appear in this section apply to fire and emergency medical services. This includes structural fire fighters, paramedics, emergency medical technicians, and advanced life support personnel. Fire fighters often provide emergency medical services and therefore encounter the exposures common to paramedics and emergency medical technicians. Job duties are often performed in uncontrolled environments, which, due to a lack of time and other factors, do not allow for application of acomplex decision-making process to the emergency at hand.

The general principles presented here have been developed from existing principles of occupational safety and health in conjunction with data from studies of health-care workers in hospital settings. The basic premise is that workers must be protected from exposure to blood and other potentially infectious body fluids in the course of their work activities. There is a paucity of data concerning the risks these worker groups face, however, which complicates development of control principles. Thus, the guidelines presented below are based on principles of prudent public health practice.

Fire and emergency medical service personnel are engaged in delivery of medical care in the prehospital setting. The following guidelines are intended to assist these personnel in making decisions concerning use of personal protective equipment and resuscitation equipment, as well as for decontamination, disinfection, and disposal procedures.

### A. Personal Protective Equipment

Appropriate personal protective equipment should be made available routinely by the employer to reduce the risk of exposure as defined above. For many situations, the chance that the rescuer will be exposed to blood and other body fluids to which universal precautions apply can be determined in advance. Therefore, if the chances of being exposed to blood is high (e.g., CPR, IV insertion, trauma, delivering babies), the worker should put on protective attire before beginning patient care. Table 39.4) sets forth examples of recommendations for personal protective equipment inthe prehospital setting; the list is not intended to be all-inclusive.

*1. Gloves*

Disposable gloves should be a standard component of emergency response equipment, and should be donned by all personnel prior to initiating any emergency patient care tasks involving exposure to blood or other body fluids to which universal precautions apply. Extra pairs should always be available. Considerations in the choice of disposable gloves should include dexterity, durability, fit, and the task being performed. Thus, there is no single type or thickness of glove appropriate for protection in all situations. For situations where large amounts of blood are likely to be encountered, it is important that gloves fit tightly at the wrist to prevent blood contamination of hands around the cuff. For multiple trauma victims, gloves should be changed between patient contacts, if the emergency situation allows.

Greater personal protective equipment measures are indicated for situations where broken glass and sharp edges are likely to be encountered, such as extricating a person from an automobile wreck. Structural fire-fighting gloves that meet the Federal OSHA requirements for fire-fighters gloves (as contained in 29 CFR 1910.156 or National Fire Protection Association Standard 1973, Gloves for Structural Fire Fighters ) should be worn in any situation where sharp or rough surfaces are likely to be encountered.[37]

While wearing gloves, avoid handling personal items, such as combs and pens, that could become soiled or contaminated. Gloves that have become contaminated with blood or other body fluids to which universal precautions apply should be removed as soon as possible, taking care to avoid skin contact with the exterior surface. Contaminated gloves should be placed and transported in bags that prevent leakage and should be disposed of or, in the case of reusable gloves, cleaned and disinfected properly.

*2. Masks, eyewear, and gowns*

Masks, eyewear, and gowns should be present on all emergency vehicles that respond or potentially respond to medical emergencies or victim rescues. These protective barriers should be used in accordance with the level of exposure encountered. Minor lacerations or small amounts of blood do not merit the same extent of barrier use as required for exsanguinating victims or massive arterial bleeding. Management of the patient who is not bleeding, and who has no bloody body fluids present, should not routinely require use of barrier precautions. Masks and eyewear (e.g., safety glasses) should be worn together, or a faceshield should be used by all personnel prior to any situation where splashes of blood or other body fluids to which universal precautions apply are likely to occur. Gowns or aprons should be worn to protect clothing from splashes with blood. If large splashes or quantities of blood are present or anticipated, impervious gowns or aprons should be worn. An extra change of work clothing should be available at all times.

*3. Resuscitation Equipment*

No transmission of HBV or HIV infection during mouth-to-mouth resuscitation has been documented. However, because of the risk of salivary transmission of other infectious diseases (e.g., herpes simplex and Neisseria meaningitidis)and the theoretical risk of HIV and HBV transmission during artificial ventilation of trauma victims, disposable air way equipment or resuscitation bags should be used. Disposable resuscitation equipment and devices should be used once and disposed of or, if reusable, thoroughly cleaned and disinfected after each use according to the manufacturer's recommendations.

Mechanical respiratory assist devices (e.g., bag-valve masks, oxygen demand valve resuscitators) should be available on all emergency vehicles and to all emergency response personnel that respond or potentially respond to medical emergencies or victim rescues.

Pocket mouth-to-mouth resuscitation masks designed to isolate emergency response personnel (i.e.,double lumen systems) from contact with victims' blood and blood contaminated saliva, respiratory secretions, and vomitus should be provided to all personnel who provide or potentially provide emergency treatment.

## V. LAW-ENFORCEMENT AND CORRECTIONAL-FACLLLTY OFFICERS

Law-enforcement and correctional-facility officers may face the risk of exposure to blood during the conduct of their duties. For example, at the crime scene or during processing of suspects, law-enforcement officers may encounter blood-contaminated hypodermic needles or weapons, or be called upon to assist with body removal. Correctional-facility officers may similarly be required to search prisoners or their cells for hypodermic needles or weapons, or subdue violent and combative inmates.

The following section presents information for reducing the risk of acquiring HIV and HBV infection by law-enforcement and correctional-facility officers as a consequence of carrying out their duties. However, there is an extremely diverse range of potential situations which may occur in the control of persons with unpredictable, violent, or psychotic behaviour. Therefore, informed judgment of the individual officer is paramount when unusual circumstances or events arise. These recommendations should serve as an adjunct to rational decision making in those situations where specific guidelines do not exist, particularly where immediate action is required to preserve life or prevent significant injury.

The following guidelines are arranged into three sections: a section addressing concerns shared by both law-enforcement and correctional-facility officers, and two sections dealing separately with law-enforcement officers and correctional-facility officers, respectively. Table 39.4 contains selected examples of personal protective equipment that may be employed by law-enforcement and correctional-facility officers.

## A. Law-Enforcement and Correctional-Facilities Considerations

### *1. Fights and assaults*

Law-enforcement and correctional-facility officers are exposed to a range of assaultive and disruptive behaviour through which they may potentially become exposed to blood or other body fluids containing blood. Behaviours of particular concern are biting, attacks resulting in blood exposure, and attacks with sharp objects. Such behaviours may occur in a range of law-enforcement situations including arrests, routine interrogations, domestic disputes and lockup operations, as well as incorrectional-facility activities. Hand-to-hand combat may result in bleeding and may thus incur a greater chance for blood-to-blood exposure, which increases the chances for blood-borne disease transmission.

Whenever the possibility for exposure to blood or blood-contaminated body fluids exists, the appropriate protection should be worn, if feasible under the circumstances. In all cases, extreme caution must be used in dealing with the suspect or prisoner if there is any indication of assaultive or combative behaviour. When blood is present and a suspect or an inmate is combative or threatening lo staff, gloves should always be put on as soon as conditions permit. In case of blood contamination of clothing, an extra change of clothing should be available at all times.

### *2. Cardiopulmonary resuscitation*

Law-enforcement and correctional personnel are also concern about infection with HIV and HBV through administration of cardiopulmonary resuscitation (CUR). Although there have been no documented cases of HIV transmission through this mechanism, the possibility of transmission of other infectious diseases exists.

Therefore, agencies should make protective masks or airways available to officers and provide training in their proper use. Devices with one-way valves to prevent the patients' saliva or vomitus from entering the caregiver's mouth are preferable.

## B. Law-Enforcement Considerations

### *1. Searches and evidence handling*

Criminal justice personnel have potential risks of acquiring HBV or HIV infection through exposures which occur during searches and evidence handling. Penetrating injuries are known to occur, and puncture wounds or needle sticks in particular pose a hazard during searches of persons, vehicles, or cells, and during evidence handling. The following precautionary measures will help to reduce the risk of infection:

- # An officer should use great caution in searching the clothing of suspects. Individual discretion, based on the circumstances at hand, should determine if a suspect or prisoner should empty his own pockets or if the officer should use his own skills in determining the contents of a suspect's clothing.
- # A safe distance should always be maintained between the officer and the suspect.
- # Wear protective gloves if exposure to blood is likely to be encountered.
- # Wear protective gloves for all body cavity searches.
- # If cotton gloves are to be worn when working with evidence of potential latent fingerprint value at the crime scene, they can be worn over protective disposable gloves when exposure to blood may occur.
- # Always carry a flashlight, even during daylight shifts, to search hidden areas. Whenever possible, use long-handled mirrors and flashlights to search such areas (e.g., under car seats).
- # If searching a purse, carefully empty contents directly from purse, by turning it upside down over a table.
- # Use puncture-proof containers to store sharp instruments and clearly marked plastic bags to store other possibly contaminated items.
- # To avoid tearing gloves, use evidence tape instead of metal staples to seal evidence.
- # Local procedures for evidence handling should be followed. In general, items should be air dried before sealing in plastic.

Not all types of gloves are suitable for conducting searches. Vinyl or latex rubber gloves provide little protection against sharp instruments, and they are not puncture proof. There is a direct trade-off between level of protection and manipulability. In other words, the thicker the gloves, the more protection they provide, but the less effective they are in locating objects. Thus, there is no single type or thickness of glove appropriate for protection in all situations. Officers should select the type and thickness of glove which provides the best balance of protection and search efficiency.

Officers and crime scene technicians may confront unusual hazards, especially when the crime scene involves violent behaviour, such as a homicide where large amounts of blood are present. Protective gloves should be available and worn in this setting. In addition, for very large spills, consideration should be given to other protective clothing, such as overalls, aprons, boots, or protective shoe covers. They should be changed if torn or soiled, and always removed prior to leaving the scene. While wearing gloves, avoid handling personal items, such as combs and pens, that could become soiled or contaminated.

Face masks and eye protection or a face shield are required for laboratory and evidence technicians whose jobs which entail potential exposures to blood via a splash to the face, mouth, nose, or eyes.

Airborne particles of dried blood may be generated when a stain is scraped. It is recommended that protective masks and eyewear or face shields be worn by laboratory or evidence technicians when removing the blood stain for laboratory analyses.

While processing the crime scene, personnel should be alert for the presence of sharp objects such as hypodermic needles, knives, razors, broken glass, nails,or othersharp objects.

*2. Handling deceased persons and body removal*

For detectives investigators evidence technicians all other who may have to touch or remove a body, the response should be the same as for situations requiring CPR or first aid: wear gloves and cover all cuts and abrasions to create a barrier and carefully wash all exposed areas after any contact with blood. The precautions to be used with blood and deceased persons should also be used when handling amputated limbs, hands, or other body parts. Such procedures should be followed after contact with the blood of anyone, regardless of whether they are known or suspected to be infected with HIV or HBV.

*3. Autopsies*

Protective masks and eyewear (or face shields), laboratory coats, gloves, and waterproof aprons should be worn when performing or at tending all autopsies. All autopsy material should be considered infectious for both HIV and HBV. Onlookers with an opportunity for exposure to blood splashes should be similarly protected. Instruments and surfaces contaminated during postmortem procedures should be decontaminated with an appropriate chemical germicide.[4] Many laboratories have more detailed standard operating procedures for conducting autopsies; where available, these should be followed. More detailed recommendations for health-care workers in this setting have been published. [4]

*4. Forensic laboratories*

Blood from all individuals should be considered infective. To supplement other worksite precautions, the following precautions are recommended for workers in forensic laboratories.

a. All specimens of blood should be put in a well-constructed, appropriately labelled container with a secure lid to prevent leaking during transport. Care should be taken when collecting each specimen to avoid contaminating the outside of the container and of the laboratory form accompanying the specimen.
b. All persons processing blood specimens should wear gloves. Masks and protective eyewear or face shields should be worn if mucous-membrane contact with blood is anticipated (e.g., removing tops from vacuum tubes). Hands should be washed after completion of specimen processing.
c. For routine procedures,such as histologic and pathologic studies ormicrobiological culturing, a biological safety cabinet is not necessary. However, biological safety cabinets (Class I or II) should be used whenever procedures are conducted that have a high potential for generating droplets. These include activities such as blending, sonicating, and vigorous mixing.
d. Mechanical pipetting devices should be used for manipulating all liquids in the laboratory. Mouth pipetting must not be done.
e. use of needles and syringes should be limited to situations in which there is no alternative, and the recommendations for preventing injuries with needles outlined under universal precautions should be followed.

f. Laboratory work surfaces should be cleaned of visible materials and then decontaminated with an appropriate chemical germicide after a spill of blood, semen, or blood-contaminated body fluid and when work activities are completed.

g. Contaminated materials used in laboratory tests should be decontaminated before reprocessing or be placed in bags and disposed of in accordance with institutional and local regulatory policies for disposal of infective waste.

h. Scientific equipment that has been contaminated with blood should be cleaned and then decontaminated before being repaired in the laboratory or transported to the manufacturer.

i. All persons should wash their hands after completing laboratory activities and should remove protective clothing before leaving the laboratory.

j. Area posting of warning signs should be considered to remind employees of continuing hazard of infectious disease transmission in the laboratory setting.

## C. Correctional-Facility Considerations

### *1. Searches*

Penetrating injuries are known to occur in the correctional-facility setting, and puncture wounds or needle sticks in particular pose a hazard during searches of prisoners or their cells. The following precautionary measures will help to reduce the risk of infection.

# A correctional-facility officer should use great caution in searching the clothing of prisoners. Individual discretion, based on the circumstances at hand, should determine if a prisoner should empty his own pockets or if the officer should use his own skills in determining the contents of a prisoner's clothing.

# A safe distance should always be maintained between the officer and the prisoner.

# Always carry a flashlight, even during daylight shifts, to search hidden areas. Whenever possible, use long-handled mirrors and flashlights to search such areas (e.g., under commodes, bunks, and in vents in jail cells ).

# Wear protective gloves if exposure to blood is likely to be encountered.

# Wear protective gloves for all body cavity searches.

**Table- 39. 5**
**Reprocessing Methods for Equipment Used in the Prehospital[1] Health-Care Setting**

| | | |
|---|---|---|
| Sterilization: | Destroys | All form of microbial life including high numbers of bacterial spores. |
| | Methods: | Steam under pressure (autoclave), gas (ethylene oxide), dry heat, or immersion in EPA-approved chemical "sterilant" for prolonged period of time, e.g., 6-10 hours or according to manufacturers' instructions. Note: liquid chemical "sterilants" should be used only on those instruments that are impossible to sterilize or disinfect with heat. |
| | Use: | For those instrumetns or devices that pen etrate skin or contact normally sterile ar eas of the body, e.g., scalpels, needles, etc. Disposable invasive equipment eliminates the need to reprocess these types of items. When indicated, however, arrangements should be made with a health-care facility for reprocessing of reusable invasive instruments. |
| High-Level Disinfection: | Destroys: | All forms of microbial life except high numbers of bacterial spores. |
| | Methods: | Hot water pasteurization (80-100 C, 30 minutes) or exposure to an EPA-registered "sterilant" chemicals above, except for as hort exposure time (10-45 minutes or as directed by the manufacturer). |
| | Use: | For reusable instruments or devices that come into contact with mucous membranes (e.g., laryngoscope blades, endotracheal tubes, etc.). |
| Intermediate-Level | Destroys: | *Mycobacterium tuberculosis*, vegetative bacteria, most viruses, and most fungi, but does not kill bacterial spores. |
| | Methods: | EPA-registered "hospital disinfectant" chemical germicides that have a label claim for tuberculocidal activity; commer cially available hard-surface germicides or solutions containing at least 500 ppm free available chlorine (a 1: 100 dilution of com mon household bleach-approximately ¼ cup bleach per gallon of tap water). |
| | Use: | For those surfaces that come into contact only with intact skin, e.g., stethoscopes, blood pressure cuffs, splints, etc. and have been visibly contaminated with blood or bloody body fluids. Surfaces must be precleaned of visible material before the |

{Cont.}......

| | | |
|---|---|---|
| | | germicidal chemical is applied for disin fection. |
| Low-Level Disinfection: | Destroys: | Most bacteria, some viruses, some fungi, but not *Mycobacterium tuberculosis* or bacterial spores. |
| | Methods: | EPA-registered "hospital disinfectants" (no label claim for tuberculocidal activity). |
| | Use: | These agents are excellent cleaners and can be used for routine housekeeping or removal of soiling in the absence of visible blood contamination. |
| Low-Level Disinfection: | | Environmental surfaces which have become soiled should be cleaned and disinfected using any cleaner or disinfectant-agent which is intended for environmental use. Such surfaces include floors, woodwork, ambulance seats, countertops, etc. |
| IMPORTANT: | To assure the effectiveness of any sterilization or disinfection process, equipment and instruments must first be thoroughly cleaned of all visible soil. | |

[1] Defined as setting where delivery of emergency health-care takes place prior to arrival at hospital or other health-care facility.

Not all types of gloves are suitable for conducting searches. Vinyl or latex rubber gloves can provide little if any, protection against sharp instruments and they are not puncture-proof. There is a direct trade-off between level of protection and manipulability. In other words, the thicker the gloves, the more protection they provide, but the less effective they are in locating objects. Thus, there is no single type or thickness of glove appropriate for protection in all situations. Officers should select the type and thickness of glove which provides the best balance of protection and search efficiency.

*2. Decontamination and Disposal*

Prisoners mayspit at officers and throw feces; sometimes these substances have been purposefully contaminated with blood. Although there are no documented cases of HIV or HBV transmission in this manner and transmission by this route would not be expected to occur, other diseases could be transmitted. These materials should be removed with a paper towel after donning gloves, and the area then decontaminated with an appropriate germicide. Following clean-up, soiled towels and gloves should be disposed of properly.

## References


1. Garner JS, Favero MS. Guideline for handwashing and hospital environmental control, 1985. Atlanta: Public Health Service, Centers for Disease Control, 1985. HHS publication no. 99-1117.
2. Garner JS, Simmons BP. Guideline for isolation precautions in hospitals. Infect Control 1983; 4 (suppl):245—325.
3. Williams WW. Guideline for infection control in hospital personnel. Infect Control 1983; 4(suppl):326-49.
4. Centers for Disease Control. Recommendations for prevention of HIV transmission in health-care settings. MMWR 1987; 36 (suppl 2S).
5. Centers for Disease Control. Update: Universal precautions for prevention of transmission of human immunodeficiency virus, hepatitis B virus, and other bloodborne pathogens in health-care settings. MMWR 1988; 37:377-382,387-88.
6. U.S. Department of Labour, U.S. Department of Health and Human Services. Joint Advisory Notice: protection against occupational exposure to hepatitis B virus (HBV and human immunodeficiency virus HIV). Federal Register 1987; 52:41818-24.
7. Centers for Disease Control. Recommendations for protection against viral hepatitis. MMWR 1985; 34:313-324,329-335.
8. Kunches L M, Craven DE, Werner BG, Jacobs LM. Hepatitis B exposure in emergency medical personnel: prevalence of serologic markers and need for immunization. Amer J Med 1983; 75:269-272.
9. Pepe PE, Hollinger FB, Troisi CL, Heiberg D. Viral hepatitis risk in urban emergency medical services personnel. Annals Emergency Med 1986; 15(4):454 457.
10. Valenzuela TD, Hook EW, Copass MK, Corey L. Occupational exposure to hepatitis B in paramedics. Arch Intern Med 1985; 145:1976-1977.
11. Morgan-Capner P. Hudson P. Hepatitis B markers in Lancashire police officers. Epidemiol Inf 1988; 100:145-151.
12. Peterkin M, Crawford RJ. Hepatitis B vaccine for police forces [Letter]? Lancet 1986; 2: 1458-59.
13. Radvan GH, Hewson EG, Berenger S. Brookman DJ. The Newcastle hepatitis B outbreak: observations on cause, management, and prevention. Med J Australia 1986; 144:461-464.
14. Centers for Disease Control. Inactivated hepatitis B virus vaccine. MMWR 1982; 26:317-322, 327-328.
15. Centers for Disease Control. Update on hepatitis B prevention. MMWR 1987; 36:353-360, 366.
16. Marcus R. and the CDC Co-operative Needlestick Surveillance Group. Surveillance of health care workers exposed to blood from patients infected with the human immunodeficiency virus. N Engl. J Med 1988; 319:1118-23.
17. Henderson DK, Fahey BJ, Saah AJ, Schmitt JM, Lane HC. Longitudinal assessment of risk for occupational/nosocomial transmission of human immunodeficiency virus, type 1 in health care workers. Abstract #634; presented at the 1988 ICAAC Conference, New Orleans.

18. Barnes DM. Health workers and AIDS: Questions persist. Science 1988; 241:161-2.

19. Gerberding JL, Littell CG, Chambers HF, Moss AR, Carlson J. Drew W. Levy J. Sande MA. Risk of occupational HIV transmission in intensively exposed health-care workers: Follow-up. Abstract #343; presented at the 1988 ICAAC Conference, New Orleans.

20. Health and Welfare Canada. National surveillance programme on occupational exposures to HIV among health-care workers in Canada. Canada Dis Weekly Rep 1987; 13-37: 163-6.

21. McEvoy M, Porter K,Mortimer P. Simmons N. Shanson D. Prospective study of clinical, laboratory, and ancillary staff with accidental exposures to blood or body fluids from patients infected with HIV. Br Med J 1987; 294: 1595-7.

22. Centers for Disease Control. Public Health Service guidelines for counseling and antibody testing to prevent HIV infection and AIDS. MMWR 1987; 36:; 509-515.

23. Centers for Disease Control. Additional recommendations to reduce sexual and drug abuse-related transmission of human T-lymphotropic virus type III/lymphadenopathy associated virus. MMWR 1986; 35:152-55.

24. Jenison SA, Lemon SM, Baker LN, Newbold JE. Quantitative analysis of hepatitis B virus DNA in saliva and semen of chronically infected homosexual men. J Infect Dis 1987; 156:299-306.

25. Cancio-Bello TP, de Medina M, Shorey J. Valledor MD, Schiff ER. An institutional outbreak of hepatitis B related to a human biting carrier. J Infect Dis 1982; 146:652-6.

26. MacQuarrie MB, Forghani B. Wolochow DA. Hepatitis B transmitted by a human bite. JAMA 1974; 230:723-4.

27. Scott RM, Snitbhan R. Bancroft WH, Alter HJ, Tingpalapong M. Experimental transmission of hepatitis B virus by semen and saliva. J Infect Dis 1980; 142:67-71.

28. Glaser JB, Nadler JP. Hepatitis B virus in a cardiopulmonary resuscitation training course: Risk of transmission from a surface antigen-positive participant. Arch Intern Med 1985; 145:1653-5.

29. Osterholm MT, Bravo ER, Crosson JT, et al. Lack of transmission of viral hepatitis type B after oral exposure to HBsAg-positive saliva. Br Med J 1979; 2:1263-4.

30. Lifson AR. Do alternate modes for transmission of human immunodeficiency virus exist? A review. JAMA1988;259:1353-6.

31. Friedland GH, Saltzman BR, Rogers MF, et al. Lack of transmission of HTLV-III/LAV infection to household contacts of patients with AIDS or AIDS-related complex with oral candidiasis. N Engl J Med 1986; 314:344-9.

32. Curran JW, Jaffe HW, Hardy AM, et al. Epidemiology of HIV infection and AIDS in the United States. Science 1988; 239:610-6.

33. Jason JM, McDougal JS, Dixon G. et al. HTLV-III/LAV antibody and immune status of household contacts and sexual partners of persons with hemophilia. JAMA 1986; 255:212-5.

34. Wahn V, Kramer HH, Voit T. Bruster HT, Scrampical B. Scheid A. Horizontal transmission of HIV infection between two siblings [Letter]. Lancet 1986; 2:694.

35. Kane MA, Lettau LA. Transmission of HBV from dental personnel to patients. J Am Dent Assoc 1985; 110:634-6.

36. Lettau LA, Smith JD, Williams D, et al. Transmission of hepatitis B virus with resultant restriction of surgical practice. JAMA 1986; 255:934-7.

37. International Association of Fire Fighters. Guidelines to prevent transmission of communicable disease during emergency care for fire fighters, paramedics, and emergency medical technicians. International Association of Fire Fighters, New York City, New York, 1988.

# 40

# Information, Education and Communication

## 1. INTRODUCTION

The pandemic of Acquired Immuno-deficiency Syndrome (AIDS) poses a unique challenge to public health planners and programme developers. With no cure in sight, we are forced to look closely at behavioural patterns and how to alter them to prevent AIDS. Since AIDS is primarily a sexually transmitted disease (STD), it is important that policy-makers, communicators and public health professionals examine the sexual behaviour patterns of the communities they are serving and develop strategies aimed at behavioural change.

Information, education and communication (IEC) plays a crucial role in bringing about this change. IEC is seen as an essential component of an AIDS prevention and care programme. However, IEC alone is not enough; it must be supported by health and social services and should be planned for in the context of the overall programme objectives and activities. One of the necessary conditions for effective implementation is the understanding of (and commitment to) the IEC framework among the key personnel in each country. Promoting this may need specific steps, including:

- Involvement of such key persons in the finalization of an overall strategy.
- Workshops that help to disseminate and clarify the strategy.

Implementation of IEC efforts in relation to HIV/AIDS requires an appropriate organizational set-up in each country and this must take place in close collaboration with other services. There are advantages in having an integrated IEC organization for all activities in the health sector. However, in such a case it is essential to have a nodal person—or even a small group—for focusing specifically on the IEC activities for HIV/AIDS. Implementation should be done in the context of the totality of the problem and the overall framework of the strategy. Thus, a 'total system' or holistic approach is essential. Not only does each of the elements—including planning, research, message design, production, dissemination, monitoring and evaluation—need attention, but the relationship between each, as also the overall process, must be addressed.

A concerted effort, through a well-planned and effectively implemented IEC strategy, should create the necessary conditions for bringing about favourable behavioural changes. It is only through this that the preventive steps will succeed and help in combating the spread of HIV/AIDS.

### 1.1 What is IEC ?

IEC is a broad term comprising a range of approaches, activities and outputs. Although the most visible component of IEC is frequently the materials produced and used, such as posters hanging on clinic walls, materials are only one component. Effective IEC makes use of a full range of approaches and activities.

Approaches may range from the use of mass media to inform or establish positive norms among the general population to the use of targeted interpersonal communication to help those at particular risk evaluate their own behaviour and develop new personal skills. IEC activities may include designing and providing training in communication skills, carrying out research on audiences to determine what information is needed and the most effective way of delivering it, as well as designing and producing the materials to support activities.

Overall, IEC must be integrated with all existing HIV/AIDS prevention and care programmes as well as with on-going training services. For example, promotion of condom use or STD treatment among individuals with high-risk behaviour will be effective only if condoms are also made accessible and STD treatment services are available and non-stigmatizing.

Similarly a positive social environment without discrimination and stigmatization will facilitate behavioural change.

### 1.2 How can this Guide Help?

This document provides guidelines for national AIDS programme managers on how to set priorities and systematically plan and implement IEC activities as part of AIDS prevention and care programmes. It describes steps for the planning, implementation and evaluation of IEC activities. To reinforce the step-wise approach, a specific example of IEC activities addressed to young people has been included in the text.

## 2. HIV/AIDS BURDEN IN THE SOUTH-EAST ASIA REGION

In the South-East Asia Region, HIV infection was first reported in 1984 in Thailand. In most other countries, HIV infection was not diagnosed until 1986 or later. Since then, however, HIV infection has spread rapidly. WHO estimates that, as of early 1995, there are more than 2 million HIV-infected people in the Region. Three-fourths of reported AIDS cases from the Region have acquired the infection through sexual intercourse and more than 80 per cent are in the age group of 15-49 years.

In view of the fact that heterosexual contact is the predominant mode of HIV transmission in the Region, the rates of sexually transmitted diseases are high and that there is considerable unprotected sexual activity, continued transmission of HIV in the general population appears inevitable unless effective measures are taken immediately. Furthermore, WHO estimates that while the annual number of HIV infections may peak in Africa by the mid-1990s, infections in Asia will continue to increase well into the early years of the next century. By the year 2000, it is probable that the cumulative number of infections in Asia will rise by 8-10 million and that the annual numbers will fat exceed those in sub-Saharan Africa (Figure-40.1).

The greatest tragedy, besides medical and health care costs, will be the loss of thousands of lives, particularly those of young adults in their most productive years and infants born to HIV-infected mothers, which will directly affect child survival rates.

## 3. THE ROLE OF IEC IN HIV/AIDS PREVENTION

All countries in the Region now have national AIDS prevention and care programmes and are organizing efforts to combat the spread of HIV which include IEC, condom programming, providing STD services, and ensuring blood safety.

The general goal of IEC is to promote and support appropriate changes in behaviour, especially among populations with high-risk behaviour. While cultural differences are likely to require different styles of presentation of material between countries and between different target groups, the desired behaviours or behavioural changes will be similar (or even the same):

- — Postponement of first sexual encounter;
- — Decrease in multiple-partner sex;
- — Increase in condom use;
- — Increased use of health services to treat STDs; and
- — Increased use of clean syringes by injecting drug users.

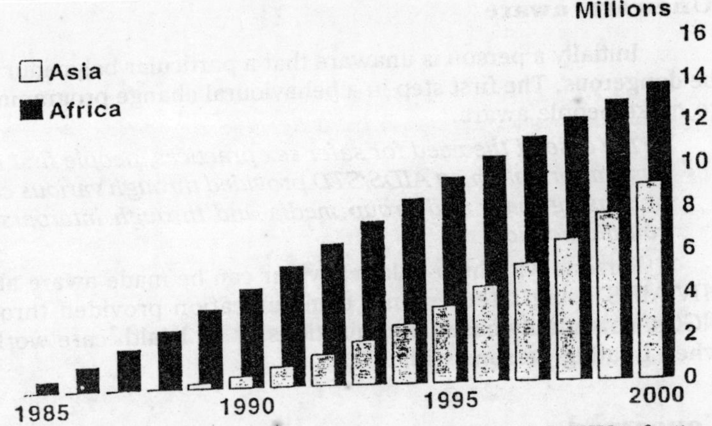


*Figure 40.1. Estimated and projected cumutative adult HIV infections in Asia and Africa*

## 3.1 Process of Behavioural Change: A Continuum

Bringing about a behavioural change is, however, a difficult process. The task is further complicated by the sensitive and personal nature of the issues, dealing as they largely do with sex and sexuality. A variety of approaches and messages will be needed to promote movement of individuals and populations along the continuum of behavioural change. The "adoption of safer sex" example below illustrates the various stages of the behavioural change model shown in Figure 40.2.

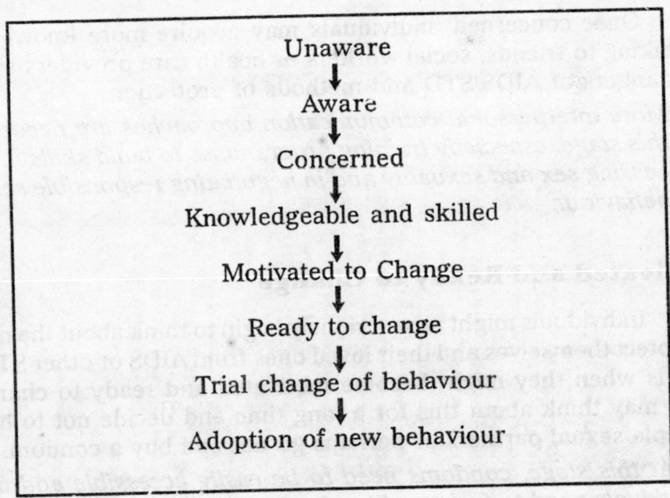


*Figure 40.2. Behavioural change model*

## Unaware- aware

Initially a person is unaware that a particular behaviour may be dangerous. The first step in a behavioural change programme is to make people aware.

*In the case of the need for safer sex practices, people first need basic information on AIDS/STD provided through various channels using mass and group media and through interpersonal communication.*

Persons with high-risk behaviour can be made aware about HIV/AIDS using interpersonal communication provided through NGOs, community-based organizations or by health care workers when treating persons with STD.

## Concerned

It is possible to be aware without being concerned. Information must be given is such a way that the audience feels it applies to them, i.e., the audience becomes concerned, and people are motivated to evaluate their own behaviour.

*Mass media approaches aimed at the general population are less likely to be effective in creating concern and overcoming denial, particularly among those at greatest risk. Targeted communication and interpersonal approaches are therefore more useful.*

## Knowledgeable and Skilled

Once concerned, individuals may acquire more knowledge by talking to friends, social workers or health care providers about the dangers of AIDS/STD and methods of protection.

*More interpersonal communication approaches are needed at this stage, especially training programmes to build skills in discussing sex and sexuality and in negotiating responsible sexual behaviour.*

## Motivated and Ready to Change

Individuals might now seriously begin to think about the need to protect themselves and their loved ones from AIDS or other STDs. This is when they might become motivated and ready to change. They may think about this for a long time and decide not to have multiple sexual partners or perhaps go out and buy a condom.

*At this stage, condoms need to be easily accessible and individuals need to feel capable of using condoms and negotiating safer sex. Mass and targeted media can help provide a supportive environment by showing role models and promoting a positive view of safer sexual behaviour. Positive messages from peers are particularly effective.*

## Trial Change of Behaviour

At a later stage individuals are in a situation where a sexual encounter could take place and they have access to a condom. They could then decide to try the new behaviour.

*The results of any trial will be evaluated. If the experience has been too difficult or embarrassing, due to lack of experience and skills, then they may not try again for a long time. Therefore, skills* to *negotiate condom use, and to use condoms correctly, are essential.*

## Adoption of New Behaviour

Finally, the individual decides to remain faithful to one faithful partner or regularly uses condoms as a source of protection from AIDS/STD.

*Assuming the new behaviour continues to be evaluated as largely positive, sustained behavioural change could take place at this stage. Continuous messages of support and access to condoms are still essential.*

Programmes must ensure that overall and individual stages of behavioural change are taken into consideration when IEC approaches and activities are being planned and implemented.

## 3.2 The Role of IEC in STD/AIDS Prevention and Control

(1) *Public education and targeted interventions:* education of the general population can best be carried out through the mass media. Additionally, while use of the mass media can be a most useful way to educate the population at large, experience indicates that more individualized, interpersonal channels of communication are needed, particularly for individuals engaged in high-risk behaviour. Efforts through the mass media may result in generating awareness and creating a positive environment, but interpersonal communication is a must for behavioural change. For this to occur, IEC efforts must be continuous.

Moreover, the mass media often do not reach those segments of a population which are most in need of information. Women, poorer communities, and those who operate on the fringes of society often have limited access to mass media. Traditional channels for communication, such as folk media including street theatres, are particularly effective in rural areas and urban slums. Other channels which also need to be explored include women's organizations and existing community networks. It is important to choose the right channel of communication for each target audience.

(2) *Advocacy:* IEC has an important role in advocacy. Policy and decision-makers have to be persuaded to take steps and/or initiate policies and services that will limit the spread of HIV infection and influence legislation. They must be made aware of the present magnitude and the frightening potential of HIV/AIDS, the consequent economic loss and the load on health services. Similarly, IEC efforts must also be directed to teachers, health and health-related workers and other intermediaries or 'influencers'. Equally important, through education programmes related to how HIV is not transmitted, IEC can assist in limiting discrimination and stigma and in promoting community acceptance of people with HIV or AIDS.

(3) *Support for various components of an AIDS Prevention and Control Programme:* IEC campaigns can promote seeking of quality STD services, which of course must be made available. IEC can also support efforts to promote voluntary blood donation and the implementation of universal precautions in health care settings.

## 4. LESSONS LEARNT FROM IEC PROGRAMME EXPERIENCES

Countries in South-East Asia can benefit from the experiences gained within as well as outside the Region. Learning from others allows programme managers to initiate more effective strategies and communication approaches to assist behavioural change. Such lessons illustrate the importance of selecting appropriate communication approaches, of targeting education and of integrating IEC with health and social services.

### 4.1 Using Appropriate Communication Approaches

Some examples of lessons learned about communication approaches early on in the AIDS pandemic in many countries include the following:

In many countries, including the U.K. and Australia, fear campaigns were initiated with the reasoning that people would be shocked into behavioural change. However, studies showed contrary results, since individuals at low risk became irrationally concerned and those at high risk turned away from the messages. Such approaches may provide short-term improvement but do not lead to sustained behavioural change.

*Fear campaigns do not work and are not effective in bringing about behavioural change*

Denial of the AIDS epidemic is a stage most countries have gone through. A slogan such as 'Do not have sex with foreigners' blames others. This slogan claims that only foreigners have AIDS and that AIDS does not exist in the home country. Denial is extremely dangerous as it allows individuals and policy-makers to lay the blame elsewhere and to block and unnecessarily delay needed action.

*Denial or blame campaigns inhibit necessary action*

In the United States, policy-makers initially believed that AIDS was a disease of gay men only and they ignored all the signs and evidence that AIDS was a sexually transmitted disease of the entire population. In India, and in some other South-East Asian countries, blame in many quarters is being placed on sex workers and drug users, when the HIV virus can already be found in many other pockets of society, for example, in clients who infect sex workers.

*Moral messages may turn away the very people you want to reach or deny lifesaving information to those in need*

AIDS education necessitates talking about sexual behaviour and methods of protection from HIV through sexual intercourse. To date, the only known method, barring abstinence, is condom use. However, in many countries, governments and religious organizations have prohibited the promotion of condom use with the argument that it would promote promiscuity. This has led to disastrous results in some countries. Studies have conclusively demonstrated that education on sex and methods of contraception in schools do not lead to an increase in sexual activity among youth; only to an increase in the use of contraceptive methods. In some cases, such education has instead led to an increase in the postponement of initiating sexual activity.

## 4.2 Designing Appropriate Audience Communications

Messages and delivery channels must be tailored for the specific target group. Consideration needs to be given to cultural acceptability, literacy levels, preferred sources of information, and available infrastructures. Communication must be gender sensitive and should be delivered through a variety of channels, packaged in different forms.

The development of messages should take place after rapid assessment of the current knowledge, attitudes, behaviour and practices (KABP) in relation to sexuality and AIDS/STDs. Population KABP studies have been found to be expensive, time-consuming and laborious. Qualitative methods have instead been found to be more useful.

Keeping all these issues in mind, guidelines which can assist in avoiding some of the mistakes of the past indicate that messages should:

— be consistent and accurate and disseminated in a continuous manner.

— be positive and aim to help people protect themselves and help those already infected to live productive and socially beneficial lives.

— be action oriented, so leading individuals to actions such as calling for more information, buying condoms, or using clean needles.

— be linked to service delivery. For exarnple, information and counselling centres must be available to help people gain knowledge about the spread of infection and methods of prevention, and to counsel those in need. If condoms are being promoted, affordable condoms must be available in the area. STD treatment services should also be made easily accessible.

— offer options. For example, when dealing with dificult-to-change behaviour patterns such as drug use, it is helpful and morc effective to provide the individual with options for action. For example 'Your chances of getting AIDS are high if you inject drugs, so don't inject: if you can't avoid injecting, don't share needles; if you can't avoid sharing, at least clean the needles before sharing'. Such behaviour options also apply to sexual transmission. For example: 'Your chances of contracting HIV/STDs increase if you have multiple sexual partners; so abstain from sex or stick to one uninfected partner; or practise safer sex such as condom use for every sexual encounter in situations of risk.'

## 4.3 Targeting AIDS Education

Another important lesson learned is the need to prioritize programme activities. Not everyone is at equal risk of contracting HIV. Identifiable groups of people who are engaged in behaviours which facilitate the spread of HIV can be targeted for priority prevention activities. These behaviours include having multiple sexual partners and sharing injecting equipment. People with a high prevalence of other sexually transmitted diseases also need to be targeted.

The groups at high risk may differ from city to city and area to area. It is important for each national or district-level programme to evaluate the risk determinants and identify the populations that may be at high risk of infection so that appropriate strategies to reach such populations can be developed on a priority basis.

Groups of individuals who share common high-risk behaviour might include, among others, commercial sex workers and their clients; injecting drug users; people with STDs; migrant workers; transportation workers—especially truck drivers; street children; and the military. Other general groups, such as women who have limited access to information and services or youth, also need special emphasis.

Targeted interventions among these populations, given the current epidemiological situation in the Region, will have the greatest impact on limiting the further spread of HIV.

## 4.4 IEC as a Part of an Integrated Intervention Package

Experience shows that IEC alone will not have a significant impact on the spread of HIV infection unless it is complemented by making available health and other services which address factors contributing to vulnerability to STD and HIV infection. Such an integrated approach among truck drivers, for example, would necessitate AIDS education in an interpersonal manner, the availability of condoms, STD services in a non-stigmatizing setting and possibly counselling services. For women, besides IEC, such an approach would entail the provision of STD services within MCH/FP and primary health care facilities along with the mobilization of women's organizations and counselling services. IEC should lead to action, and the means to facilitate that action must be in place and easily accessible.

No single organization can carry out all these activities. AIDS prevention and control activities need to draw on the wide range of multisectoral expertise and skills required for intervention development and implementation. This means close collaboration between government services and NGOs working with particular groups. If such programmes do not exist, it is essential that these be initiated urgently.

## 5. STEPS IN IEC PLANNING, IMPLEMENTATION AND EVALUATION

Effective IEC programmes are based within the overall context of the programme goals and can be developed following a systematic assessment of the target audiences and with their participation. The steps which need to be taken for the development of an effective IEC programme are as follows:

— Planning;
— Preparatory Activities and Materials Development;
— Dissemination and Utilization, and
— Monitoring and Evaluation.

A framework for IEC is presented in Figure 40.3.

### 5.1 Planning

First, the current situation must be reviewed. This will include a thorough assessment of the programme's IEC needs and existing IEC activities, identification of target audiences, formulation of achievable objectives, and identification of activities to be carried out as well as potential partners for implementation.

#### 5.1.1 Situational Analysis

(a) The first step of a situational analysis is examination and analysis of existing national policies, especially those relating to Health, Education and Communication, and laws which can impact on AIDS/STD prevention efforts. For example, a national policy against condom promotion would need to be revised in the light of the AIDS pandemic. The organizational structure and manpower available for AIDS prevention should be analysed, while communication and outreach networks, both within the government as well as among NGOs, should be assessed for use in AIDS educational activities.

(b) Another task in situational analysis is examination of existing epidemiological, cultural and behavioural data and exploration of the existing situation from a number of points of view, including: past/present preventive actions and their effectiveness; the extent of spread of HIV in different groups and areas; assessment of vulnerable populations; and any information relating to particular groups of interest such as demographic data, social structure, the status of women and literacy levels. Every effort must be made to fully utilize existing data from studies in various fields, particularly including those in

*Figure 40.3 IEC Framework*

SITUATIONAL ANALYSIS (5.1.1)
a) NATIONAL POLICIES AND ORGANIZATIONAL STRUCTURE
b) PHILOSOPHY/APPROACH TO IEC FOR AIDS PREVENTION
c) AVAILABLE EPIDEMIO-LOGICAL AND BEHAVIOU-RAL DATA
IDENTIFY TARGET GROUPS (5.1.2)
ESTABLISH GOALS/OBJECTIVES OF IEC (5.1.3)
DEVELOP LINKAGES WITH OTHER ORGANIZATIONS AND CARRY OUT ADVOCACY (5.2.1)
CONDUCT TRAINING (5.2.3)
ARRANGE SUPPORT SERVICES (5.2.2)
· ADVOCACY
· CONDOMS
· STD SERVICES
· COUNSELLING
PLAN FOR MONITORING & EVALUATION (5.4)
CONDUCT TARGETE D RESEARC H (5.3.1)
DESIGN/P RETEST TARGETE D MESSAGE S. CHOOSE MEDIA AND CHANNEL (5.3.2)
DEVELOP IEC MATERIALS (5.3.3)
DISSEMINATE AND USE MATERIAL (5.3.4)
MONITOR ACTIVITIES AND EVALUATE IMPACT (5.4)
Planning (5.1)
Preparatory activities Including material development
Implementation of IEC activities (5.3)
Monitoring and Evaluation

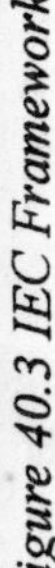

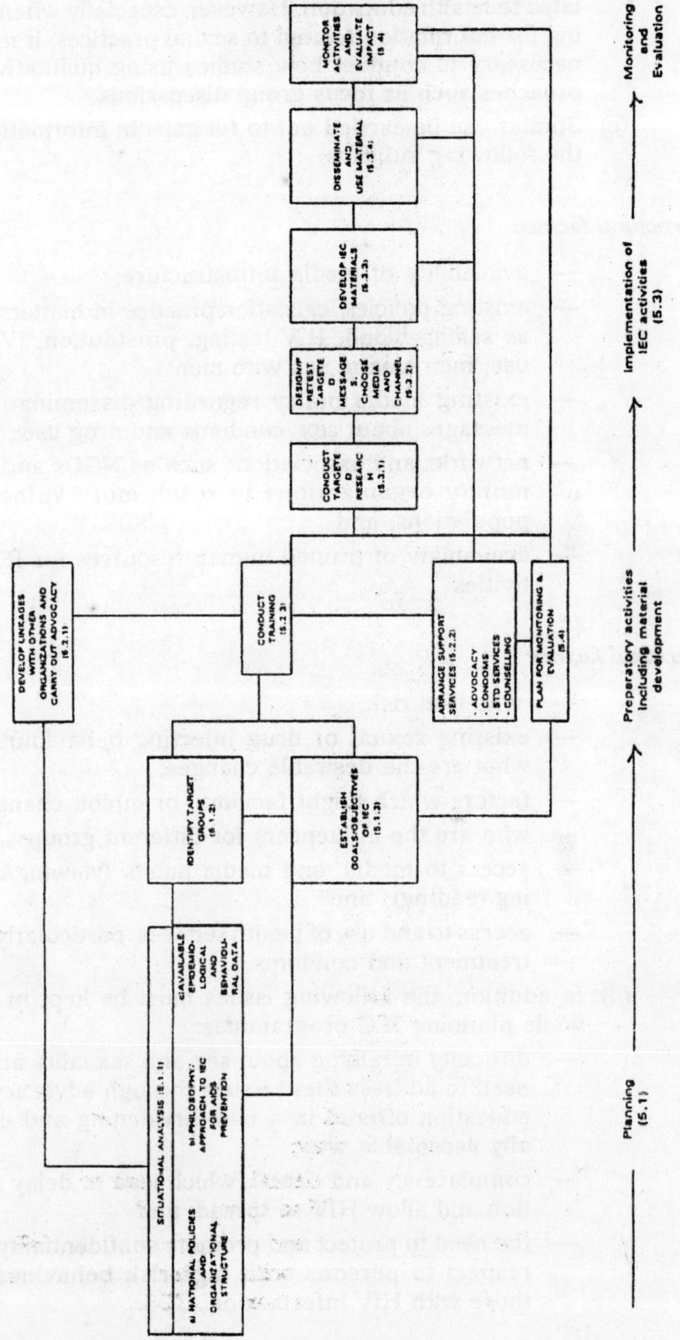

sociology, social anthropology, psychology, and fields related to health education. However, especially when looking for information related to sexual practices, it may be necessary to conduct new studies using qualitative approaches such as focus group discussions.

(c) Studies can be carried out to fill gaps in information on the following subjects:

*Structural factors:*

— availability of media infrastructure;
— existing policies/legislation/practice in matters such as selling blood, HIV testing, prostitution, IV drug use, men having sex with men;
— existing media policy regarding dissemination of messages about sex, condoms and drug use;
— networks and associations such as NGOs and community organizations to reach more vulnerable populations, and
— availability of trained human resources for IEC activities.

*Personal factors:*

— who is at risk;
— existing sexual or drug injecting behaviours and what are the desirable changes;
— factors which might facilitate or inhibit changes;
— who are the influencers for different groups;
— access to media, and media habits (viewing/listening/reading); and
— access to and use of health services, particularly STD treatment and condoms.

(d) In addition, the following issues must be kept in mind while planning IEC programmes:

— difficulty in talking about sex and sexuality and the need to address these issues through advocacy and education offered in a non-threatening and culturally acceptable way;
— complacency and denial, which lead to delay in action and allow HIV to spread; and
— the need to protect and promote confidentiality with respect to persons with high-risk behaviour and those with HIV infection or AIDS.

### 5.1.2 Identify Targets Groups

Identification and prioritization of target groups for the overall IEC programme is of great importance. In the absence of specific targeting, IEC messages tend to be very general, non-focused and, while they may provide information, they do not foster either change or action. Setting priorities is also necessary since resources are inevitably limited and their optimal use requires a clear understanding about which groups are to be the focus of attention.

Target groups for intervention should be identified according to criteria such as risk behaviour, population size, potential for contributing to spread of infection and accessibility. In South-East Asia, populations at high risk or vulnerable to HIV infection might include:

- adolescents and youth, especially street children;
- women in the reproductive age group (15-45 years); and
- known populations with a high prevalence of risk behaviour such as sex workers and their clients, injecting drug users, truck drivers and migrant populations.

### 5.1.3 Establish Goals, Objectives and Targets

IEC programme goals for each target group should describe the desired behavioural changes, while the specific objectives for each target group should be stated in measurable terms. This means that it will be possible to observe and measure progress towards meeting the objectives. For example, 'Within 12 months, 50 per cent of injecting drug users in one urban slum will stop sharing the injection equipment'; and, for IEC,' Within 12 months, 80 per cent of injecting drug users will be reached with accurate information on safer injecting practices'.

Realistic targets must be set taking into consideration the characteristics and situation of the target groups involved, the extent of communication infrastructure and the access that various groups have to information and services (e.g., radio and TV ownership/access in the case of education for the general population, or the presence of an NGO in the case of a population with high-risk behaviour); and the support services available.

Overall programme objectives for most of the target groups would include:

- decrease in number of sexual partners;
- increase in safe injecting practices (for injecting drug users);
- increase safer sex practices including condom use;
- enhance negotiating skills on sexual decisions;

— increase STD treatment-seeking behaviour;
— increase in health care-seeking behaviour (especially for women).
— reduction in STD rates.

## 5.2 Preparatory Activities

Essential preparatory activities include developing linkages, establishing co-ordination for essential services and ensuring availability of trained manpower.

### 5.2.1 Develop Linkages

Linkages for implementation of IEC activities within the government may be with the ministries of education, youth, women and child welfare, tourism, information and broadcasting, and transportation. Integration with MCH/FP programmes is an important strategy to reach women and should be a major priority. Collaboration with various ministries is also needed for advocacy to establish the sound policies needed for planning and implementation of effective IEC programmes.

NGOs are also important. While conducting the assessment and looking closer at identified vulnerable groups and high-risk behaviour groups, nongovernmental partners for implementing integrated programmes can be identified. Governments cannot do this work alone as they do not often have the close contact with vulnerable/high-risk populations that NGOs or community-based organizations may have. The national programme must provide technical and material support to NGOs in these activities.

### 5.2.2 Arrange Support Services

Planning in advance for provision of health services and supplies is essential for facilitating behavioural change and in generating an impact (effect) of IEC programmes. This includes physical inputs such as availability of condoms, bleach or needles, and also services such as counselling. Also included are allied health services such as the provision of STD clinics and primary health care facilities which are prepared to manage STDs. The services and availability of inputs will influence the objectives and targets set for the overall programme and for specific groups.

### 5.2.3 Conduct Training

Effective implementation of the IEC strategy requires that manpower needs are reviewed to ensure that personnel involved in implementation have the requisite knowledge and skills. Training is vital for ensuring that personnel have the ability to carry out programme activities as required. Development of appropriate training materials should be part of the total material development for IEC and training in communication skills needs to be emphasized. Long-term measures could include the incorporation of an HIV/AIDS IEC component into the curricula of basic training programmes for health and health-related workers, or workers in other sectors who will be providing STD/AIDS information. Short-term measures could include the promotion of inservice training and ensuring that all existing training materials dealing with AIDS/STD give consistent, correct information. The categories for training where special attention needs to be devoted are:

- Health and health-related workers
- Teachers
- NGO workers/volunteers, and
- Leaders or peers from high-risk populations and vulnerable groups.

## 5.3 Materials Development

Suitable partners should be identified to assist in materials development. This is especially important if ministries of health do not have the in-house capacity for development of IEC materials appropriate to meeting the needs of the programme. As a general strategy, it is suggested that the actual development of materials be contracted out to appropriate professionals, if available. The demands of targeting materials to produce sexual behaviour change may require skills beyond what is normally available.

*When developing communication tools for a programme, it is important to call in communication professionals, if available, for every step in the process.*

In this case, the manager's responsibility is to ensure that the contracting agency carries out all important steps. The following steps are essential:

### 5.3.1 Conduct Targeted Behavioural Research

Rapid research among specific target groups is needed for information during the development of appropriate communication strategies and tools. This entails a series of rapid qualitative studies to test relevant concepts and areas of perceived threat and needs of the targeted group. For example, one group may feel that AIDS is only spread by visiting sex workers and they may feel safe even though they habitually have multiple partners. They may use condoms with some partners and not with others.

Understanding behaviours and beliefs is essential for formulating effective, targeted IEC. This research, carried out when specific communication strategies and tools are being developed, will identify keys to behavioural change and help developers to tailor communication messages and materials to meet the needs of the identified population.

Maintaining confidentiality is essential; care must be taken to ensure that the research does not lead to the stigmatization or marginalization of any group.

### 5.3.2 Design Messages, Choose Media and Channels

Data and inputs from target groups can be used to determine the messages, and the medium and channels needed for conveying them (such as radio, TV, posters, interpersonal approaches, traditional media,) to each segment of the audience. This is the culmination of the conceptualization, analysis and planning exercise. Targeted IEC research, including an analysis of existing data, and a knowledge of the target group, plays an important role in selecting and defining the message, format, presentation, medium, etc., for each identified target group. At the design stage, the exact types of media, the channels for communication and the style should be determined. A balance between passive (e.g. posters, print or video) and interactive media must be created. In many cases, folk media such as puppetry, drama and story telling, can be used quite effectively to support interpersonal communication and should be actively considered as part of the overall IEC plan.

### 5.3.3 Develop IEC Materials

Development of draft materials is based on decisions about messages, media and channels to be used for delivery to each target group. Materials may consist of radio/TV spots, booklets, posters, handouts or hoardings, but these are not all. IEC also involves tools for use in interpersonal communication. It must be kept in mind that materials are a support tool for activities which lead to the achievement of goals and objectives. IEC materials alone will not produce behavioural change.

Pretesting of materials is one of the most important steps in materials development. Pretesting allows the evaluation of messages and materials with regard to acceptability and potential impact before large amounts of resources are used in production and distribution. Although it adds to the cost and time of producing materials, it prevents wastage of resources by ensuring that materials are effective.

Once draft materials are developed, they are carefully reviewed with groups selected from the specific target audience. For example, a TV spot providing general information on AIDS should be tested with samples from the general public using a rough story board or outline of the pictures and text, before even beginning to film the spot. This process should continue once the rough film has been shot. In this way, planners can be assured that, as much as possible, the spot will convey the information desired as effectively as possible. Pretesting should take place with every material from TV spots to more specific outreach materials being developed for non-literate audiences. Pretesting is cost-effective in the long run.

A summary of the steps to be followed in materials development is shown below:

**MATERIALS DESIGN STEPS**

Design prototype material

↓

Pretest

↓

Revise material

↓

Pretest again and produce

Setting up a resource centre where all materials (communication products) related to HIV/AIDS/STD are available would also be very helpful and cost-effective. These materials can be used as they are, if appropriate, or adapted and used as prototypes for new materials.

*Cost and cost-effectiveness of materials.* Determining affordability and cost effectiveness is important, as resources are always scarce. Cost-effectiveness of materials (in terms of development, production and dissemination costs as compared to their reach and effectiveness) is, therefore, an important consideration. In this context, it would be well to judiciously and selectively use expensive media such as film and TV. The glamour of these media often results in an overemphasis on their use, even though the cost of production and dissemination is extremely high. On the other hand, traditional media (including puppetry, traditional theatre and songs) and interpersonal communication tools (such as flip-charts and flash cards) are often neglected, though they are generally very cost-effective. Special efforts must, therefore, be made to use traditional media wherever they are more suitable.

**What will it Cost?**

Each step in the IEC development process can be reviewed to identify items and activities that will have to be contracted for. Items that are important to include in overall costing are:

— costs of targeted behavioural research
— costs of development of prototype or draft materials
— costs of pretesting
— costs associated with each type of medium: availability of in-house capacity for any aspects of production, the quality desired
— costs of producing sufficient copies for intended use
— costs of distribution or dissemination—whether it be freight or postal charges, trucking or buying air time on radio or TV
— costs of storage. Materials produced in quantities will require dry, secure storage space
— costs of reprints and revisions. All materials have a 'lifet' and will need replacement and updating.

### 5.3.4 Disseminate and Utilize Materials

Planning effective ways to make sure that materials reach their target audiences is as important as producing effective materials. It is often the case that good quality materials never reach those who need them or who could most effectively use them. Planning a distribution strategy and setting up a distribution network at the beginning is important.

Using materials to support IEC activities, through mass media or for interpersonal communication requires knowing how to use them effectively. Ideally, users will become familiar with different types of materials and methods for using them during communication training. At the very least, instructions and suggestions for use must be supplied along with the materials.

## 5.4 Monitoring and Evaluation

Monitoring and evaluation provide inputs for guiding and improving programme implementation, for appropriate redefinition or fine-tuning of messages and materials, for reworking objectives/goals and for the overall IEC approach.

Monitoring and evaluation must be built into the overall programme process. Monitoring and evaluation are essential parts of the overall IEC programme and must be planned for from the beginning. Monitoring and evaluation are, however, different.

Monitoring is a continuous activity, and provides immediate feedback so that timely corrective action can be taken. Evaluation, on the other hand, is carried out at regular intervals to assess programme effectiveness and impact.

### 5.4.1 Monitoring

Monitoring can be defined as the ongoing process of collecting and analysing information about implementation of the programme. It involves regular checking to see whether programme activities are being carried out as planned so that problems can be discussed and dealt with. It allows managers to follow the progress of planned activities, identify problems, give feedback to staff and solve problems before they cause delays.

Monitoring can answer questions such as:

- Have relevant health care workers and others received training?
- Are the appropriate services in place?
- Have the IEC materials been distributed to those they are intended for?
- Are the IEC materials being utilized?

#### (a) What to Monitor

Deciding what to monitor can begin by preparing a list of programme and activity targets and indicators as well as important tasks, performances and outputs.

A task is one of a set of actions required to carry out an activity. Examples are 'identify partners for work with vulnerable populations' or 'identify organizations for materials development'. Performance refers to how well a task is carried out. The quality is assessed by comparing current practice with established standards of performance. Examples are 'training health workers to give appropriate health education sessions on STD' or 'advising women at antenatal clinics on the risks of HIV infection and pregnancy'. Output refers to the quantity of items used to carry out activities or to the quantified result of carrying out a task. Examples are numbers of brochures printed or distributed, numbers of personnel trained, and numbers of condoms distributed.

#### (b) Adoption of Monitoring Methods, and Development and Adoption of Appropriate Tools for Monitoring

Programme activities can be monitored through checklists

of observations to be made during supervisory visits, regular checking of workplans, and use of reporting forms. Some monitoring methods for collecting data to measure indicators/progress are outlined below.

— Routine reports are reports of certain information submitted on a regular basis by all or most reporting sites in an area. Useful periodic records and reports that can be reviewed for monitoring IEC activities might include those on dissemination of print materials, training sessions held with NGOs and community organizations, advocacy meetings, new partners identified to reach vulnerable populations, and number of TV spots aired.

— Supervisory visits/reports are reports of visits by supervisors to oversee tasks and performances of workers, identify problems and help solve performance and output problems. Supervisory activities may include observation, exit interviews, record reviews, or other ways of monitoring performance and output. When supervisory visits are carried out with appropriate checklists, the information gathered can be very useful for monitoring the programme. Regular supervisory visits are difficult to achieve, and transportation costs arc difficult to sustain. However, frequent supportive supervision is an indispensable monitoring method.

### (c) Use of Monitoring Results

It is important to use what is learned from monitoring as feedback to the programme so that necessary corrective actions can be taken. Feedback should be quick and action oriented and aimed at making immediate changes to improve effectiveness. It will in particular, provide key inputs to modify the messages and media used to reach specific target groups and to make improvements/changes in services. Feedback assumes even greater importance in the context of the proposed strategy, since it has been suggested that implementation begin immediately, without waiting for the results of detailed research or large-scale surveys. Thus, IEC messages/products will be based on existing data/studies, which may not be fully adequate. Needed corrections and adjustments will have to be based on monitoring efforts which feed back into the redesign of the programme.

A system based on a short, quick and reliable feedback mechanism is essential. Such feedback will cover, with regard to IEC material, aspects such as target group interest in the material, comprehension of it, reaction to the format, language and characters used (if any), and visual appeal (where relevant).

### 5.4.2 Evaluation

Evaluation is the process of collecting and analysing information at regular intervals about the effectiveness and impact of either particular parts of the programme or the programme as a whole. A variety of different evaluation methods is possible depending on programme needs. Regardless of method, planning for evaluation, including development of programme indicators and planning for information collection, should take place at the beginning of the programmer to ensure that essential data will be available when needed.

Impact is measured against the programme objectives. Baseline data will be needed, and methods for collecting the information need to be spelled out so that the amount of change can be assessed.

At a given point in time, evaluation can answer such quantifiable, impact-related questions as:

— Are access to condoms and information on correct use-increasing?
— What proportion of health workers are providing health education?
— What proportion of prostitutes report the correct and consistent use of condoms?
— What proportion of the general population can cite at least two acceptable ways to protect themselves from HIV infection?
— What proportion of women who have been advised on the risks or HIV infection and pregnancy at antenatal clinics can cite two risk factors for HIV infection?
— What proportion of the general population who are sexually active can report that they are practising safer sex?
— Has the incidence of STDs declined?

*Collection of appropriate baseline data is essential if an evaluation of impact is to take place*

Evaluation can also be designed to help a programme manager understand why a programme is where it is. Did certain types of activities have bigger impacts than others? What types of problems occurred? How can such problems be solved or prevented in the future? Periodic programme reviews provide more qualitative or descriptive information on the status of the programme.

Evaluation should include not only the impact on the target audience, but must also cover an evaluation of other activities, such as training and/or utilization of services.

Some evaluation methods are outlined below:

*Community surveys, such as the general population survey:*

These are usually regionally (and sometimes nationally) focused investigations. They can be conducted as household surveys, which collect information from a representative sample of a population and are conducted by trained interviewers who go to the dwellings in a selected geographic area for face-to-face interviews, or targeted population surveys, which collect information about a population of particular interest, and are carried out in locations where these populations can be found.

*Comprehensive programme reviews:* These are carried out primarily for management purposes. They assess the relevance and adequacy of the national plan and existing policies including those related to IEC. They assess adequacy and appropriateness of the structure of the national AIDS programme, progress toward targets, and the efficiency of prevention and control activities. The objective of a review is to identify achievements and problem areas, including recommendations for solutions. Reviews also assess the adequacy of management information systems. Reviews are done at regular intervals; internal reviews are done by country staff every year and external reviews are done every two to three years by staff outside the programme.

*Accumulation of monitoring results:* This is a collection of monitoring data gathered over time that is judged valid and useful for evaluating certain components of programme activities that require repeated assessment.

*Special studies and surveys:* These are studies that assist in understanding specific operational issues. For example, a pilot study of a prevention strategy such as 'Use of peer educators for HIV prevention in prostitute populations' will eventually assist managers in deciding whether or not to expand the approach to a national scale. HIV or STD surveillance in antenatal clinics help the national AIDS programme to better understand trends in disease prevalence.

Depending on the methods selected, evaluation will provide an in-depth, integrated feedback, covering a longer time-scale and at a broader level than that provided by monitoring. It svill indicate the extent of success in meeting the behavioural objectives/goals of IEC, and provide inputs for changes or modifications in these, and possibly even the overall approach/philosophy of IEC.

## 6. IEC FOR SPECIFIC TARGET AUDIENCES - YOUTH AS AN EXAMPLE

This section illustrates the use of the IEC planning and implementation process with one target group: young persons - adolescents and youth—from 10 to 24 years of age. This group will need to be divided into segments due to the wide range of developmental stages and cultural norms.

## 6.1 PLANNING

### 6. 1.1 Situational Analysis

*(1) National policy and organizational structure*

In the case of youth it is important to know what policies are in place for: the health of youth of each segment, including children in school, condom use and sex education in schools. In light of the AIDS pandemic, the need for advocacy to change policies should also be assessed. An analysis should take place on how best to utilize the government structures for Youth and AIDS.

*(2) Philosophy/approach to IEC for youth*

At the central level a decision needs to be made on how to approach the topic of Youth and AIDS. This will entail a decision on sex education or life-style education in schools; how to handle discussion on condoms; and other issues. It is necessary to strike a delicate balance between the promotion of traditional values and a practical programme to meet the needs of young people who may already be sexually active.

*(3) Examining existing data*

The factors that need to be examined as part of the situational analysis have already been discussed. It is on the basis of such an analysis that one can identify youth as a priority target group. The situational analysis will also provide details that will help to further identify the target group and how to reach them, involvement with youth/sports or other organizations and key 'influencers' (e.g. teachers). Existing research reports may indicate the habits, preferences and effectiveness of different media, etc. for this target group. All this data will be crucial in:

- Further/finer stratification of the target group;
- Developing suitable messages;
- Ensuring participation and involvement of youth in the process (message design) and-where possible—in developing communication tools;
- Identifying and using peers as communicators;
- Identifying suitable media and means of reaching the

target group (including through influencers);
— Development of appropriate school curricula on AIDS; and
— Development of co-curricular activities for AIDS.

### 6.1.2 Target Group Identification

Youth, both male and female, can be further segmented in most countries as follows:

— Youth in school (urban and rural);
— Youth out of school in the urban setting;
— Youth out of school in the rural setting;
— Street youth or street children; and
— University students.

Each group has different levels of literacy and may have different behaviour patterns as well as information and service needs. It is also important to target parents and teachers.

*The role of teachers and parents in informing and educating youth must be explored thoroughly. Often a well intentioned programme will fail because the important role of teachers and parents has been ignored.*

### 6.1.3 Goals/Objectives/Targets/Indicators

For the specific target audience, it is now necessary to define the behavioural goals on the basis of the philosophy or approach and the situational analysis. In this, one also has to take note of the communication infrastructure that is available and the access that the target group has to various channels of communication such as mass media, print media and interpersonal channels.

For this target group (youth), the desired behavioural goals may be stated as follows:

— Delay sexual initiation (relevant for adolescents and younger people);
— Provide safer intimacy options;
— Reduce the number of sexual partners;
— Increase condom use;
— Discuss sexual matters openly;
— Actively seek information on sexual matters and seek counselling;
— Seek STD services; and
— Develop 'enabling skills' to promote healthy lifestyles.

In the Region as a whole, these would be the primary goals, since almost all the HIV infection is sexually transmitted. However, in certain parts of some countries (e.g. India, Thailand, Myanmar), injecting drug use is also a major problem. In such areas, the behavioural goals will have to emphasize sterilization and non-sharing of needles and other injecting equipment, while simultaneously attempting to reduce drug injecting itself. These messages should be integrated into promoting and supporting a positive life-style.

As noted in the previous section, the goals and objectives should be quantified or expressed in measurable terms as far as possible, and targets set. These will differ from country to country, depending upon the situation prevailing there. Specific indicators should be developed and a system to collect the appropriate information designed.

## 6.2. PREPARATORY ACTIVITIES AND MATERIALS DEVELOPMENT

### 6.2.1 Linkages with Existing Organizational Structure and other Organizations

Close and active collaboration with other agencies and programmes is vital for the success of any IEC strategy. In the case of youth, collaboration should be established with educational authorities and institutions (ministry of education, schools/colleges, universities, etc.) and with youth organizations (Ministry of Youth Services, scouts/guides and social service organizations, student bodies, etc.). Links should also be sought with youth cubs and sports organizations.

NGOs and voluntary organizations can play important roles because of the commitment and dedication of those involved. Also, they are generally able to establish a better rapport with young people and high-risk behaviour groups than official agencies, while their ability to reach out-of-school youth and street children is particularly high. The entertainment industry is geared largely to attracting young people. They would, therefore, be appropriate partners for many IEC activities.

In addition, strong linkages must obviously be established with other relevant health programmes) especially with STD and family planning services, for condom distribution.

### 6.2.2 Services

Services play an important role in supporting behavioural

change and facilitating the adoption of appropriate safe/preventive practices and behaviour.

For this target group the services include:

— Counselling, which is of special relevance for this age group;
— Condom distribution;
— STD/health services; and
— Information service ('hotline' through telephones, or a 'post box') providing relevant information on an anonymous basis.

### 6.2.3 Training

The categories to which special attention needs to be devoted for training in youthrelated activities include teachers, health workers, NGO workers and volunteers, youth leaders and peer groups.

### 6.2.4 Targeted Behavioural Research

IEC research can play a major role in designing the right messages. Such research will indicate the target audience's current level of knowledge including any misconceptions. Focusing IEC research on youth will help to find keys to overcoming the perceived invulnerability of youth - the 'it can't happen to me' syndrome.

### 6.2.5 Design of Targeted Messages and Media

The basic or core messages are:

— Delay sexual activity;
— Single sex partner (mutual faithfulness);
— Avoid penetrative sex; and
— Use latex condoms.

Some specific messages for this target group (youth and adolescents) would be:

— How HIV is transmitted and also how it is not;
— How to protect oneself and one's sexual partner from HIV;
— Seeking appropriate treatment for STDs;
— The STD and HIV relationship, i.e. recognition of how STD increases the risk of HIV;
— Proper condom use;

— Hazards of drug use, particularly injecting;
— Existence of support/counselling services and where to go for these; and
— Knowledge about human sexuality (development, behaviour, relationships), especially for adolescents.

The choice of medium for each message will depend upon the extent of access that the target group has to the medium. The situational analysis and IEC research should provide crucial data on this. In general, however, one may list the general products which might be appropriate for a general youth population:

— Broadcast media—especially targeted youth programming: audio and video cassettes;
— Books (including textbooks), magazines, newspapers;
— Films/movies;
— Street theatre, especially for street children and college students;
— NGOs and voluntary agencies; not necessarily those working on AIDS, but many others who are basically working with youth in areas such as health, women, development and water supply;
— Entertainment shows and sports—these are a very effective way of reaching urban youth;
— Exhibitions;
— Peer group—this generally makes for the best and most effective communication. It will require the training of a few selected individuals from each institution/organization. This may be particularly useful for street children, since their access to other media is limited and distrust of people in authority is likely to be strong, and
— Teachers—again some training will be necessary. This is obviously only for in-school/college groups. Some countries have adolescent/sex education as part of the curriculum, and messages on AIDS/HIV must be integrated into this.

Some of these, or a combination, can be used, depending upon the target audience, the situational analysis and a cost analysis. Among the settings or locales for conveying IEC messages, appropriate ones for this target group include:

— The classroom, for school and college students;
— Youth clubs;
— 'Video Parlours', which, in most places, draw a large number of young people; and
— Youth festivals, youth camps, sports events, etc.

### 6 2.6 IEC Materials Development

It is essential to develop appropriate communication tools to support the approaches that have been decided upon. IEC research inputs have already been indicated as being essential at the message design stage. Similar inputs are required in developing appropriate materials such as radio/TV programmes, posters and booklets. Pretesting, in particular, is a vital element of materials development.

When designing communication materials, experienced communicators should be involved. This is not something that should be left to medical experts or health workers. Further, the involvement of the target group (in designing the material) is essential and has been found to be very effective in terms of the final impact of the product. This particular target group (young persons) provides great scope for direct involvement in the development and even production—of materials. It is possible to tap student groups and to work through schools of art/communication/journalism, in particular, to evolve materials that are most appealing and suitable for the target group.

The materials produced must obviously be within the framework of the overall approach/philosophy and the messages identified for this specific target group. Special care needs to be taken to avoid any contradictions or ambiguities in the messages.

Full use must be made of textbooks for in-school/college groups. The materials developed for these books must be interesting, clear, and provide sequential graded learning. Since the 'printed word', especially in a textbook, carries great sanctity, this material must be thoroughly pretested to eliminate any possible misunderstandings or ambiguities.

## 6.3 Dissemination and Utilization

In examining the considerations outlined in the previous section, it is crucial to keep the target audience in mind In each country/situation, it is necessary to determine which message through which medium will most effectively **reach** (in this case) young persons.

Choice of the means of dissemination is therefore linked to the target audience and the message. Some channels for dissemination of messages include:

— Broadcast media. In many countries, the broadcasting organizations make some air-time available free of cost for social messages which may require strong advocacy efforts. Efforts need to be made to obtain such allocations everywhere. Care should be taken that spots or programmes aimed at youth are aired when young people are watching, which is usually during prime time. When free air-time is not possible, or more is needed, good planning is required to buy time in a cost-effective manner, trading off between costs and (target) audience size.

— Integration with on-going TV programmes/features. For example, some messages could be appropriately woven into a popular 'soap-opera'.

— Message dissemination through peer groups. NGOs can play a major role in this. Training of peer-leaders (mentioned above in the section on Training) thus assumes even greater importance. The possibility of organizing such groups is obviously higher for that segment of the target audience which is in school/college. However, attempts have been successful in organizing groups among street children and employed persons.

— Anonymous methods to gather queries from young people and disseminate accurate information. In some countries, schools have set up post boxes where students can place sensitive queries, to which answers can be given in a newsletter or in general discussions. Another method is to set up a telephone information hotline.

Curriculum. Where 'dissemination' takes place through the curriculum (in school or college), it is essential that the teacher does not shy away from confronting the issues. A discussion after each lesson is the ideal way of maximizing learning and aiding behavioural change by clarifying all doubts, etc. (see matrix presented in Table 40.1).

At the receiving end, utilization of media products is a vital, and unfortunately, much-neglected aspect. The impact of any communication is increased many-fold if it is discussed among receivers, if their questions are answered and if their doubts clarified. Steps must be taken to ensure this, either through inter-personal communication as follow-up, or through supporting printed material, where appropriate.

## 6.4 Monitoring and Evaluation

As discussed in the text of this document, it is essential to plan for monitoring and evaluation at the outset. Monitoring activities may include collecting reports from teachers or NGOs working with youth out of school, collecting data on the distribution of IEC materials and the airing of radio and TV spots aimed at youth, along with listener surveys. Evaluation can be accomplished if

*Table 1. Matrix: Youth*

| Target group | Desired behaviour change | Approach | Media channel | Interpersonal channel (Networks) | Support services |
|---|---|---|---|---|---|
| Youth in school | Responsible sexual behaviour<br>↓ Drug use (injecting)<br># Condom use<br># Health care seeking behaviour | Mass media<br>Peer education<br>Curriculum development<br>Co-curricular activities | TV, Radio<br>Press Interpersonal | Schools<br>School organizations<br>Ministry of Education<br>Ministry of Youth | Counselling<br>Condoms<br>STD services |
| Youth in college | # Responsible sexual behaviour<br>↓ Drug use (injecting)<br># Condom use<br># Health care seeking behaviour | Mass media<br>Peer education<br>Curriculum development<br>Co-curricular activities | TV, Radio<br>Press Interpersonal | Schools<br>School organizations<br>Ministry of Education<br>Ministry of Youth | Counselling<br>Condoms<br>STD services |
| Youth out of school (urban) | # Responsible sexual behaviour<br>↓ Drug use (injecting)<br># Condom use<br># Health care seeking behaviour | Peer education outreach<br>Mass media | TV, Radio<br>Interpersonal<br>Street theatre | NGOs<br>Ministry of Youth | Counselling<br>Condoms<br>STD services |
| Youth out of school (rural) | # Responsible sexual behaviour<br>↓ Drug use (injecting)<br># Condom use<br># Health care seeking behaviour | Peer education outreach<br>Mass media | Peer education<br>Traditional media<br>Street theatre | Rural outreach networks<br>NGOs<br>Ministry of Youth | Counselling<br>Condoms<br>STD services |

{Cont.}..........

| | | | | | |
|---|---|---|---|---|---|
| Street children | # Responsible sexual behaviour<br>↓ Drug use (injecting)<br># Condom use<br># Health care seeking behaviour | Peer education Outreach<br>Mass media | Interpersonal<br>Street theatre<br>Traditional media | NGOs<br>Department of Child Welfare<br>Ministry of Social Welfare/Youth | Counselling<br>Condoms<br>STD services |

TABLE 40.2. Matrix: Target Populations and Communication Approaches

| Target group | Desired behaviour change | Approach | Media channel | Network | Support services |
|---|---|---|---|---|---|
| Brothel-based workers | Condom usage<br>Seeking treatment for STD | Outreach<br>Peer education | Target print and audio-video material<br>Street theatre | NGOs<br>Health workers<br>Local GPs | Condoms<br>STD services<br>Counselling |
| Street sex workers | Condom usage<br>Seeking treatment for STD | Outreach | Target print and audio-video material<br>Street theater | NGOs<br>Health workers<br>Local GPs | Condom<br>STD services<br>Counselling |
| Madams of brothels | Condom promotion<br>Condom usage | Outreach<br>Peer education | Target print and audio-video material<br>Street theatre | NGOs | Condoms<br>STD services<br>Counselling |
| Pimps | Condom promotion<br>Appropriate treatment for STD | Outreach | Target print and audio-video material<br>Street theater | NGOs | Condom<br>STD services<br>Counselling |
| Truck drivers/ transport workers | Condom use<br>Appropriate treatment of STD | Outreach<br>Peer education | Target print and audio-video material | NGOs<br>Peers<br>Trucking Association<br>Ministries of Transport | STD services<br>Condom<br>Counselling |
| Men who have sex with men | Condom use<br>Appropriate treatment of STD | Outreach<br>Peer education | Target print material | NGOs | STD services<br>Condoms<br>Counselling |
| Migrant workers | Condom use<br>Appropriate treatment of STD | Local media<br>outreach Peers | Street theatre<br>Traditional media<br>Target print material and audio-video | NGOs<br>Intercountry Cooperation Labour Unions<br>Ministry of Labour | STD services<br>Condoms<br>Counselling |

TABLE 40.3. Target Population and Communication Approaches

| Target group | Desired behaviour change | Approach | Media channel | Networks | Support services |
|---|---|---|---|---|---|
| Injecting drug | Cleaning needles<br>Condom use<br>Appropriate treatment of STD | Outreach<br>Peers | Targeted print and<br>Audio-video material | NGO<br>De-addiction programmes<br>Prisons | Counselling<br>STD services<br>Condoms |
| STD patients | ↑ in condom use<br>↑ in health care seeking behaviour<br>↑ treatment compliance | Interpersonal<br>Mass media | TV Radio<br>health workers | NGO s<br>health Services | Counselling<br>Condoms |
| General population | ↑ inability to discuss<br>↑ sex and sexuality<br>↑ Seeking of information on STD/AIDS<br>↑ empathy for HIV and people with AIDS<br>↑ in condom use | Mass media | TV, Radio<br>Press<br>Billboard<br>Exhibition<br>Cinema slides | Associations<br>Community organizations<br>Workplace settings | Counselling<br>Condoms<br>STD services<br>Information Services (Hotlines) |
| Policy-makers | ↑ in support to AIDS prevention programme<br>↑ in understanding of communication needs | Mass media<br>Interpersonal | TV, Radio<br>Press<br>Seminars<br>Meetings | | |
| Women | ↑ in health care seeking behaviour<br>↑ in knowledge of STD & AIDS<br>↑ ability to negotiate sexual behaviour | Mass media<br>Peer education outreach | TV, Radio<br>Press<br>Traditional media | NGOs<br>Associations<br>Existing government programmes<br>Health workers<br>Women's organizations | Counselling<br>STD services |

baseline data are collected on knowledge and practices. Key indicators of the desired behavioural change can be measured through repeat surveys. It is important to evaluate process and outcome if results are to be fedback into programme planning. Monitoring and evaluation must be planned before activities are conducted.

## 7. PLANNING A MASS AWARENESS CAMPAIGN

Mass awareness campaigns are recommended for reaching the general public with basic information on AIDS/STD, for articulating the general philosophy behind the overall programme, and for providing an umbrella message network for the entire programme. A mass awareness campaign is the utilization of all mass media channels (TV, radio, press, general print materials) to disseminate a sequence of basic messages on HIV/AIDS/STD in a co-ordinated fashion aimed at a loosely segmented target population. Often *ad hoc* media activities, such as individual TV spots, are mistaken for mass awareness campaigns. It is important that a campaign is recognized by the general population as a cohesive programme no matter which channel of the mass media is used.

Most national AIDS programmes do not have the infrastructure to develop such a campaign in-house and the development of the design and media plan is often contracted out to communications professionals/organizations. Understanding of the elements which go into planning a mass awareness campaign is, however, useful for a programme planner and a concise overview of the elements and steps necessary for an effective mass awareness campaign therefore follows.

*Segment Target Population:* A decision should be made on what segments of the general population should be targeted. For instance, if segmenting for youth, men and women between 15 and 49 is suggested, then messages directed at women, men, and youth in general should be developed.

*Market Research:* Before developing a campaign it is essential to conduct some rapid research among the identified segments of the general population to ascertain current levels of knowledge, general practices, sexual health care seeking behaviour and perceptions of AIDS and STDs. A combination of quantitative and qualitative data collection is recommended. Qualitative research should be conducted first, after which a broader quantitative study for a larger sample size can be implemented. The quantitative study can provide baseline data for future evaluation of impact. Marketing research firms and large social science institutions can be contracted to carry out this work. It is essential that the programme planner works closely with the contractor on questionnaire development and sampling.

*Message Development:* Specific messages for the segmented populations should be developed on the basis of the philosophy, the research and the availability of services.

*Concept Development and Media Plan:* The overall tone and theme of a campaign should be developed on the basis of the philosophy and the results of research. This will entail designing a logo and signature line or tune to unite the various media used. Some samples are 'Prevention is the only cure' with an identifiable graphic for use in all visuals. At this stage the mix of media will be identified ands for each audience segiment, a detailed plan for dissemination will be developed. This will include identifying appropriate air time and broadcast channels for TV and radio; identifying which press would be used for which segment listing out the support print materials which should be developed and where they would be disseminated; and sequencing messages. It is recommended that, for print materials, emphasis be given to visuals; even a literate audience will look at a visual before reading a text.

Professional advertising agencies, working closely with national AIDS programme staff, or other identified communications professionals should be recruited for the development of the overall campaign.

*Prototype Development, Pretesting and Revision:* Software for TV, radio, press advertisement and print materials must be developed in a cohesive fashion. It will be based on research, but will probably cover basic information on AIDS and materials to address the common misconceptions of each target group. For example, research among youth might show that they:

— have low levels of knowledge;
— perceive themselves to be not at risk;
— watch TV and listen to pop radio programmes; and
— do not read newspapers.

Based on this a decision could be made to develop TV and radio spots and a comic format brochure to disseminate in schools. A similar process would take place for each identified segment of population. All spots and materials. however, would share a common logo and signature line to identify each material as part of the campaign, reinforce messages and provide legitimacy for the information.

The overall concept and individual prototypes need to be thoroughly tested with the target audience. This can be done, for example, through focus group discussions, or through stopping people in the street or at a bus stop. If a large number of individuals do not understand the message, then it should be redesigned. After the pretesting process, revisions should be made and additional pretests conducted as appropriate.

*Implementation:* A campaign can run for a period of three months to one year depending on audience exhaustion and comprehension of the messages. All media materials should be ready and disseminated at the same time.

*Monitoring*: it is essential to carefully monitor the implementation and impact of the campaign to ensure that materials have been disseminated, and to assess audience participation through listener surveys, spot interviews, and analysis of letters and requests for information in an on-going fashion during the life of the campaign. If a particular material or software is clearly unacceptable, then it can be taken off the air immediately. An advertising agency will have the capability to professionally monitor the progress of the campaign.

*Evaluation and Reprogramming:* After the completion of the campaign cycle, a repeat baseline evaluation should be conducted along with a study to produce some qualitative data on the impact of the campaign. The data should be analysed and fed into reprogramming of the next cycle of the awareness campaign. Messages will change from straight information to more specific behavioural change messages based on the greater knowledge of the target audience. The next cycle of the campaign will probably tackle issues related to empathy for those afflicted and queries which have been raised in the first cycle. Awareness campaigns must be continuous.

Finally? a mass awareness campaign will begin the process of making people aware of the problem and the methods of prevention. It is only one component of an overall IEC programme and does not replace interpersonal approaches.

*(This document was developed based on a consultation meeting held in WHO-SEARO, New Delhi during 20-22 March, 1994.)*

# 41

# Behaviour Change

(Summary Report of the Informal Consultation on Behaviour Change: a Central Issue in the Response to the HIV Epidemic Dakar, Senegal, 12-15 December 1991)

---

The consultation was structured around six specific questions. This report summarizes the discussion around these questions and the responses.

Q 1. What behavioural and attitudinal changes limit the spread of the epidemic?

Q 2. What is the basis of our shared belief and hope that the epidemic can be overcome?

Q 3. How do the required changes come about?

Q 4. How can community-based organizations assist individuals and communities to change?

Q 5. How do programmes expand and develop to assist these changes to come about?

Q 6. How can these changes be documented and why do we want to do this?

## Q 1. What Behavioural and Attitudinal Changes Limit the Spread of the Epidemic?

Behaviour change happens in the context of the individual, the group and the community. It is not just an event, but a process taking place over a long period of time, ranging from a stage of unawareness through awareness and trying out new behaviours, to reaching sustained change. Important facilitators of change include stories, role models and the support of the community and peer groups. Behaviour change is first of all a personal responsibility, but it is very difficult to achieve alone. Community support and help are essential for sustained changes in behaviour.

This process of behaviour change begins from birth and continues throughout one's lifetime. Individuals determine and shape their identities in relation to their immediate communities. Behaviour is a part of individual identity and is, therefore, strongly influenced by community values. People are constrained by their belief systems which reflect the community beliefs, and individuals need to learn how to explore alternative options. Individuals are able to change when and if the community recognizes that specific behaviours need to be changed and creates its own strategy to achieve this. But a supportive community atmosphere alone cannot always generate change: there is also the need for a positive approach to suggesting alternative behaviour (for example, young women may engage in sex to gain money or popularity, so alternative behaviour which also achieves these objectives needs to be identified). Resources may be needed to sustain behaviour change.

## Q 2. What is the Basis of our Shared Belief and Hope that the Epidemic can be Overcome?

The influence of people living with HIV is a major factor in the belief that the epidemic will be overcome: respect for people with HIV is enhanced by their involvement with others working in the field and the way they have been able to teach others so much about the effect of the virus. The response of people with HIV has also reinforced the belief that human nature is essentially good.

There is evidence that people are able to change their behaviour and that communities are acting collectively to organize themselves to change, to care and to cope. We already know a great deal about the virus, and we have technical knowledge on how to prevent transmission. Lessons have been learnt from coping with previous epidemics. Stories of activities and achievements help to motivate and sustain others working in the field. There is increasing conviction of the need to support one another at the local, national and international levels. There is a great potential for change, compassion, consensus, involvement and collaboration.

Motivation also comes from a fundamental belief in people's capacity to change, and recognition that the response to the epidemic has reflected a range of human values such as trust, respect, dignity and solidarity. There is a strong desire for group survival, and recognition that there is no alternative to behaviour change. Concern for those affected and for the next generation was recognized as a major motivating factor.

## Q 3. How do the Required Changes Come About?

Influences on an individual's capacity to change include: faith, religion, education, economics, and environmental influences. Some of these influences cannot be changed by the individual- such as family, time and place of birth, mobility, psychosocial dependence, peer pressure, and environmental changes. The media, membership in organizations involved in change, fashion and trends affect individuals. Traditional media (i.e. storytelling) are also an influence. Such factors can either be constraints or strengths in that they can either help or inhibit behaviour changes.

Working in the field of HIV is itself a factor in change. We are changing ourselves in the process of changing others. Organizations may need to change in order to accommodate our need to bring about change.

### 1. Personal Behaviour Change

Individuals in the group changed because they gained knowledge of the transmission and prevention of the disease, and because of various individual experiences of, for example, being infected, caring for someone who is infected, losing someone close or interacting with organizations involved with HIV.

They have received support and positive reinforcement from peer groups, family and friends. The desire to survive and the hope for a better future have both influenced individual behaviour, and this has included the re-evaluation of spiritual faith and values, which have in turn been able to sustain change. Finally, concern and respect for others have been important elements in determining behaviour.

### 2. Organizational Experiences

Change in an organization can be initiated by a variety of stimuli whose effects vary according to the type and situation of the organization, for instance:

The motivation for change may come from within the organization:

* Changes are driven by need and the recognition of need - projects run by an organization may move from simple to complex and from small to large as the people within the organization gain deeper understanding of the problems with which they work.
* Financial considerations may determine how programmes move. Increased resources may bring expansion or extension of services. Resource constraints may bring streamlining of activities or reorientation.
* Leadership determines how programmes progress. This may be through managers or through other influential individuals.

External influences can also result in change:

* Governments can be changed in response to community needs if they are identified and articulated.
* In certain communities in Africa, religious groups play a role which can be either a constraint on, or a catalyst for, change. In addition, some social and cultural agents can determine the way the programmes evolve.
* The severity of the epidemic and changes in the perception of its seriousness can lead to changes in programmes.

## 3. How is Change Initiated by People Living with HIV (PLWH)?

Individuals who are able to provide a role model by publicly avowing their status as HIV positive give others the courage to come out. But before change can come about, whether it is change in behaviour or the change in attitudes which allows people to be open about HIV infection, information is essential. This has to be available in the form of facilities for testing, supportive counselling and the development of the capacity in every individual to examine the options open to him or her. Changes in attitude are necessary before changes in behaviour at an individual or community level can take place.

Nomalizing HIV is necessary—exposing the myth of the hidden enemy and giving a human face to AIDS.

Active participation and leadership from PLWH is necessary in all our work. For this to happen, it is important to recognize that while PLWH are well, there is no distinction between them and anyone else. While they are sick, they need care and facilities, exactly the same as for any other illness.

However, while recognizing the vitas importance of role models and stories of people who are affected themselves, issues of confidentiality must be carefully thought through. PLWH need to be able to publicize their stories without losing their privacy. Loss of privacy often takes place at an enormous personal cost. Activist groups need to discipline themselves not to be casual about revealing identities.

In a discussion of openness about being HIV positive, the following points were made:

* There should be concern about the price of openness.
* It takes time to get a large enough number of people who will state openly that they are infected or affected.
* Openness should be planned and gradual; it needs a supportive environment.
* Secrecy also has a price, and a balance has to be found between the need for privacy and openness: an example

was given of a woman who died without having had appropriate treatment because her daughter did not know the nature of her illness.

* Secrecy can perpetuate the stigma attached to HIV, especially in relation to the media.
* If we recommend personal story-telling to people with HIV, we need a social contract to protect them from discrimination.
* Those who are not themselves infected with HIV can have stories to tell.

We are all potentially positive but public attitudes towards AIDS service organizations is often prejudicial and leads to a them and us syndrome.

## 4. Community Agents of Change and Role Models—how do they Initiate Change in Communities?

Community agents of change can be anyone who is motivated by:

* being infected or affected.
* caring for someone who is infected.
* knowing and understanding about HIV and its consequences.

Belief leads to conviction which leads to commitment which leads to change.

Change is affected by:

* modelling and using examples,
* sharing experiences and telling stories,
* challenging peers to take notice and act at every opportunity,
* organizing and supporting practical activities,
* facilitating community ownership, and
* changing the attitudinal environment within the community.

## 5. Interaction Between Communities: can this be a Catalyst for Change?

Belonging to a community is a prerequisite to change for individuals because of the esteem which the sense of belonging brings, and because of the support which the community provides. Change within communities involves the belief that change is possible.

Once communities have generated change, empowerment allowing obstacles to be overcome can follow. The dynamic which leads to change in a community creates the desire to carry the changre beyond the immediate community.

This can be carried out via a bridge to another community when there is an individual who belongs to overlapping communities; for example, the experience of the gay community in Malaysia was transferred to women's groups.

Some communities lack the sense of community identity to operate effectively. Established communities are able to help loose networks of people to become effective community members, and thus a base for change.

Comrnunities can act by example to other communities, proving that change is both possible and beneficial. The process of change is strengthening and desirable for that reason.

## 6. How do Communities Recognize that Change has taken Place and how do they use this to Sustain Change?

The tools currently used for looking at behaviour change are: seropositivity, clinical prognosis, levels of sexually transmitted infections and use of condoms. These are not necessarily valuable, because they measure factors which may not be related to behaviour change. By involving the community, it may be possible to make causal links. To do this, communities must be involved in the process of evaluating change. They need to be involved in determining indicators of change, identifying the information to collect, and at which stages of planning, implementation, measurement and evaluation. So far, monitoring behaviour change has not been done properly, and has not received enough attention.

Some of the indicators of change identified included:

* communities no longer condoning travel for sex;
* increased usage of condoms (but this can result in more sexual activity);
* villages becoming suspicious and unwelcoming towards strangers because they are thought to be to blame for the infection;
* marrying earlier—this is difficult because the bride price for young women is too high and because young men cannot afford any bride price; in one community the bride price was reduced;
* males have stopped running with the girls, i.e. having many sex partners;

* development of sex education in schools based on a concept of family life.

## Q 4. How can Community-based Organizations Assist Individuals and Communities to Change?

Presentations from six of the participating organizations highlighted some of the ways in which behaviour change is initiated and sustained through community action. Brief descriptions of the organizations represented are attached to the end of this report.

1. **Counselling has a significant role to play:** The AIDS Support Organization, TASO (Uganda), reaches the community through counselling within the family, through the participation of the person with HIV. The communities identify themselves to TASO, and TASO is able to respond with training workers selected by the community to counsel and care. TASO is able to provide back up if the care cannot be managed within the community. This leads to community-based education programmes.
2. **The same holds for Chikankata (Zambia),** where the community itself is the initiator, and requests training and education. Two teams, one carrying out the home-based care programme and the other carrying out the community counselling training programme, build on the process of diagnosis and care in hospital, and an assessment of the appropriateness of home care. The community counselling team holds meetings with the community and initiates a file for each community, allowing for progress and strategies to be followed. Entry points to the community are from the experience of another community, from the acceptance of homebased care, or following recognition of the problem and the need to know more. WAMATA has observed an attitude change, in that people are becoming more willing to share information and experience; membership of the organization is growing.
3. **The recognition that members of WAMATA** (Tanzania) are HIV-infected brings about a change in attitude toward HIV and PLWH. Most of the counselling is done by volunteers and this is leading to wider participation in the community.
4. **The Victorian AIDS Council** (Australia) has found that education, carried out according to the principles of community development, has been successful in bringing about behaviour change and in involving a large num-

ber of people. Individuals are mutually supportive, and through campaigns with which they identify, come to participate in and control the services being offered. All the work has been done by gay men, but there has been no pressure for disclosure. Counselling facilities were available, but it was some time before these were used. The strength of the programme lay in the mutual support and respect for the people witnin it.

5. Kitovu Hospital (Uganda) has programmes covering hospital-based and home-based care. To assist behaviour change in the hospital itself, and recognizing that change is most effective in a group, a hospital community was established in order to encourage behaviour change in all aspects of life, including the spiritual aspects of change. The home-based care in the Masaka District, where there are high levels of sickness from AIDS, builds on community involvement to promote positive living and self-reliance. This includes income generation activities and focus group discussions.
6. Women and AIDS Support Network, WASS (Zimbabwe), has concentrated on the problems of women, particularly those who are in occupations where they are vulnerable to discrimination such as domestic workers. Change has been encouraged through close links and networking with other agencies and by drawing attention to some of the problems specific to women who are not protected by law(s) in their employment or in their relationships. Behaviour change which is positive for one individual may be detrimental for another, for example a second or third wife has no legal protection, and if her husband decides to return to monogamy, he can reject her.

The presentations highlighted the fact that communities need to define their own methodology and monitor their own progress. This depends on the capacity to agree within the community and through agreement to establish community norms which express what is acceptable to the whole community, developed through a process of discussion and consensus. Counselling, in various forms, is crucial to behaviour change - information is necessary before people can make choices. Research by outsiders may be irrelevant to the needs and experience of the community. Community organizations and communities need to set their own agendas.

Discussion brought up the following points:

1. Behaviour change is related to attitude change and it is difficult to evaluate attitude change; some indicators highlighted include:
   * Families are changing, getting involved with caring, and using the opportunity of having an infected family member to learn more about HIV.
   * Increasing numbers of people with HIV are coming forward to be educators.
   * Communities are becoming more open and involved.
   * People are joining organizations which are identified with infected people.
   * People are living longer with HIV and leading happier lives.
2. The discussion on research reflected the controversy of this issue.
   * Research should be action-oriented and participatory.
   * Research should always be accompanied by intervention.
   * Research has often been mistakenly seen as intervention.
   * Community-based care is a long-term process, but research results on this are demanded in the short term.
   * The importance of recognizing both the diversity of cultures in different regions and the commonality of regions was acknowledged. The need to present research in a particular way, in order for its value to be understood, causes frustration to community groups who know their work is valid but who have difficulty in getting it accepted as such. We all need to work towards legitimizing the research methods and the results coming from community groups. Terminology is important; for example, anecdotes can also be case histories.
   * Research methods to evaluate behaviour change have not been acceptable to the scientific research mainstream.

## Q5. HOW DO PROGRAMMES EXPAND AND DEVELOP TO ASSIST THESE CHANGES TO COME ABOUT?

Several different stimuli to expansion were identified:

* Kilamanjaro Christian Medical Centre's, KCMC

(Tanzania), motivation came from individuals who were concerned about a need to know more and take action after they realized the high level of seropositivity in the community.

* Chikankata (Zambia) responded to requests from the community, following their realization that the traditional methods were not working and that more realistic approaches were needed.
* Programmes change if it is established that a strategy is not successful and that another must be developed.
* Increasing involvement of volunteers leads to a change in strategy because they represent community involvement.
* Community participation and involvement can change the direction or the plans of the programme.
* Evaluation may precede a decision to expand or alter direction.

Expansion may also be influenced by a need to complement services provided by governments, or by what other organizations are doing; it is important to avoid duplication. Equally, expansion may be affected by factors outside the control of community-based organizations: one example is that international NGOs can attract resources and staff from local NGOs, thus inhibiting their development.

## Q 6. HOW CAN THESE CHANGES BE DOCUMENTED AND WHY DO WE WANT TO DO THIS?

Community organizations continually change, refine, revise and expand their programmes. They do this on the basis of observation, intuition, feedback. Their closeness to the community within which they were formed guarantees that this is a participatory process.

This is a process of continuing analysis, evaluation and redesign which occurs in response to (and in order to sustain) changes taking place in the community. This process can provide the basis of the documentation of change.

To overcome the epidemic, both attitudes and behaviour must change. This occurs through ongoing interactions between individuals and their communities.

Changes are taking place in attitude and behaviour. Both individuals and communities are changing. There is a need to record and share these processes. Systematic recording of processes needs thought and training. for the benefit of both community volunteers who play a crucial part within the community as well as professional workers.

## Summary of Methods and Indicators of Change in the Community

Indicators of change are already being used informally by community organizations represented at the consultation. The indicators identified were illustrative rather than exhaustive. But they do identify ways in which change is being determined and identified, and this could form the basis of a more endogenous methodology.

## Changes in Attitude

Change in attitude was seen as not only a vital first step in individual and community behaviour change, but also as a legitimate and very important end in itself in leading to an environment in which behaviour change is encouraged and supported.

Indicators of attitudinal change:

1. Establishment of HIV-related community organizations, which can be measured as:
   * Number of groups formed
   * Membership of such groups
   * Total membership
   * Involvement of people not themselves infected
   * Involvement of people not directly affected by HIV.
2. Involvement of people living with HIV (PLWH) in changing behaviour in the community, which can be measured by:
   * Number of PLWH trained as educators
3. Involvement of PLWH in decision-making at all levels, local to national, which can be measured by:
   * Consultation by decision makers with infected individuals and communities
   * Number of PLWH on management boards of community organizations, national HIV/AIDS committees, etc.
4. Acceptance of PLWH within communities, which can be measured by:
   * Number of families a) willing to care for their infected members and b) interested to find out more about HIV

* Number of PLWH prepared to:
  — tell their stories
  — become educators
  — participate on boards, in consultations, etc.
5. How community leaders talk about HIV/AIDS and PLWH, which can be measured by;
   * Language used
   * Concern and respect shown
   * Openness of discussions
6. Support for affected families, which can be measured by:
   * Number of people visiting an affected household
   * Care given to survivors—elderly parents or children
7. Talking about illness and death, which can be measured by:
   * Number of funerals where it is said that the person died of AIDS

## Behaviour Change

The problems of research methodologies for measuring behaviour change are well known. However, communities can and do define their own strategies and targets, and can be helped to measure their own successes (or failures) against these. Doing this means identification of high risk behaviours (which is in itself an indicator of attitude change).

Indicators which have been observed or heard of by programmes at the consultation include:

1. Talking about change of behaviour, which can be measured by:
   * Reports to counsellors, educators, etc.
   * Information from men and women prepared to talk openly about how they have changed
2. Choosing to be counselled and tested, which can be measured by:
   * Attendance records for men and women at voluntary testing and counselling centres
3. Changing patterns of sexual behaviour, which can be measured by:
   * number of adultery disputes or divorce proceedings in traditional courts
   * Changes in sex-worker population
   * Changes in patterns of sex-worker clients.

Indicators of change in norms set by community:

Communities assist and sustain people in changing their behaviour and attitudes. Communities reach a consensus on strategies or behaviours which are acceptable or which are judged to achieve a certain aim. These changes in community norms often precede or accompany individual behaviour change. The monitoring may be done by the community as a whole or by individuals or organizations within it.

Indicators could include:

1. Acceptance of talking about sexuality and HIV infection, which can be measured by:
   * Education on sexuality and HIV in schools.
2. Changing of cultural practices which put people at risk, which can be measured by:
   * Number/proportion of spouses cleansed by non-sexual means.
   * Age of marriage and bride price.
3. Changing patterns of alcohol consumption, which can be measured by:
   * Opening hours of bars.
   * Number of people drinking in bars.
   * Sale records of alcohol in bars.
4. Communities seeking help for prevention and care, which can be measured by:
   * Number of communities requesting help
   * Number of families accepting home-based care for people with AIDS
   * Willingness to raise local funds for people affected
   * Identification by communities of high-risk behaviours
   * Identification by communities of behaviour-change indicators
   * Identification by communities of strategies for behaviour change.
5. Changes in community customs relating to sex and marriage, which can be measured by:
   * Greater stability of marriages
   * Resumption of teaching on taboos
   * Marriage patterns and pre-marital counselling

**BEHAVIOUR CHANGE:**

*A Central Issue in Responding to the HIV Epidemic*

Agenda for the Future

1. Carry back the message that behaviour change is a critical strategy for overcoming the epidemic.

   *There is a need to influence governments and community groups to focus on behaviour change.*

2. Incorporate the knowledge and insights of the informal consultation into the daily work programme of each organization.

   *To do this, there is a need for increased understanding of the processes of attitudinal and behaviour change, as well as a need to learn from one another's experience in programme development.*

3. Value the processes and knowledge by which individuals and community organizations identify needs in order to design, evaluate and redesign their programmes.

4. Feed back insights, intuitions, stories and research findings to communities, educators, outreach workers and programme managers.

5. Give value to what communities and their organizations are doing by documenting and sharing their experience.

6. Increase the sharing of experience among countries and regions.

   *This can be done through the strengthening of existing linkages, the exchange of material, consultation, visits to other organizations and through meetings.*

7. Bring about a partnership based on respect, trust and support between community organizations and governments.

   For communities and organizations to continue to function effectively, their initiatives must be complemented and supported by government policies and programmes. This requires a balance of support between government and community.

8. Establish a means or structure which would enable communities to share experiences, work collaboratively, provide credibility to community organizations, provide an agreed means of community representation at local and national levels and be a means of communication between communities and governments, particularly

in national HIV/AIDS programmes.

9. Create awareness that the resources needed to address the epidemic are already scarce, and that they must continue to come from within communities and nations.
   *Community initiatives always draw on community resources - volunteers, financial and political support. These form the basis of a self-sufficient response.*
   *Community resources need to be complemented by government resources. This will require policies in support of community initiatives, the reallocation of national budgets and the selection of critical priority areas for supporting community initiatives. Communities can assist individuals in bringing about and sustaining behaviour change, but they may not themselves have the capacity to establish services requiring regular and sustained input of materials or technologies.*
10. Report to one another widen six months on progress made in the implementation of this agenda.

*Informal Consultation, Dakar, Senegal, 12-15 December, 1991*

## THE AIDS CARE AND PREVENTION DEPARTMENT THE SALVATION ARMY HOSPITAL CHIKANKATA, ZAMBIA

Chikankata Hospital has been implementing field-based AIDS care and prevention programmes since March 1987.

On-going home based care (HBC) is provided to an average of 250 patients, their families and their immediate communities each quarter. The team goes out three days a week and is committed to attending to the total needs of the patient. Two members focus on the physical, social and spiritual needs of the HIV-infected individual and his or her family while another concentrates on educating the family and the community on the facts about HIV and how to prevent its transmission. One of the team members travels with the Primary Health Care team to the schools in the catchment area twice a year to present the facts about HIV.

The objectives of the HBC teams are multiple. They visit people with HIV infection in their homes in order to assess their physical, psychological, social and spiritual needs, and to provide for these needs where possible. They carry out contact tracing. They carry out counselling and education within families and communities, providing personal support, and promoting sustained behaviour change through community counselling. They also assess the educational impact of AIDS management on people with HIV and their families. One of the team members is the school's educator. The team also tries to provide material support, giving milk. On occasion the hospital receives donations of blankets and clothes which are given out.

On the remaining two days of the week, a second team goes out to work with communities—clarifying facts about HIV, helping communities identify activities which put them at risk and coming up with strategies that will keep them from engaging in these high risk activities. This process is called community counselling. This is defined as an activity, focusing on groups and communities, which promotes responsibility transfer for behaviour change from others, including health care personnel, to the community.

Principles of counselling as applied in a one-on-one relationship have been transferred to counselling a large group or a community. After a community has been selected, the process of counselling communities, as in any counselling situation, follows the process of relationship-building, problem exploration, understanding and decision making, implementation and evaluation.

Different types of communities are concerned: kinship-based-village; occupation-based—industrial towns, commercial farms; religion-based—churches; and party systems-based.

Village health workers and other volunteers who are part of the PHC structure will be trained so that they will be part of the network working on AIDS care and prevention.

The aim of the home-based care and community counselling programmes is to transfer responsibility for care and prevention to the family and the community.

The hope for the future is to activate families and communities.

Families and communities need to have a sense that HIV is their problem and if it is going to be stopped, and if people are going to get the care they need to deal with being HIV+, it will because they, the family and community, have done something about it. Not because the hospital has done something.

The hospital's management plan consists of diagnosis/counselling; planned discharge; home-based care and hospital admission when required. Although the focus of this plan is to get the patient back into the home where he will be cared for by his extended family the hospital plays a vital part in diagnosis, stabilization and readmission for additional treatment.

From July 1989, the Chikankata AIDS care and prevention department has been conducting a five-day seminar each month.

The seminar is for health professionals and others who are currently involved in or need to start an AIDS care and prevention programme. The seminar provides an integrative approach covering such disciplines as counselling, clinical care, education, pastoral care and administration. The content is based on the practical, field-based AIDS care and prevention programmes at Chikankata.

## WOMEN AND AIDS SUPPORT NETWORK (WASN)-ZIMBABWE

WASN was established in 1989 following the international Society for Women and AIDS in Africa (SWAA) conference held in Harare. It is a group of volunteers working on the fundamental principle that women will only be able to overcome consequences of HIV through improving their self esteem and confidence. It was recognized that people needed to change their attitudes and behaviour in order to stop further transmission of HIV infection. However, in many situations women were unable to make demands that their partners change their behaviour and felt helpless to prevent infection to themselves. They also wanted to publicly display solidarity with those of us who are PLWHIVs.

WASN works to share information about how HIV affects women, to encourage women as organized groups and clubs to support women living with HIV and AIDS, and to support each other in protecting themselves against becoming infected. They target organizations working with women so that the messages are carried through to more women than WASN can reach itself. Also it is desirable that the issues be included in more permanent fashion through programmes and curricula.

WASN analyzes the quarterly statistics released by the National AIDS Control Programme to emphasize the vulnerabilities of women in the AIDS epidemic. These figures encourage young school girls targetted by programmes to understand the consequences of early sex, and to be more assertive in refusing unwanted attentions. WASN published a booklet called 'Why Should Women be Concerned About AIDS?'. It emphasizes the importance of women talking to each other in all kinds of fora so that issues about sex, condoms, HIV and AIDS become less taboo. It also emphasizes women supporting each other rather than competing with each other.

Although legislation exists to protect the rights of workers in the formal sector, many workers in the informal sector are not covered. This includes women who work as domestic workers and child minders who are often dismissed if their HIV status becomes known. To organize employers, Women and AIDS Support Network organized phone-in radio programmes (the accessible media nationally) and print media articles on transmission of HIV—emphasizing how HIV is not spread by social contact.

WASN was concerned that women were often depicted as prostitutes in harsh judgmental images, shown as reservoirs of infection. This reinforced many male attitudes that HIV is a women's disease as it is caught from women, and women were blamed for spreading the disease. WASN makes input into several drama groups to encourage them to be more progressive and in particular to be more positive in the roles women play. They can be shown supporting each other, organizing to change attitudes and behaviour in the communities.

## WAMATA (THOSE IN TANZANIA IN THE FRONT LINE AGAINST AIDS)

WAMATA began with FIVE families as a voluntary, non-sectarian and non-governmental grass-roots organization based on the spirit of solidarity, love and hope. Its mission is to provide medical and nursing home care, counselling and, to some extent, material assistance to people living with HIV. In its work WAMATA collaborates with the National AIDS Control Programme of the United Republic of Tanzania.

WAMATA provides a forum for grassroots-based organized action targeted at individual and community behaviour change; open and frank discussion of HIV as a socio-economic problem; sharing of experiences and knowledge about the epidemic among the members; planning, organizing and carrying out activities that not only comfort those living with HIV but also contribute something toward awareness of the need for individual and community behaviour change at least in the course of time of continued counselling work.

One of WAMATA's principle aims and objectives is 'To campaign against discrimination of HIV affected individuals and their families and involve the general public to institute and maintain behaviour change as a necessary step towards HIV prevention and control.' Its major activities are consciously based upon this objective.

WAMATA and other organs through campaigns, counselling, medical and home care activities have made it possible for positive and supportive attitudes to develop in the community towards those living with HIV. WAMATA members living and dying with HIV identify themselves as HIV positives. Some who were already terminally ill in 1989 have since sustained life, presumably partly because of the solidarity, support, care and hope they have been accorded by their organization (WAMATA). They are leading elements in the WAVIU (coined by the group living with HIV/AIDS to mean: People Striving to Control the Spread of the HIV Transmission).

WAMATA is involved in training of volunteer counsellors and provision of volunteer counselling, medical and home service. Indeed, most of the counselling and support is done by families and community members on a voluntary basis. Trained volunteer counsellors take on cases where the need for monitoring, supervision and follow up action has been identified.

WAMATA makes provision of material support to: HIV-affected families in need; children of HIV-affected families; and those affected families and individuals able, ready and willing to engage in income-generating activities.

WAMATA attempts to increase the participation of the wider community in the activities of the organization: in meetings, funding, publicity, etc.

## THE AIDS SUPPORT ORGANISATION (TASO), UGANDA

TASO (The AIDS Support Organization) is an indigenous, non-governmental organization based in Kampala, Uganda.

In Kampala headquarters which houses training activities, support is given to the development and co-ordination of a community-based AIDS programme, and to the development of TASO and TASO-type activities in other areas. With its theme 'Positive Living with AIDS', TASO provides a package of counselling services to people with HIV and their families. The package includes counselling, medical support and day-centre activities. To strengthen its hospital/clinic-based service, TASO has initiated a community-based HIV programme.

TASO has established seven counselling centres in seven districts along the Trans-African Highway where high prevalence of HIV has been reported. An eighth centre is planned in Arua.

TASO has periodically undertaken a critical assessment of its work to deduce lessons learnt from its experience and determine the most suitable direction for the organization over the foreseeable future. The key task has been to balance the competing demands of helping as many people as possible and providing a high quality service of training and counselling.

To facilitate project planning and implementation, TASO has established a structure where, as an organization, it will concentrate on its role of training HIV/AIDS counsellors for TASO and other organizations, will directly administer two 'model' counselling centres (Mulago and Musaka), and offer technical and management advice and financial control to the other 6 affiliate centres.

TASO recognizes that HIV education and prevention is the best weapon available to fight against HIV infection and disease.

At the same time, TASO recognizes the need to care for those already infected. To meet these very demanding needs, TASO has approached the problem directly, through those infected persons. They are the entry point to the family and community. By involving people with HIV and those who are not infected (including those who think they are not infected) in the care of people with AIDS, TASO is offering not only AIDS care, but also HIV education and prevention. Face-to-face contact and practical experience are what counts.

In response to the enormous problems caused and aggravated by HIV, TASO has the following strategic board activities:

1. Training AIDS counsellors for TASO and other organizations to offer counselling services.
2. Offering counselling services to people with HIV and their families in all TASO-established counselling centres.
3. Complementing available medical service for PWA/HIV.
4. Promoting positive attitudes in families and communities toward people with HIV.
5. Building and strengthening community-based efforts in response to the HIV epidemic.

A total of 6,000 people with AIDS have received TASO services at these centres. TASO also supports primary education of 800 AIDS orphans, though over 6,000 have been identified.

Over 25,000 family members have received HIV information and education. And millions have been reached through the TASO video—Living Positively with AIDS - which has been distributed worldwide by WHO/GPA and other organizations.

## KITOVU MOBILE AIDS HOME CARE AND EDUCATION PROGRAMME AND PASTORAL CARE AND COUNSELLING PROGRAMME, UGANDA

Kitovu Hospital is a Catholic, private hospital in Masaka District, Uganda. It has 185 beds, an out-patient department, a nutrition centre and a community-based health care programme. The hospital trains enrcled nurses and midwives.

In 1987, more than 60 per cent of patients in the general wards were HIV-positive, and the staff saw many children and adults with signs of HIV infection in the primary health care clinics. The AIDS programme at Kitovu Hospital was started in May 1987 as a part-time pastoral care programme. In October 1987 it became a fulltime programme, and it was decided to concentrate home care services on specific areas in Rakai and Masaka Districts.

The areas selected were chosen because they had the highest concentration of AIDS patients; people living in them could not visit the hospital because public transport was not available; the attitude of the local people to the team was one of openness and receptivity; the parish priest, health personnel, etc. had asked for help; and they were near enough to Kitovu for hospital vehicles to be used to bring patients to the hospital.

The AIDS programme consists of the following five interlinked components:

- hospital care;
- home visiting, including pastoral care;
- education in schools and villages;
- out-patient treatment;
- hospital pastoral care.

The main emphasis in the programme is on the Mobile AIDS Home Care Team and the Pastoral Care and Counselling Programme.

Clients are referred to the Home Care Team from the wards, the out-patient clinic and the Pastoral Care Programme. All persons with HIV infection and AIDS in the areas selected are eligible for home care.

Very ill patients and those requiring special aftercare are taken home from the hospital by the Pastoral Care and Counselling Team, which also visits patients who live near the hospital and who are too weak to come to the out-patient clinic.

Home care of persons with AIDS was chosen because it was known that people in the area prefer to die at home. In addition, it was assumed that the programme would make it easier to provide effective health education in the community.

## VICTORIAN AIDS COUNCIL/GAY MEN'S HEALTH CENTRE, COLLINGWOOD, AUSTRALIA

The Victorian AIDS Council / Gay Men's Health Centre provides education, support, advocacy and other necessary services to people affected directly or indirectly by HIV. These services are provided regardless of gender, sexual preferences or health status, but the organization acknowledges that these services will be primarily designed to meet the needs of all gay and bisexual men in Victoria.

The organization is based upon the principles of community development. Policy and programming is designed by members of the community in conjunction with employees. Education strategies are designed acknowledging that sustained behaviour change is facilitated by peer support. Support services are designed to meet people's needs in an empowering fashion.

# 42

# HIV/AIDS in South-East Asia

(Report of the Meeting of the National Programme Managers, New Delhi, 8-12, November 1993)

## I. INTRODUCTION

HIV/AIDS continues to spread in South-East Asia. The infection is not only increasing among individuals with high risk behaviour but now starting to spread to the general population as well. The countries in the Region are gaining considerable experience in the planning and implementation of activities in the fight against HIV pandemic within the framework of their national or medium-term plans. These experiences must be shared. The National AIDS Programme Managers, during the eighth meeting in November 1992, discussed interventions targeted among individuals with high risk behaviour. From 8 to 12 November 1993, the WHO Regional Office for South-East Asia organized the 9th Regional Meeting of the National AIDS Country Programme Managers at New Delhi to share the country experiences on various areas of the AIDS programme. The objectives of the meeting were:

1. To review the implementation of AIDS prevention and care activities in the countries of the Region with a view to facilitating the exchange of experiences including the successes, constraints and lessons learned;
2. To identify policies, interventions and approaches from selected countries which have proven to be successful and discuss how these could be transferred and applied, with appropriate modifications, in other countries of the Region;
3. To select priority interventions and activities for the national AIDS control programmes to be included in the 1994-95 comprehensive work plan; and
4. To finalize the 1994-95 work-plan on activities to be supported by WHO;

Twenty-three participants from ten countries were present at the meeting. Representatives of international agencies such as UNDP, UNICEF, UNESCO, ILO, USAID and the Ford Foundation were also invited to participate in the meeting.

The meeting was opened by Dr. U Ko Ko, Regional Director, WHO, SEARO. After welcoming the Programme Managers and other participants, the Regional Director highlighted the dangers posed by the HIV pandemic in the South-East Asia Region. He invited the participants to use the workshop as a forum for exchange of country experiences and ideas for the prevention and control of HIV infection and to see whether such experiences could be replicated in their own countries. He urged the Programme Managers to think of programme priorities in the light of the limited financial resources available. The external financial resources are already shrinking, and hence efforts are to be made to raise financial resources locally and to make programmes sustainable. Mr. Bayani, Acting Resident Representative, UNDP, stressed on the need for all UN agencies to work together in assisting the countries of this region in combating the HIV/AIDS epidemic. He emphasized on the WHO/UNDP alliance to combat the disease and its relevance at this juncture to merge the technical and financial support for combating the pandemic which has already reached an alarming situation.

Mr. P. R. Dasgupta, Project Director, National AIDS Control Organization (NACO), was nominated as Chairman, Dr Wiput Phoolcharoen, Director, AIDS Division, Ministry of Public Health, Thailand, as Co-Chairman, and Dr U Myo Thet Htoon, Programme Manager, Myanmar as Rapporteur. The workshop sessions consisted of plenaries, general. discussion and group work,_. Background materials on relevant subjects were provided to the participants during the opening ceremony.

## 2. REGIONAL HIV/AIDS SITUATION AND EPIDEMIOLOGICAL SURVEILLANCE

### 2.1 Current Situation of HIV/AIDS in South-East Asia

In the South-East Asia Region, AIDS was first diagnosed in 1984 in Thailand. In most other countries, HIV was not diagnosed until 1986 or later. Since then, however, HIV infection has spread extremely rapidly and WHO estimates that currently there are more than 1.5 million HIV-infected people in the Region (Table 42.1).

**Table 42.1.** ***AIDS and HIV infections in SEAR countries***
**(as of 30 June 1993)**

| Country | Reported AIDS cases | Estimated HIV Infections |
|---|---|---|
| Bangladesh | 1 | < 20, 000 |
| Bhutan | 0 | < 300 |
| DPR Korea | 0 | < 1, 000 |
| India | 336 | 1, 000, 000 |
| Indonesia | 31 | < 20, 000 |
| Maldives | 0 | < 100 |
| Mongolia | 0 | < 200 |
| Myanmar | 47 | 1, 50, 000 |
| Nepal | 18 | < 5, 000 |
| Sri Lanka | 24 | < 1, 000 |
| Thailand | 1, 569 | 4, 50, 000 |
| Total | 2, 026 | > 1, 500, 000 |

As of 30 June 1993, a total of 2, 026 cases of AIDS have been reported in South-East Asia. However, it is estimated that about 20, 000 AIDS cases have occurred till now. Thailand and India have reported the largest number of cases—1, 569 and 336 respectively - accounting for more than 95 per cent of the cases reported from the Region to date. Two countries, namely, Bhutan and DPR Korea, have not yet reported HIV infections (Table 42.2).

Trend data based on seroprevalence surveys confirm the alarming increase in HIV infection rates in selected high-risk populations. In Thailand, HIV rates of 0 to less than 1 per cent among Injecting Drug-Users (IDU) in Bangkok were found in various *ad hoc* surveys from 1985 to 1987. However, HIV rates increased sharply to 40 per cent by September 1988, and has now stabilized almost at that level. Rates similar to Bangkok were also seen in various other provinces of the country. This wave of HIV epidemic in IDU was followed by that among female prostitutes and, by successive waves of transmission, to male clients of the prostitutes, and from them to the wives and girl friends of these men in the general population. Nationally, the prevalence rates in June 1992 were 38.2 per cent in IDUs, 22.9 per cent in low-charge prostitutes, 5.7 per cent in male STD (sexually transmitted disease) patients and 1 per cent among pregnant women. Based on the currently available data, it is estimated that there are at present 450,000 HIV-infected persons in Thailand. The Thai working group projects that given that HIV transmission would continue, there would be 2-4 million cumulative HIV infections by the year 2000. In Myanmar, explosive increases in HIV seropositivity have been documented among IDUs—from 17 per cent in 1989 to 59 per cent and 71 per cent in 1990 and 1991 respectively. In addition, the rates

Table 42.2. *Number of HIV Positives Among the That male Population (low and high prevalence)*

| Age Group | Population | Male Pop. | Prev. Low | Prev.+ Low | Prev. High | HIV+High |
|---|---|---|---|---|---|---|
| Less 5 | 5, 743, 000 | 2, 871, 500 | | | | |
| 5-9 | 5, 802, 000 | 2, 901, 000 | | | | |
| 10-14 | 6, 275, 000 | 3, 137, 500 | 0.1 | 3, 137.5 | 0.2 | 6, 275 |
| 15-19 | 6, 071, 000 | 3, 035, 500 | 0.6 | 18, 213 | 2 | 6, 0710 |
| 20-24 | 6, 071, 000 | 3, 035, 500 | 3.1 | 94, 100.5 | 3.5 | 1,06, 242.5 |
| 25-29 | 5, 125, 000 | 2, 562, 500 | 3.1 | 79, 437.5 | 3.5 | 89, 68,7.5 |
| 30-34 | 5, 125, 000 | 2, 562, 500 | 1.1 | 25, 625 | 1.5 | 38, 437.5 |
| 35-39 | 3, 600, 000 | 1, 800, 000 | 1.0 | 18, 000 | 1.5 | 27, 000 |
| 40-44 | 3, 600, 000 | 1, 800, 000 | 0.5 | 9, 000 | 0.5 | 9, 000 |
| 45-49 | 2, 261, 000 | 1, 130, 500 | 0.5 | 5, 652.5 | 0.5 | 5, 652.5 |
| 50-54 | 2, 261, 000 | 1, 130, 500 | 0.1 | 1, 130.5 | 0.2 | 2, 261 |
| 55-59 | 1, 434, 000 | 7,17, 000 | 0.1 | 717 | 0.2 | 1, 434 |
| 60-64 | 1, 434, 000 | 7,17, 000 | 0.1 | 717 | 0.2 | 1, 434 |
| more 65 | 2, 240, 000 | 1, 120, 000 | 0.1 | 1, 120 | 0.2 | 2, 240 |
| Total | 57, 789, 000 | 28, 894, 500 | | 2,56, 850.5 | | 350, 374 |

among STD patients have registered an increase from 1.9 per cent in 1990 to 15.9 per cent in 1991 and from 8 per cent to 15.9 per cent among female prostitutes during the same period. About 1,50,000 persons are currently estimated to have been infected with HIV in Myanmar. Sequential infection was noted in Thailand starting with IDUs, and followed by female sex workers, STD patients and the community. This was also observed in Myanmar. In a study in the north-east Indian State of Manipur, none of the 2,322, IDUs seen from 1986 to 1989 were seropositive for HIV. However, the rate increased to 54 per cent during the period October 1989 to June 1990, and at present it is almost at the same level. Sequential infection, as observed in Thailand and Myanmar, is apprehended to occur in Manipur. In Bombay, the HIV seropositivity rate among prostitutes has increased from 2 per cent in 1988-1989 to nearly 40 per cent in 1991. Although there is evidence of increase in HIV prevalence among blood donors and women attending antenatal clinics, the rates are still less than 0.5 per cent. It is estimated that currently there are about one million HIV-infected persons in India.

Given the prevailing sexual behaviour and experiences in the three countries described above, there is a possibility of a similar scenario being repeated in other countries of the South-East Asia Region. Risk behaviour which promotes the spread of HIV, such as injection of drugs, male patronage of prostitutes, high rates of STD and low condom usage, are present in all countries. In view of the fact that heterosexual contact is the predominant mode of HIV transmission in the Region, that the rates of STD are high, and that there is considerable unprotected sexual activity, continued transmission of HIV in the general population appears inevitable. Predictions about AIDS tend to be unrealistic, but the current estimate of more than 1.5 million HIV infections in South-East Asia is nearly 12 per cent of the global total, while the proportion of reported AIDS cases is less than 1 per cent.

Furthermore, WHO estimates that while the annual number of HIV infections will peak in Africa by 1995, infections in Asia will continue to increase well into the early next century (Figure 42.1). The annual number of HIV infections by the year 2000 would far exceed that seen in sub-Saharan Africa. Given the mean progression time for initial HIV infection to develop into AIDS, now estimated to be ten years, it can be concluded that AIDS cases in the Region will continue to increase well into the next century, and close to two million cumulative cases of AIDS will occur by the year 2000.

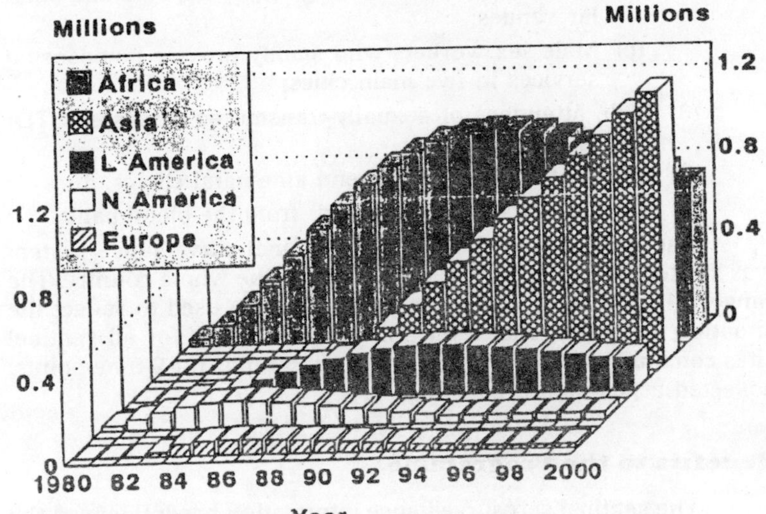


*Figure 42.1. Estimated/projected annual adult HIV infections*

## 2.2 HIV Sentinel Surveillance and Estimations in Thailand

The major objective of the HIV sentinel surveillance system in Thailand is to monitor high-risk groups in order to target intensified HIV intervention programmes and to provide early warning that the epidemic will soon reach the lower-risk general population. The latter assumes that high-risk groups are effective sentinels of future HIV infection in the general community. If this is true, local public health officials would have more time to organize control activities to safeguard the general public.

### Surveillance Methods

The sentinel surveillance started in 14 of the country's 73 provinces in June 1989. Six months later the surveillance was expanded to 31 provinces, and again expanded six months later to include all 73 provinces. The semi-annual surveys are mainly focused on selected target populations in the city areas of the provinces, which include:

(1) Injecting Drug Users (IDUs) who attend drug abuse treatment clinics;

(2) Commercial Sex Workers (CSWs) which are subclassified as:

(a) Female CSWs in brothel settings;

(b) Female CSWs not based in brothels but in establishments such as massage parlours, bars and similar venues;

(c) Male sex workers who mainly provide homosexual services in five main cities;

(3) Male attendees of sexually-transmitted diseases (STD) clinics;

(4) Pregnant women who attend ante-natal clinics, and

(5) Blood donors (donated blood) from the blood banks.

The trends from the time the sentinel surveillance system was started in June 1989 are presented for the whole country. The ranges of prevalence and mean prevalence are used to reflect the situation at the national level. The median values for all sentinel sites combined are used to show temporal trends for 9 time-points, collected at six-month intervals.

## Benefits to the Programme

The sentinel serosurveillance information has influenced the Government and public to realize the severity of the situation and to plan for action to combat the HIV epidemic. These are:

1. *Political will.* The evolving surveillance system provided information essential for taking rational action based on the prevalence of HIV infection in various segments of the society. The Thai Government established the National AIDS Committee chaired by the Prime Minister to respond to the HIV epidemic in 1991. The budget for the National AIDS Control Programme rose from 182 million bahts (approx. 7.2 million US$) in the fiscal year 1991 to 359 million bahts (14.4 million US$) and 1,125 million bahts (45 million US$) in the fiscal years 1992 and 1993 respectively. It will again rise substantially in the fiscal year 1994.
2. *Education for the general public.* Before 1989, the news on the AIDS epidemic in the country had never reached the first page of any newspaper. It was felt rumours about AIDS in the country would damage its image and hence the tourist industry. Since the last half of 1989, television and radio spots on AIDS have been aired on prime time. These spots warn the general public about the dangers of AIDS and explain exactly how to prevent it. The advertisements are explicit. In addition, the school curriculum on health education has been modified to include AIDS prevention messages.
3. ***Guidance in the development of the prevention programme development.*** **According to the results of the**

sentinel surveillance, over the last two years the IDUs and female CSWs have become the sources of HIV infection and are not the only high risk groups any more. The HIV epidemic has invaded the family; men, (pregnant) women, and their infants. Preventive actions, which focused on commercial sex activities such as the 100 per cent condom use programme, were changed to put the emphasis on the more difficult and complicated task of strengthening social norms to reject promiscuity and prostitution.

4. *Medical services safety.* In 1989, the Ministry of Public Health established the first decisive and effective intervention to prevent HIV transmission through blood transfusion. Since then, a total of 700,000—800,000 lots of donated blood are mandatorily screened for HIV antibody annually. Universal precaution techniques, practiced by public health providers, were strengthened through budgetary and technical support.
5. *Differentiating the action base on the epidemic pattern.* The epidemiological patterns of HIV infection in each part of the country are different. The northern epidemic wave has reached the family, while the north-eastern HIV epidemic is still confined to the IDUs and female CSWs. The southern and east-coast epidemics are spreading among the fishermen communities. The approach and response to these different epidemiological patterns should be strategically formulated by the local level, the so called provincial level.

## Estimations of HIV Infection

The estimation of the number of HIV infected persons in Thailand is computed from the following data sources:

1. The demographic projection estimated by sex at five-year intervals from the National Statistics Bureau;
2. The donated blood surveillance;
3. The sero survey of military conscripts, and
4. Sentinel surveillance at antenatal care clinics.

The tables (42.2 and 42.3) seen here are an example of the estimation of HIV infected persons in early 1992. The projection of the population in each cell is derived from the census data of 1990. The estimation of male HIV prevalence is derived from the calculation of low and high prevalence. The low prevalence is derived from the distribution of the age specific prevalence rate from the

*Table 42.3. Number of HIV positives among the Thai female population (low and high prevalence)*

| Age Group | Population | Female Pop. | Prev. Low | HIV+ Low | Prev. High | HIV+High |
|---|---|---|---|---|---|---|
| Less 5 | 5, 743, 000 | 2, 871, 500 | | | | |
| 5-9 | 5, 802, 000 | 2, 901, 000 | | | | |
| 10-14 | 6, 275, 000 | 3, 137, 500 | | | | |
| 15-19 | 6, 071, 000 | 3, 035, 500 | 1.0 | 30, 355 | 1.96 | 59, 495.8 |
| 20-24 | 6, 071, 000 | 3, 035, 500 | 1.0 | 30, 355 | 1.82 | 55, 246.1 |
| 25-29 | 5, 125, 000 | 2, 562, 500 | 1.0 | 25, 625 | 1.82 | 46, 637.5 |
| 30-34 | 5, 125, 000 | 2, 562, 500 | 1.0 | 25, 625 | 1.12 | 28, 700 |
| 35-39 | 3, 600, 000 | 1, 800, 000 | 1.0 | 18, 000 | 1.12 | 20, 160 |
| 40-44 | 3, 600, 000 | 1, 800, 000 | 0.5 | 9, 000 | 0.64 | 11, 520 |
| 45-49 | 2, 261, 000 | 1, 130, 500 | 0 5 | 5, 652.5 | 0.64 | 7, 235.2 |
| 50-54 | 2, 261, 000 | 1, 130, 500 | 0.1 | 1, 130.5 | 0.1 | 1, 130.5 |
| 55-59 | 1, 434, 000 | 7,17, 000 | 0.1 | 717 | 0.1 | 717 |
| 60-64 | 1, 434, 000 | 7,17, 000 | 0.1 | 717 | 0.1 | 717 |
| more 65 | 2, 240, 000 | 1, 120, 000 | | | | |
| Total | 57 789 000 | 28 894 500 | | | | |
| Grand Total | | | | | | 404 028 |

donated blood samples. The high prevalence is derived from the sero survey of conscripts in 1992 and then proportionally adjusted by the age specific prevalence of the donated blood samples. The estimation of the female high prevalence group is derived from the age specific prevalence rate of the antenatal care clinic sentinel surveillance. The number of infected cases in each age group and sex are calculated and then combined to present the total number of HIV infected persons in Thailand.

## 3. EFFECTIVE INTERVENTIONS FOR HIV/AIDS PREVENTION

As experience with HIV/AIDS prevention increases in the Region, it is becoming possible to highlight what comprises the key elements of success for interventions to change the behaviour. These elements include the use of mass media, peer-to-peer approaches and condom programming, which National AIDS Programme should consider while planning their intervention programmes to change risky behaviour. At the district or local level, a need exists to develop interventions that address local needs and are tailored to local constraints. The district-level health of ficers who wish to develop locally-based interventions for HTV prevention or to assist non-governmental organizations in doing so should focus on organizational capacity and management, situation assessment, development and planning of the intervention and on monitoring and evaluation. The intervention activities should either motivate people in changing their behaviour or assist in changing the structure or environment that either puts people at risk or inhibits their ability to change.

Examples of innovative and effective interventions in South-East Asia are highlighted below:

### 3.1 Promoting Safer Sex Behaviour—Innovative Approaches Among Individuals with High Risk Behaviour

#### 3.1.1 100 per cent Condom use Initiative in Thailand—an Update

Heterosexual intercourse is the most common mode of HIV transmission in Thailand. As of 30 September 1993, 75.5 per cent of 3 436 cumulative AIDS cases contracted the disease heterosexually. The most important factor relating to the rapid heterosexual HIV transmission is the sex entertainment industry. The total number of female sex workers in entertainment services in the whole country is estimated to be around 100, 000. They are the main sources of STD infection among male STD patients (i.e. over 96 per cent of male STD cases reported that they had contracted the disease from sex workers). Those infected acquired the HIV virus from their clients and then transmitted the virus to other clients who will further spread the disease to their wives and newborns. This trend is apparent from the increasing prevalence rate of HIV infection among sex workers, male patients attending STD clinics and pregnant women attending antenatal clinics.

Health education is the most important component in Thailand's AIDS programme. However, it is believed that the programme may be too slow to prevent effectively the spread of AIDS. Therefore, an effective programme to promote a higher degree of condom utilization is urgently required. In the past, efforts to promote condom use in Thailand relied mainly on information, education and communication activities. Reports from sentinel surveys showed that, as of December 1990, the average condom utilization rate among commercial sex workers was around 60 to 70 per cent and that among STD-clinic clients was under 50 per cent. As a result, the HIV infection rate among them still continued to increase.

It has been consistently observed that the majority of the sex workers want their clients to use condoms. However, they are unable to enforce such safety precaution regularly because a considerable number of clients refuse to use condoms. In some cases, even the owners of sex establishments pressure the sex workers to yield to the demand of their customers, that is to have sex without condom use. Therefore, increasing condom use within the sex industry was considered an arduous task.

In order to meet this challenge, the 100 per cent condom programme was initiated in August 1989 with the objective of promoting the use of condoms in sex establishments in Ratchaburi, a province in the central region, south of Bangkok. This will prevent heterosexual transmission of HIV among commercial sex workers and their clients, which will result in further prevention of HIV transmission to the general population.

*Objective and strategies.* The overall objective of the programme was to increase the rate of condom use in the sex establishments to 100 per cent. This is envisaged to be achieved through the co-operation of the government authorities and owners of the sex establishments in the province in order to instruct or require their sex workers to use condoms in all sexual encounters. If their customers refuse to use a condom, they are urged to withhold service and refund those customers' money. It is important that these measures be taken by all sex establishments in the area so that sex seekers will not be able to purchase sex services without using condoms in any sex establishment in the Province.

***Methods of implementation.*** The programme began with a joint meeting between the government sector (comprises three main agencies: health, police and local administration) and owners of all sex establishments (both direct and indirect sex facilities). This was to declare the initiation of the programme in the Province.

In the meeting, the owners of sex establishments were educated about the severity of AIDS, the current AIDS situation in Thailand and in the Province, and problems associated with AIDS control. They were encouraged to prevent the disease by instructing or ordering their sex workers to use condoms in all sexual encounters and to withhold sex service to customers refusing to use condom. These measures were to be taken by all sex establishments in the area so that sex seekers will not be able to purchase sex services without condom use in any sex establishment in the Province.

Also, at this time, the owners were made aware of the methods of investigation into condom use among sex workers that would be employed as a part of the programme monitoring process. The penalties administered to those establishments found to be uncooperative included temporary and indefinite closure of their establishments by the police. Methods of follow-up and investigation of the extent of condom use among sex workers included:

(a) Questioning male clients attending STD clinics concerning the use of condom in recent sexual encounters with prostitutes and the location of these entertainment places.

(b) Collecting information from STD contact notification forms sent from STD clinics outside the area.

(c) Sending volunteers to randomly test the sex workers' level of adherence to the "100 per cent-condom-use-only" policy in the local sex establishments.

(d) Observing STD infection rates among sex workers receiving routine examinations at local STD clinics. According to the provincial STD control programme, sex workers are motivated to have regular weekly check up at minimum or no cost.

(e) Monitoring the number of condoms provided to each sex establishment in the area. The owners as well as the sex workers were also informed about the benefits resulting from their co-operation. These benefits included the maintenance of their previous level of income and the lack of detrimental consequences associated with HIV infection among their employee population.

***Progress to date.*** The programme was satisfactorily run in the Province. The programme evaluation was performed by monitoring four factors which indicate progress and problems within the programme. These were (a) the prevalence of STD in the Province, (b) the prevalence of HIV infection in different target populations of each province from the sentinel serosurveillance, (c) attitude and practice relating to condom use among general population and groups at higher risk of STD infection, and (d) the provincial supply of condoms as well as the rate of condom use in sex establishments. The initial evaluation revealed satisfactory results especially in sex workers.

After successful implementation in Ratchaburi, the 100 per cent condom programme has been expanded to cover many nearby provinces since 1990. On 14 August 1991, the National AIDS Committee approved the nationwide expansion of the 100 per cent condom programme by issuing the following resolution: "The governor, the provincial chief of police and the provincial health officer of each province will work together to enforce a condom-use-only policy that requires all commercial sex workers to use condoms with every customer. All concerned ministries will issue directives that comply with this policy. In the case of Bangkok, the Bangkok Metropolis Administration and the Police Department are the operating agencies."

Since April 1992, all 73 provinces have reported the implementation of the programme to the Ministry of Public Health. It is still early to detect any decrease in HIV infection rate due to the 100 per cent condom programme. However, some promising results have been observed in most provinces. There has been *a marked increase in condom use in sex establishments* to a level as high as 90 per cent in June 1992. The *incidence of STD has decreased from* 6.5 per 1 000 population in 1989 to 4.48, 3.21 and 2.07 in 1990, 1991 and 1992 respectively. *The 1992 incidence is the record low in the last 20 years* (Figures 42.2 and 42.3).

***Elements considered crucial for the success.*** The following are considered as key elements for the success of the 100 per cent condom programme:

— High level commitment.

— Reduction of political, legal and social barriers.

— Participation and co-ordination of all responsible parties.

— Facilitative social pattern of target population, i.e. organized form of sex establishments.

— Efficient STD control system.

— Efficient condom promotion programme as well as logistic management and quality control.

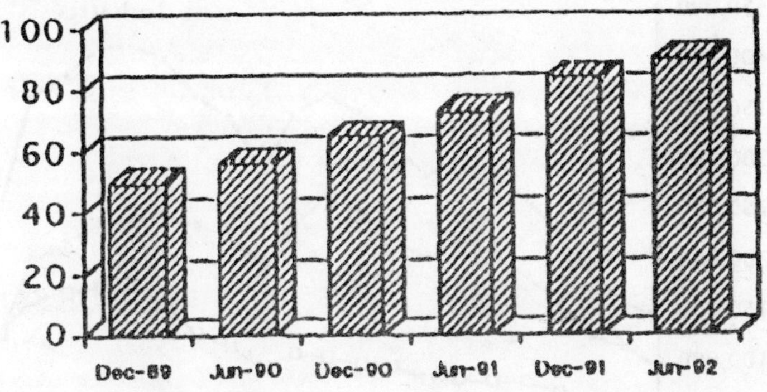


*Figure 42.2. Trends of condom use rate among clients of sex-workers in brothel settings*

— Benefit sharing nature of the programme.
— Lack of effective alternative strategies.

In conclusion, prevention of sexual transmission of HIV requires the active participation of both partners. However, such social and economic realities as poverty, inadequate education and subordinate social status may leave some individuals with little power or freedom to refuse intercourse or insist on the use of a condom. Sex workers in particular tend to be at higher risk of acquiring HIV infection through sex engaged in for economic survival. *The 100 per cent condom programme is an intervention to support and empower sex workers to be capable of controlling the action.* This will lead to the prevention of HIV infection among them and, thus, preventing the spread of HIV to the general population. With the implementation ofthe 100 per cent condom programme, the sexual transmission of AIDS will be greatly reduced nation-wide.

### 3.1.2 Peer Education and HIV Prevention Among Sex-Workers in Calcutta

In 1992, a community based sample survey of STD/HIV infections was carried out among the commercial sex-workers (CSW) of Sonagachi—a red light area in Calcutta. Sonagachi is one of the oldest and biggest red light areas in Calcutta having a population of 5,000 CSWs. The objectives of the study were to ascertain the prevalence of sexually transmitted diseases, to obtain

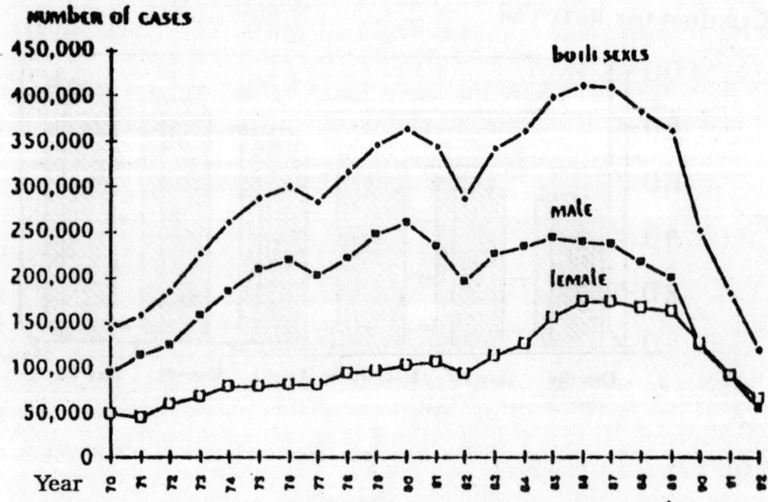


*Figure 42.3. Case report of STDs by sex (Thailand, 1970-1992)*

socio-economic information, to gather information about sexual behaviour and practices, to assess the extent of HIV infection, if any and to develop an intervention strategy of HIV/STD control. The survey was conducted jointly by All India Institute of Hygiene and Public Health and School of Tropical Medicine, Calcutta, 26 April to 6 June 1992. A sample of 450 CSWs were selected randomly and they were motivated to attend a clinic organized in the same area. CSWs were examined clinically to detect genital ulcers, genital warts, swelling of inguinal lymph nodes and signs of other STDs. Laboratory tests were conducted for four pathogens namely, *I.* pallidum by VDRL, TPHA & RPR, *N.* gonorrhoea - and *C.* albicans, by Gram stain and culture and *T.* vaginalis through wet mount in saline preparation.

An alarmingly high prevalence of STD was found among the CSWs. Seropositivity of syphilis was very high (62.97 per cent), followed by vaginal candidiasis (25.24 per cent), gonorrhoea (13.24 per cent), and trichomoniasis (11.11 per cent). It was also revealed from the study that about 81 per cent of CSWs are infected with one or more STD pathogens.

On the other hand, among 450 sex workers surveyed, 84.89 per cent were in the age group 15 - 29 years and about 84.44 per cent of the sex workers were found to be illiterate. It was also found that the majority of sex workers did not take any precaution against pregnancy. Clients of only 1.11 per cent of sex-workers were found to use condom regularly. Fortunately the HIV prevalence found among these sexworkers were very low (1.11per cent). Another positive aspect of this project was that during our survey work we were able to draw support from different sections of the community.

*Methods of implementation.* A batch of skilled field workers from a non-governmental organization assisted in the project and established good rapport with a large number of CSWs within a very short span of time. Though the study was completed by the early part of June 1992, the clinic continued to function as there was a great demand for the quality medical services provided by the project. The intervention programme of STD/HIV among the CSWs was started in September 1992 with assistance from NORAD, which is still continuing. Two non-governmental organizations, namely, Health and Eco-defence Society and Human Development and Research Institute, are active partners in this intervention programme. The programme components include early diagnosis and treatment of STDs, promotion of condoms and educational activities. To spearhead IEC and condom promotion activities, a batch of peer educators were identified and trained for a period of six weeks. The training curriculum included both technical and theoretical aspects of AIDS and STDs. They also received on an average 2-1/2 hours field training each day, six days a week for six weeks. At present there are 61 peer educators, who are the backbones of this intervention programme. House to house visit is the major communication strategy adopted in Sonagachi. Peer educators are divided in 12 groups. Seven of these groups are headed by one field supervisor - a social worker. Each group visits seven to eight brothels daily communicating with around 40-45 sex-workers and 5-6 "madams" (employees of the CSWs). They discuss different issues related to STD and AIDS, educate them regarding condom use with the help of flip charts and with other IEC materials and provide condoms according to the need and demand of the sex workers. They revisit the same brothel after a gap of six or seven days, assess the extent of condom use, collect information about non-compliance and complaints about quality of condoms.

*Progress to date:* At the start of this intervention programme, only 2,500 condoms were distributed throughout the month of September 1992. At present, roughly 62,000 condoms are being distributed to the CSWs every month, and it satisfies only 80 per cent of their demands. The use of condoms by the clients of the sex workers has been rapidly increasing as has been assessed by sentinel surveillance conducted in the month of May-June 1993 (Figure 42.4). The condom use has increased to 44 per cent compared to only 1 per cent about nine months ago.

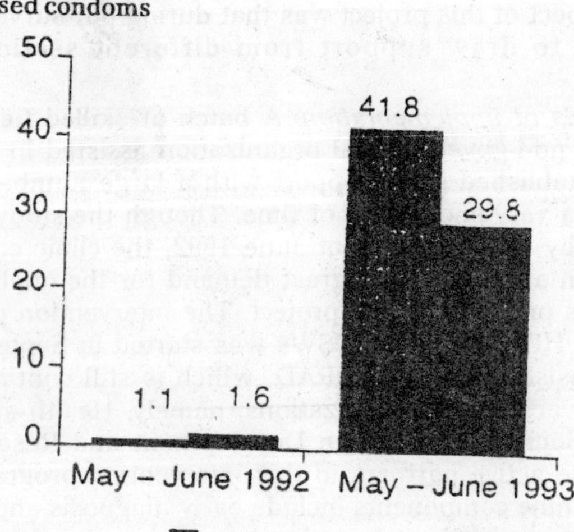


*Figure 42.4. Peer education among commercial sex workers, Calcutta*

It is true that the results placed above based on clinic attendance is not comparable qualitatively with the results of the community-based study conducted one year previously in the same population. However, it can provide some idea about the progress of activities in the area and it provides definite indication of changes in the sexual behaviour of clients. CSWs are being trained to develop skills to motivate clients on condom use through peer educators and field supervisors.

In the sex market, it is the buyer who dictates the norms and types of services that they would like to buy. So, various agencies involved in the trade need to be involved in the programme so as to motivate the clients to use condoms. At present, the intervention strategies include involvement of pimps, madams and landowners, and youth-club members. The twelve youth clubs of the area have been drawn into the fold of the intervention programme. Many youth-club members are actively involved in these activities. In fact both the clinics (one run in the morning and the other in the evening) are situated in the club premises. The morning clinic caters to 30-35 patients per day and the evening clinic (which is also attended by clients) caters to 15-20 patients per day. Through this clinic, we are providing medicine, counseling services, etc. Treatment is provided for all categories of illnesses. We provide the diagnosis of STD cases with laboratory support and also its management. These three-pronged activities have helped to increase the condom use of the clients and utilization of medical services by CSWs offered through those clinics. The impact of these activities is indicated by the decline in STD rates among the sex workers.

In conclusion, this project demonstrates the effectiveness of peer education in bringing about a behaviour change. *The commercial sex workers not only educate their peers and distribute condoms but provide the support necessary for behaviour modifications to occur.* The project also shows that implementation of such programmes among individuals with high risk behaviour can bring down STD rates and lead remarkably to maintaining HIV infection levels low. *Such programmes are essential and should be adapted for use in other parts of India and elsewhere.*

### 3.1.3 Targeted AIDS Campaign Among Transvestites in Indonesia

In Indonesia, studies show that upto 39 per cent of transvestites in many provinces are infected with syphilis, compared to less than 8 per cent of the prostitutes. During 1991/1992, HIV and STD serosurveys were carried out in 14 provinces with support from WHO. Results based on 18 194 individuals tested showed the STS (Serologic test for syphilis) positivity rates of 5.8 per cent among registered prostitutes; 7.5 per cent among unregistered prostitutes and 38.9 per cent among transvestites. A similar survey in 26 provinces conducted in 1992/1993, showed STS positivity rates of 7.7 per cent and 41.2 per cent among prostitutes and transvestites respectively.

Transvestites have a variety of occupations including hairdressing, beauty saloon management, entertainment, etc. As a matter of fact, they also engage in prostitution. Based on the above summary results, the Indonesian Public Health Association (IPHA) launched a health education campaign targeted at transvestites in Jakarta. A field study assessment of condom usage and availability among 59 commercial sex workers carried out in Jakarta in May 1992 by a consultant found that the transvestites in Jakarta were more likely to carry and use condoms when participating in penetrative sexual intercourse for payment than female and male CSWs in the city.

By the end of 1993, WHO-sponsored behavioural intervention projects—one in Jakarta to minimize HIV transmission among groups of Waria (transvestites) and the other in Surabaya by Perwakos (The Association of Surabaya Warias) to prevent HIV infection among transvestites had already been launched. These two transvestite projects are developed to be the prototypes of transvestite AIDS campaign, which can be replicated later in many other priority areas in Indonesia.

**The objectives** of these projects were to: (1) increase HIV/AIDS awareness and risk reduction practices among warias and their sexual partners (in Jakarta and Surabaya), (2) provide pre-test and post-test counselling for H1V seropositive and seronegative transvestites, their family members and partners, (3) provide a confidential HIV testing service, and (4) encourage the active participation of the waria community in preventing H1V transmission. Methods of implementation consist of training of peer group educators, designing and pretesting health education materials, condom promotion, establishing a clinic for Waria and outreach peer health education activities.

> **Results so far.** Under the project, 2,000 warias in Jakarta have already been given health education on HIV/AIDS. Blood samples from 500 warias in Jakarta and 400 warias in Surabaya were tested for H1V antibody, and in July a blood sample from one of the warias in Jakarta was found seropositive for H1V. The H1V seropositive waria was successfully persuaded to stop involving in prostitution and then become an owner of a beauty saloon. The important activities of the project are regular counselling, health services including laboratory examination (free of charge) and persuasion to change high risk behaviour/employment. Condom promotion is carried out through health education and social marketing. Each waria after having health education, including demonstration on how to use condom properly, is given 100 condoms. Whenever they need more condoms they can either buy them from condom sellers or request them from 1PHA. 1PHA has also launched a health education campaign targeted at transvestites.

An independent field assessment of condom usage and availability among 59 commercial sex workers (CSWs) carried out in Jakarta in May 1992 found that the transvestite CSWs in a location in Jakarta were more likely to carry and use condoms when participating in penetrative sexual intercourse for payment than female and male CSWs in the city. Moreover, the repeated observation that none of the transvestite CSWs would agree to unprotected receptive anal intercourse despite being offered twice the asking price (while all the male CSWs agreed to unprotected receptive anal intercourse at their initial asking price) highlights the marked difference in the attitude of these two CSW groups to condom use. There are anecdotal evidence to suggest that the transvestite CSWs were more knowledgeable and accept more readily safe sex practices. Another study showed that *condom use by Surabaya transvestites had increased from less than 5 per cent a year ago to 35 per cent in 1993, thereby demonstrating the effectiveness of the approach used among transvestites in Indonesia.*

## 3.2 PROMOTING SAFER SEX BEHAVIOUR: INNOVATIVE APPROACHES AMONG YOUTH

### 3.2.1 Universities Talk AIDS (UTA) in India: An Educational Experiment for Student-Youth

The National Service Scheme (NSS)—a student association for social welfare as part of its commitment to combat AIDS launched a project called "University Talk AIDS" (UTA) in 1991 in selected universities and colleges. The project has been designed and implemented by NSS with technical assistance from the World Health Organization (WHO) and the Ministry of Health and Family Welfare (MoHFW).

**The objectives.** The key objective of UTA was to raise awareness among university students of AIDS and STD. The project was directed towards creating desirable beliefs and attitudes towards AIDS and STD by providing accurate information on the subject and addressing the misconceptions that exist in the minds of the target audience. UTA's immediate objective is to raise the existing knowledge levels of university students and teachers on AIDS and STD. It was envisaged that the correct knowledge on AIDS and STD would slowly and gradually promote positive attitudes, which would, in turn, in the long run translate into a healthy and positive life-style. Thus, the long-term objective of UTA is to change the behaviour of today's youth.

**Methods of implementation.** In view of the communication objective of the Ministry of Health and Family Welfare, India, to reach appropriate information on AIDS to all young people in the age group of 15-30 years, the National Service Scheme identified the student community to be the primary target audience for the project. Positive attitudes among this target group could ensure a decelerated trend of students indulging in risk taking behaviour such as sharing of needles and syringes by drug users. The UTA programme is being implemented by the vast NSS network in the country. The key communication agents in the programme are the NSS volunteers. The project planners identified these volunteers to be both key informants and key influencers. They were identified as key informants or key communicators because this vast task force already existed in respective colleges and was engaged in implementing the other activities of NSS. Therefore, it was recognized that if this task force was trained on the subject, they could effectively reach out to the student and teaching community in their colleges.

The campaign was implemented step by step in the following manner:

## Step 1: Establishing Project Objectives

The social marketing approach has been used to conceptualise and design the project. The UTA programme planners recognized that the first step was to equip the NSS student volunteers with correct information and knowledge on AIDS. To this end, four regional training workshops were organized in the third week of November 1991. These were organized at New Delhi, Calcutta, Baroda and Madras. All the four training workshops were initiated with focus group discussions. These focus group discussions were conducted by an independent research agency called Social and Rural Research Institute. This is a specialist unit of the Indian Market Research Bureau. The objective of conducting focus group discussions was two fold:

1. The organizers (NSS and WHO) wished to explore attitudes to AIDS, extent of understanding of the subject and attitudes to matters that have a bearing on AIDS such as sexual practices, use of drugs and safe sex; and
2. To provide an opportunity to the participants to recognize their own beliefs, attitudes, inhibitions and misconceptions.

The first objective was crucial because, if the communication was to have any favourable impact, it was important to ensure that the medium itself (in this case the NSS volunteers) was geared to disseminate correct knowledge and attitudes. Ideally, the entire training programme should have been devised on the basis of the feedback received from the group discussions. However, due to constraints of time, it was not possible to delay the training of the initial batch of volunteers. Nevertheless, the inputs of research were utilized for subsequent trainings.

Focus group discussions were extremely useful for the volunteers because they helped them to shed their inhibitions and exposed them to the type of difficulties they would encounter while communicating on the subject. It also triggered a process of evaluating their own perceptions and that of their "peer group". Such sensitization helps to create a favourable atmosphere for programme intervention, by overcoming the resistance of people to change. In the UTA programme, this process helped in sensitizing the participants to the reality of the AIDS threat that was facing India. Thus, in this manner the NSS volunteers could be effectively mobilized to initiate a dialogue with their "peer group" on AIDS and its prevention.

The participatory approach which was adopted during the training workshops also ensured an environment in which the volunteers could unhesitantly seek clarifications for dispelling their own doubts and mis-conceptions on the subject. In order to assess the similarities and differences among NSS volunteers and the non-NSS students who formed the bulk of the target audience, group discussions were also conducted among non-NSS students in all the four centres. This was necessary because it was important to know the frame of mind of the target audience before planning any communication intervention.

## Step 2: Development of Campaign Strategy

The first phase of the UTA project focused on the development of the communication campaign strategy for the project. During the regional workshops, not only was information gathered about the knowledge, attitude and practice (KAP) of university students regarding sexuality and AIDS and awareness of HIV/AIDS generated among the communicators, but a series of targeted messages were also identified. On the basis of these messages communication materials were developed and designed for the project.

A unique approach was employed here. The communication materials were developed by the university students themselves. A nation-wide message and materials development contest was organized covering 65 universities across the country. After producing the initial draft of the materials they were pre-tested by the students themselves to ensure the efficacy of the materials. Based on the pre-test, necessary modifications were made to produce the prototypes which were again pre-tested and subsequently modified and refined. These materials were then collected, screened and judged at the state level in 20 states. A state-level ceremony was held at each of these venues to felicitate the winners, exhibit all the entries, involve the press and media to highlight the efforts of the students in the area of AIDS awareness and to generate interest among the general population. The prize-winning entries at the state-level were sent for the regional level competition where the two best entries were selected. A national ceremony was organized at New Delhi, where all the winning entries at the statelevel and the best eight entries (two from each region) were exhibited.

The material development contest was highly successful due to the following reasons:

1. Effective Communication materials were developed by the target group themselves. These materials were tested to ascertain that they actually conveyed what they were designed to convey.
2. The student community, i.e. the beneficiaries of the programme were mobilized and enthused .
3. A socio-anthropological content analysis of the communication materials was undertaken. This provided insights into the students perceptions about AIDS and

helped in identifying their biases and fears. This helped in identifying the existing perception and the desired perceptions.

Thus, the material development contest created a favourable tempo and environment for expanding the project activities. The participatory approach which was followed during the material development contest helped he creating a sense of involvement and "ownership" of the UTA programme. The empathy that was generated made the task of awareness generation and attitude change much simpler. Thus, the target audience was favourably disposed to further project intervention and this ensured a committed target audience.

## Step 3: Implementation of Pilot Campaign

In order to sustain the tempo created during the first phase, NSS launched another countrywide mass awareness campaign entitled "AIDS AWARE college campaign". It was a week long campaign, which was launched last year on World AIDS Day. During this week a variety of activities were organized such as blood donation campaign, poster exhibitions, quiz on AIDS, public rallies and discussions, games and street plays. During this, demonstrations on correct use of condoms were also organised. The objectives of organising the World AIDS week were: (1) to assess the existent level of knowledge on AIDS/HIV, (2) to increase the level of awareness on AIDS/HIV, (3) it aimed at increasing the level of commitment of the target audience (University students) towards UTA, and (4) to create centres of consciousness on AIDS, thus providing launching pads for extending the coverage of UTA.

The objectives (3) and (4) were essentially directed at sensitizing and mobilizing students for playing a positive role both as receivers and providers of communication. This signifies the chain reaction where, over a time, the receiver of communication becomes the provider of communication. Thus, the requisite information reaches the entire target community. The UTA programme has various research components woven into it. This helps in both evaluating the performance of the programme and providing effective guidance and direction for the future. Thus, integrated targeted research has helped in ensuring pragmatism in the UTA programme.

**Progress to date.** During phase II of UTA, a evaluation study was also conducted. A brief questionnaire was given, both prior to and after the World AIDS Week, to the participants, to assess their level of knowledge and attitudes towards AIDS and related issues. This approach also helped in ascertaining the impact of the week-long campaign.

After the World AIDS Week, more than 200 colleges were declared "AIDS AWARE". In the UTA programme, specific criteria had been laid out for declaring a college "AIDS AWARE". In order to meet these criteria the colleges had to organize specific activities, and weightage was also given to the level of participation of its students he each activity.

The above approach ensured that messages were disseminated to the concerned target audience, through their active participation. It also created an atmosphere, where issues which were only joked about or were discussed in hushed tones could be discussed he the open. The momentum that had been set also helped the target audience to realize that AIDS was not distant. Therefore, it was in their own self-interest to know about AIDS and methods of its prevention. Moreover, the strategy of declaring colleges as being "AIDS AWARE" also helped generating a "sense of pride" and "ownership" of the programme among its students all of which went a long way in ensuring a more lasting impact of the communication intervention.

*The first two phases of UTA covered around 250 colleges across 65 universities in the country. The target of covering 100 universities by 1994 and all the universities and higher secondary schools by 1995 has been set.*

### 3.2.2 AIDS/STD Education in Schools in Mongolia

The reporting of the first HIV infected case in the country in 1992 provided an impetus for AIDS/STD education ha schools. In the absence of a cure for AIDS or a vaccine against HIV infection and in view of the increasing rates of STD among youth, education is recognized to be critical in prevention and reducing the transmission of both AIDS and STD in Mongolia. *Since considerable proportion of young people can easily be reached through schools, colleges and universities and may learn in the classroom the facts, values and skills they need to protect themselves from HIV infection, the Government, by issuing in 1992, decree No.18 entrusted the Ministry of Science and Education (MSE) and the Ministry of Health (MoH) with the task of integrating AIDS education within existing curricula in schools and postgraduate institutions at all levels.*

Objectives. The objectives of AIDS/STD education in schools are to impart appropriate knowledge, skills and attitudes to young people in order to form a basis for safe sexual behaviour that would permit them to protect themselves and others from infection before they have their first sexual experience, permit effective communication, responsible decision-making and the development of healthy human relationships.

*Progress in promoting AIDS/STD education in schools.* As part of the ongoing education reform programme, a new curriculum for the ten-year secondary education course has been developed by the Institute of Curriculum and Methodology under the National Pedagogical University and issued in 1991 by the then Ministry of Education. In 1992 the Ministry of Health submitted to the Ministry of Science and Education some proposals on a broad health education programme, including modules on HIV/AIDS/STD in the curricula of formal and non-formal (adults) education.

Keeping in mind the WHO guidelines, attention is paid in Mongolia to AIDS/STD education in schools by:

(1) developing a good curricula with substantial classroom time and environment for social and behavioural skills development,
(2) training teachers and preparation of guidelines and manuals,
(3) preparation and making available for children and students educational printed and audio-visual materials and textbooks,
(4) using all forms of education (mass or in target groups, formal or non-formal, use participatory or didactic methods, curricular or extra-curricular like role plays, etc.),
(5) creating an awareness on how AIDS is easily acquired, and the relevance of social, cultural, and behavioural contexts in the country,
(6) involving parents,
(7) monitoring and evaluating AIDS education, and
(8) ensuring that the subject can be taught.

Because of the new and sensitive nature of AIDS issues and their association with sexual behaviour, questions like what (content), how (styles), when (in what age) should be taught in schools with regard to AIDS/STD and who is to do it need a careful approach. The Ministry of Science and Education has decided to incorporate within the subjects "biology" and "physical education and health", the following modules in the existing (partly renewed) curriculum of secondary schools:

1. 4th grade (11-12 years of age): danger of HIV infection and AIDS to humankind
2. 8th grade (15-16 years of age): HIV/AIDS, STD, routes of transmission, role of immunity, ways of protection from HIV/AIDS/STD, anatomy and physiology of sexual organs
3. 8-10th grades (16-18 years of age): human relationships,

sexuality, healthy sexual behaviour, HIV/AIDS/STD and their prevention.

In October 1993, a one-day seminar was held for school teachers in charge of teaching "biology" and "physical education and health" in the capital city's secondary schools with the aim of providing information on global and country HIV/AIDS/STD situation and guidelines based on WHO recommendations in developing a curriculum for AIDS/STD education at the school level. In aimaks (provinces) and other cities, epidemiologists in charge of HIV/AIDS problems are assisting in developing and adapting modules on AIDS/STD education at local school level. Activities facilitating AIDS education in schools, such as preparation, printing and distribution of guidelines and manuals for school teachers, textbooks for children, conducting national workshops to train trainers of school teachers who will be responsible for AIDS education, have been included in the 1994 draft working plan for implementation of MTPII for AIDS Prevention and Care in Mongolia. These activities will be implemented by the Ministry of Science and Education in co-operation with the Ministry of Health keeping in mind WHO recommendations.

With regard to AIDS education at postgraduate institutions, lectures on the subject are being regularly given to students in order to sensitize and create awareness among them about HIV/AIDS/STD. Modules on etiology, pathogenesis, clhlical features, and consequences of HIV/AIDS have been aded newly to curricula of the National Medical University, National University and Pedagogic University. In some universities and colleges, some student organizations have started to deal with AIDS through condom promotion and promotion of safer sex behaviour.

## 3.3 CONDOM PROGRAMMING

### 3.3.1 Condom Social Marketing—a Major Priority

Social marketing is marketing through existing commercial outlets, a consumer good that fulfils a public health or a social need. It is subsidized by donors and/or governments to keep retail costs down and to increase access to the product by low income target audiences. Condom Social Marketing (CSM) is an approach that has been used in many developing countries to promote and distribute condoms for family planning, and for *STD/AIDS* prevention.

In South-East Asia, 396 million condoms were distributed in 1992 through CSM in 6 countries (Bangladesh, India, Indonesia, Nepal, Sri Lanka and Thailand), with India and Bangladesh contributing 67 per cent and 30 per cent respectively.

## How Does Condom Social Marketing Work?

CSM is powerful because:

(1) people are more likely to use a condom purchased, even at low, subsidized prices rather than one that is given away free of charge by the government;

(2) it utilizes an existing distribution infrastructure of private retailers such as pharmacies, drug stores, food stores, hotels, and non-traditional outlets such as street vendors, bars, bazaars, barber shops, taxis, gasoline stations, vending machines and other;

(3) campaigns draw upon a wide range of communication techniques, including:

   (a) mass media advertising;

   (b) traditional media such as street theatre troupes and folk bands, especially in rural areas;

   (c) information, education and communication materials including comic books, leaflets, flyers, posters, videos and other;

   (d) face-to-face communication and peer outreach;

   (e) product promotion such as sponsored events, point-of-sale promotional items such as 2-for-the price of l or free samples of condoms; and,

(4) it uses public relations techniques to generate wide support among government and political leaders, the general public and the media.

## CSM Increases Competition and Reduces Dependency on Public Sector Support

Marketing and product costs are subsidized so that condoms can be offered to consumers at a price that more people find affordable; while at the same time, some of government and donor costs of providing condoms are defrayed through revenue generated by the increased sale of the products.

There is a convincing evidence that condom social marketing promotional efforts stimulate the entire condom market. This means that other commercial condom marketers tend to increase promotion and advertising and sometimes even lower their prices in response to social marketing programmes. The increased competition enhances condom promotion and helps build a broader and more viable commercial condom market. CSM however tend more to be urban based, its implementation is initially costly, and serving rural areas is an expensive proposition.

In summary, *condom social marketing (CSM) programnle* channels providing broad access to attractive (commercially-developed), affordable (subsidized price) products for low income people at risk. While using private sector marketing techniques, CSMs are not-for-profit, socially-motivated programmes which generate income that can be used to offset the costs of operating the programme.

### 3.3.3 Condom Social Marketing in Bangladesh: Experiences from Family Planning

In Bangladesh, a country with 110 million people, the CSM programme has been in existence since 1974, funded by USAID and run by the parent organization Population Services International (PSI). CSM is a nonprofit-making concern engaged in providing low cost health and family planning products and services to lower income people. *The CSM has an extensive network reaching remotest parts of the country.* Four brands of condoms are being promoted and sold in the country. However, the public media such as television and radio have been prohibited from promoting condoms, and the words 'sex' and 'condoms' cannot be used in the television or radio broadcasting.

Despite such socio-cultural and religious constraints prohib iting condom promotion, particularly in the public broadcasting media, condom sales since 1983 have increased significantly, both in urban and rural areas; (but particularly more so in urban areas). The 25,000 family welfare centres and personnel of the non-governmental organizations account for nearly 70 per cent of condom distribution in the country.

## 3.4 STD PREVENTION AND CARE

### 3.4.1 STD prevention initiatives in Bhutan

Sexually transmitted diseases (STD) are a substantial problem in Bhutan. There has been reports of high prevalence STD he certain areas, and in antenatal clinic attenders the prevalence of STD and Chlamydia have been found to be quite high. Genital ulcers, urethral discharge and vaginal discharges are the most commonly seen STDs. The sluggish healtll-seeking behaviour of the peoplc, especially among women, due to shyness and lack of symptoms, and lack of diagnostic facilities, are some constraints he assessing the actual situation, and contribute to the spread of the diseases. With the initiation of AIDS prevention activities ha 1988-89, STDs have come under the umbrella of AIDS/STD control programme. The programme is fully integrated in the existing health system, and there are no special STD/VD clinics

**Strategies.** The strategies that were adopted to strengthen the ongoing STD control activities included the establishment of the AIDS/STD control programme office, providing a management structure, and STD awareness activities targeted at the general population as well as special population groups such as students, armed forces and opinion leaders. Awareness campaigns focused on sensitizing about condom use and increasing awareness of how to prevent transmission.

Awareness activities were also intensified in high STD prevalent areas and border towns. In a high STD prevalent area, a mass education campaign was carried out to cover all the people. The campaign covered a gewog (block) with intensive information on STD/AIDS and their prevention. People in a locality were gathered by giving them prior information, and documentary and health education films were screened. This strategy drew a near 100 per cent crowd as films are a powerful media. After the gathering was fully settled and put at ease, slide presentations on STDs followed by condom promotion were carried out. The discussions that ensued clarified many issues and tried to clear the misconceptions people had about STDs. This mass education activity was also utilized to train the health personnel including health in-charge and village health workers in the district to carry out similar activities in their respective blocks. Therefore, the campaign not only aimed at educating the people about STD/AIDS but also trained the health personnel so that they could carry out similar activities in their areas, thus spreading awareness throughout the district.

*Standardization of case management.* A case management guideline based upon syndromic approach was prepared and distributed to all health facilities. The guidelines emphasize adequate and appropriate treatment, proper follow up and the importance of individual health education on disease transmission and risk reduction.

*Training of health care personnel.* To prepare the health workers for disease surveillance, management and prevention of STDS, almost all staff of the basic health units and a few hospital-based staff have been trained.

*Research.* A *KABP* (knowledge, attitude, behaviour and practice) survey and a Chlamydia prevalence study were conducted. A preliminary study to determine the prevalence of PPNG is under way. Pilot activities are being undertaken to improve the availability of condoms.

*In conclusion,* initiatives for the prevention of STDs in Bhutan have endeavoured to reduce the transmission of STDs and prevent the morbidity and mortality associated with it by establishing an integrated STD/AIDS control programme, extensive IEC campigns, standardization of management of STDs, development of laboratory capacity for early case detection and quality control, and training of health personnel to improve the quality of care.

Though no studies have been conducted as yet to assess the impact of the initiatives, *it is generally felt that the initiatives have succeeded in increasing the awareness about STDS, increasing the use of condoms, and reducing the incidence of STD in certain areas.* However, there are many constraints in further pursuing the achievements. It will be crucial to overcome these constraints for the success of the prevention initiatives in Bhutan, which include low literacy rate, lack of manpower resources, and lack of financial resources.

### 3.4.2 STD Control Activities in India

In India, a country with the second largest population after China, STD problem in the past has not been taken up as earnestly as it should have been. Precise information on the magnitude of STD as a public health problem is not available. It is however estimated that only 5 per cent-10 per cent of STD cases in the country take treatment from government STD clinics. No information is available with respect to the remainder of the STD patients who may be taking treatment outside government clinics.

In the first half of 1992, a number of STD baseline surveys were conducted in Jaipur, Madras, a rural area in Tamil Nadu, and in a red light area in Calcutta. In Jaipur 519 males were selected from transport and industrial workers, and 250 patients attending ante-natal clinics (ANC) for inclusion in the survey. On clinical examination 2.1 per cent of the males suffered from urethral discharge, while 0.8 per cent had a genital ulcer. Of the ANC attenders 58 per cent had a vaginal discharge, 27 per cent complained of lower abdominal pain, and 18.4 per cent complained of dysuria.

In Madras and Tamil Nadu study VDRL positivity ranged from 0.8 per cent among the industrial workers to 10 per cent in female remand prisoners, with relatively high rates in ANC attenders (1.74 per cent) and the rural population (3.3 per cent in females and 3.6 per cent ha males). The STD baseline study in a red light area in Calcutta was the first population based STD survey among sex workers, based on a cluster sampling technique. Not surprisngly, the study showed that only 25 per cent of the sex workers did not have any STD; 52 per cent suffered from a single infection, while 23 per cent had two or more infections. A repeat survey was conducted in 1993-94, 12 monthes after a comprehensive intervention project had been initiated. The initial analysis of the results of the repeat survey showed that the prevalence had declined for gonorrhoea by 66 per cent, from 13.2 per cent to 4.4 per cent, for trichomoniasis by 31 per cent, from 11. 1 per cent to 2.5 per cent, while the VDRL positivity declined by 20 per cent. The HIV prevalence increased by only 53 per cent, from 1.3 per cent to 1.6 per cent. Antenatal-clinic attenders are in principle screened for syphilis. The prevalence of positive syphilis serology ranges from 1.2 per cent to 4.8 per cent in various groups of ANC attenders.

The policy adopted by the Technical Advisory Sub-Committee on STD for the control and prevention of STD, emphasizes the syndromic approach for the management of STD patients. A training module for "STD case management for first level doctors" is currently being developed. This module will form the basis for the training of first level doctors, in both the public and the private sector for STD case management. It is envisioned that the specialized STD clinics will play an important role in providing services for referral, training and supervision, and research. Monitoring of antibiotic susceptibility and the efficacy of the syndromic approach will also be done through these centres.

The existing guidelines for diagnosis, treatment and laboratory diagnosis of STD patients have been reviewed and "Simplified STD Treatment Guidelines" have been published. These provide treatment guidelines for syndromic management of STD patients. *In recognition of the fact that women have little access to non-stigmatizing services for STD care, an attempt is made to incorporate STD prevention and control in the existing family welfare services, as part of the reproductive health services.* A number of pilot projects are under development, to assess the feasibility, the cost and the outcome of such an integrated service.

One of the main strategies of the National Plan for the Prevention and Control of AIDS in India is the prevention and control of STD. Planning of STD control activities is a responsibility of the state AIDS officers, or where applicable the state STD officers. Plans have been received from a number of states, although not in all cases do these plans prioritize sufficiently for identified high-risk behaviour groups. A number of STD planning workshops have been organized, and further training will take place during the programme managers' training, which is planned for the second half of 1994. Technical assistance for the planning of state and municipal level STD control activities is provided from the centre, as is regular supervision. A management information system for the AIDS programme is currently under development. This includes a number of key indicators to monitor the implementation of the STD control component. An STD surveillance system is also being developed, with a first draft of an STD surveillance/protocol currently being reviewed.

## 3.5 BLOOD SAFETY

### 3.5.1 Blood Transfusion Services in Sri Lanka

In Sri Lanka, blood safety is one of the major activities in prevention and control of HIV/AIDS. All blood donations are screened for HIV, prior to transfusion. The blood safety is the responsibility of the National Blood Transfusion Services and the Central Laboratory for STD/AIDS control which come under the Ministry of Health.

Blood is declared as a drug in some parts of the Region, hence it must be carefully managed. Among important activities is provision of safe blood transmission. There must be a correct assessment of the demand and mobilization of the voluntary agencies for collecting blood through voluntary blood donation camps. Blood transfusion must be kept as a last resort and blood should be transfused only if it is a must to save life. Testing of pooled sera assists in cost-saving in Sri Lanka because HIV prevalence is still very low.

### 3.5.2 Rational Use of Blood in Nepal

Nepal Red Cross Society is responsible for providing the entire quantity of blood required for use by various hospitals and institutions in the country. The blood donation is a part and parcel of the activities included in the HIV/AIDS control programme and the blood donation is on a non remunerative basis. Prior to 1992, facilities for screening of blood were poor; after 1992, the programme embarked on a plan to go for universal screening of donated blood. Some of the policies and strategies which were formulated by the Kingdom of Nepal include:

1. Blood will be collected *only on* non-remunerative basis;
2. all collected blood meant for transfusion will be screened for HIV and VDRL;
3. Rational use of blood will be advocated and promoted throughout the Kingdom.

The government has started a targeted programme of regular training for medical personnel with regard to safe blood services through rational and judicious blood transfusions. These measures are expected to improve tremendously the blood safety situation in Nepal.

## 4. HIV/AIDS CARE

### 4.1 Development of Community and Home-Based Care for People with HIV/AIDS in Thailand

The concept of providing effective and humane care to people with HIV/AIDS must extend beyond the provision of acute, in-patient hospital care. Appropriate medical and social support services need to extend and include the community and families of people with AIDS. The characteristics of various difficulties and problems affecting AIDS patients might be divided into two types:

*Underlying Structural Problems.* The beginning of the AIDS epidemic is that of the silent HIV epidemic. The three modes of HIV infection may not be known equally well among all members of society, and certain groups may, by their very social status, be placed at greater risk of acquiring HIV infection. These individuals and clusters of groups may include isolated hill tribe villagers, low income urban slum-dwellers, illiterate and poorly educated hldividuals (particularly women), male and female sex workers, as well as injecting drug users. National efforts to reach out and inform all members of society about HIV/AIDS may first reach the higher to middle income groups, with greater access to information, communication and health services. Such underlying structural differences within the population place certain individuals at greater risk of infection. These same differences will also affect the delivering and availability of community care.

*Problems associated directly with HIV infection:* Persons with HIV will face additional problems, which may be classified into three stages:

1. *Asymptomatic stage:* During the asymptomatic stage, a person with HIV may face no new particular problem. However, should his or her HIV status become known to others, very real problems can soon develop. Healthy people with HIV may be tested without voluntary consent in many circumstances. In some countries, patients attending STD clinics as well as sex workers may be required to undergo mandatory testing. In other countries, medical staff may routinely test all patients. As a result of such testing, people with HIV may experience considerable fear and anxiety. These fears may include the fear of dying, social discrimination, loss of employment and rejection by friends and family.
2. *Symptomatic stage.* As HIV infection progresses to AIDS disease, individuals find it increasingly difficult to continue with daily-life activities. A person may no longer be able to work, and entire families may be placed into

economic crisis. Physical strength disappears and leaves individuals dependent on other care givers.

3. *Terminal stage.* At the final stage before death, PWAs require even more spiritual support and compassion. If they have children, they may also want someone to take care of their children.

The problems that PWAs face are complex and tend to become more severe as time passes. In order to provide care for AIDS patients and family, the services must be comprehensive and integrated at every level from household to community to institutional.

The care should include:

1. *Medical and nursing services:* in-patient and outpatient care, home nursing, hospice care, etc.
2. *Psychosocial support:* counselling, information and education, establishment of self-help groups, etc.
3. *Practical support:* social welfare services, housing, meals, transportation, recreation, child care, etc.
4. *Legal, ethical services:* protection of human rights, health and life insurance, access to medical care, etc.

The care should be continuously provided. At household and community levels, community based and home-based care should be provided.

*Activities so far.* To achieve the objective of establishing community-based and home-based care of AIDS patients he Thailand, efforts were made to compile ideas from experts in the area of community-based and home-based care among governmental and non-governmental agencies in early 1992. The idea was then translated into two projects. One was to develop a network of social services which will co-ordinate support for AIDS patients, and the second was to develop models of community-based and home-based care for AIDS patients in northern Thailand, where the epidemic is more advanced.

The first project which started in late 1992 for a six-month duration, emphasized the development and strengthning of networks among various social service agencies (public welfare offices, counselling clinics and the social welfare section in hospitals) in twelve selected provinces. Participating social workers realized the importance and need for providing care and social support to people with HIV and AIDS. It is shown that the project could provide services for 3,107 people with HIV/AIDS (3,670 service-episodes) during the study period. Among all episodes, 2,502 (68.2 per cent) were counselling, 1,050 (28.6 per cent) were financial support, and the rest were referral service and others. However, there is a need to train more social workers to increase understanding of the concept of confidentiality and counselling, as well as ways of assessing the problems of clients and home-visit techniques. One of the recommendations from this project was to allocate financial assistance for people with HIV and AIDS.

The second project focuses on the development of a manual on home-based care for AIDS patients. A workshop was conducted for representatives of 25 organizations (government and non-governmental) from the northern provinces. All participating agencies were requested to conduct a community-based and home-based care project in their local area. The project is going on. The feasibility will assessed and the lessons learned from each project will be studied at the end of this year. The home-based care manual will be evaluated. Training in and implementation of, community-based and home-based care will be expanded to cover more areas next year.

Other activities that will enable the possibilities of community-based and home-based care is to support non-governmental organizations working in the area of care. Since the beginning of the AIDS prevention and control programme, the Ministry of Public Heath (MOPH) has supported many non-governmental organizations working with AIDS patients, both technically and financially. Most non-governmental organizations provide comprehensive care in collaboration with other government and non-governmental organizations. The MoPH is also interested in setting up rehabilitation centres for AIDS patients who need basic physical and psychological support before returning back to the community. These rehabilitation centres will also serve as training sites for AIDS patients and their families. The first centre is expected to open early next year. Seven more centres throughout the country are planned to be opened during 1994-1995.

*Obstacles.* The major obstacle is the attitude of the public towards AIDS patients. There is still irrational fear of HIV/AIDS. Some groups of people do not understand and do not want to accept people with HIV/AIDS to live within the same community. The community-based and home-based care programme should also look into ways of changing the public attitude from fear, stigma and ignorance to acceptance, compassion and support for AIDS patients and their families. In this respect, educational messages now need to focus more on how to live with HIV/AIDS in society.

*In conclusion,* as the epidemic becomes more evident, *Thailand is beginning to develop strategies for communities to live with HI V and AIDS by integrating community-based and home-based care into the existing primary health care network.* It is important to acknowledge that community care requires an integrated joint effort by all concerned institutes, organizations and people. *In order to develop successful programmes to support people with HIV/*

*AIDS, stigma and fear about HIV and AIDS must be overcome.*

## 4.2 Development of Counselling Services in Myanmar

Myanmar's experiences of counselling services at the beginning have been very limited. Very few competent counsellors were available to provide the counselling service, and these were available only to the urban population, none of the non-governmental organizations worked in this area, and services were available largely in specialized service hospitals. However, since HIV/AIDS is now appearing in urban as well as rural areas, hospitals in both urban and rural areas have to provide the counselling services. The objectives of the counselling service in Myanmar are to:

1. provide psycho-social support for people who are infected with HIV:
2. provide information regarding the danger of high-risk behaviours in order to prevent them from becoming infected with HIV and to prevent transmission from them to the community.

The strategy for the development of counselling services in Myanmar included training of health workers especially in the areas where HIV/AIDS patients would most likely come for care; inclusion of counselling in the training courses of basic health workers so that they understand the importance of counselling. They can also, where possible, refer cases to a well-equipped hospital where specialists' services are available. The Government of Myanmar during 1992-1993 took the following steps in the development of counselling services:

(1) establishment of a counselling team and the AIDS prevention and control programme. The team conducts trahaing courses for people to become counsellors, and to monitor services provided to cases which were referred to the nearby referral centre;

(2) with financial assistance from WHO, several training courses for counsellors were conducted from September 1992 and during 1993; as well as an advance course for conllsellors who had undergone the counsellor's training previously;

(3) arrangements were made for counsellors to attend the monthly meetings to share their experiences and also get technical support from the experts;

(4) The Government issued directions to the department of health and superintendents of major hospitals to provide necessary support for counsellors to carry out their work.

In spite of these steps which the National AIDS programme

in Myanmar took for developing counselling activities, there still remain several constraints which need to be overcome. These include lack of money for conducting training courses, difficulty in selecting health workers who have the right attitude to undertake counselling, inadequate monitoring of the work being performed by the counsellors in the remote peripheral areas; and difficulties in distributing the health education material to counsellors in the rural areas.

## 5. PROGRAMME MANAGEMENT AND CO-ORDINATION

### 5.1 Multi-Sectoral Collaboration and Co-ordination:

#### Thailand's National AIDS Programme

As our understanding and knowledge has grown over the last decade in terms of the scope and impact of the HIV/AIDS pandemic, it is clear that the response to the epidemic transcends the responsibility of the health sector, thus requiring a multi-sectoral response. In recognition of this, Government of Thailand has taken decisive steps to encourage and enhance participation by various sectors and groups involved in AIDS work.

Collaboration among and co-ordination between various sectors and participating parties poses a great challenge for the country to facilitate involvement by all concerned parties in a way that will improve the overall national response to the AIDS epidemic as well as in making the most effective and efficient use of limited resources available to an ever-increasing number and wide-range of organizations becoming involved. The parties involved that are increasingly playing a more active role in AIDS efforts in Thailand include government ministries and offices, private sector, non-governmental organizations and multilateral and bilateral agencies (see Table 42.4).

Collaboration among various sectors and groups occurs through both formal and informal co-ordination mechanisms, which have been established and adapted to meet the rapidly changing nature of the AIDS situation in Thailand.

*Formal-Co-ordination Mechanism and Structure.* At central level, the National AIDS Committee (NAC) chaired by the Prime Minister with the Ministry of Public Health (MOPH) as the secretariat, serves as the national policy and broad co-ordination body of Thailand's National AIDS Programme. Included as members of the National AIDS Committee are representatives from all government ministries, special public agencies, non-governmental organizations, private sector and eminent experts. Sub-committees to consider various technical issues with regards to AIDS are appointed as appropriate and revised from time to time. AIDS policies are approved by the Cabinet and endorsed by the Parliament. These policies have been articulated within the Seventh Five-Year National Social and Economic Development Plan of the country and have been expounded in a Five-Year National AIDS Plan (1992-1996), providing the framework and guidelines within which HIV/AIDS activities are planned and implemented. The National AIDS Plan serves as an important co-ordination tool.

*Each ministry has developed implementation plans for AIDS prevention and control activities consistent with the National AIDS Plan.* In addition, each ministry has established an AIDS committee and assigned focal persons for co-ordination.

The provincial structure of the Ministry of Public Flealth and the Ministry of Interior plays a very important role he country-wide co-ordination. AIDS committees have been set-up at provincial and district levels, witil representation from local ministries, government and health offices and in some cases non-governmental organizations. They are responsible for developing AIDS implementation plans. STD/AIDS centres and clinics have been established at provincial and district levels and serve as co-ordination nodes for activities. At the primary health care level, village volunteers are active in disseminating AIDS information.

Thailand is currently in the early stages of a multi-sectoral planning exercise to revise the present Five-Year National AIDS Plan in order to develop further the implementation plan for 1995-1996, addressing the rapidly changing circumstances. In August 1993, all ministries, various government offices, non-governmental organizations, United Nations agencies and the private sector participated in a National Formulation Workshop of the implementation Plan for 1995-1996,organized by the National Economic and Social Development Board. This was a brainstorming exercise for various actors to contribute to an open participatory process by expressing views and experiences and to suggest revisions and additions to the current plan for consideration by a multi-sectoral working group. These inputs are being compiled and formulated into a policy framework which will include guidelines and measures to implement strategies. This plan will be endorsed by the National AIDS Committee and the Cabinet. A revised plan is expected by the end of the year in time to mobilize resources for the remaining two years of the Plan. Every ministry as well as non-governmental organizations will be requested to submit their plans/programmes for considerating the budget allocation from the Bureau of the Budget.

**Table 42.4.**
**Role of Agencies in Prevention and Control of AIDS, Thailand**

| Agencies | Programmes | | | |
|---|---|---|---|---|
| | Public Information | Treatment and Care | Human Rights | Research and Evaluation |
| I Office of the Prime Minister | ... | ... | ... | ... |
| 2. Ministry of Public Health | ... | ... | ... | ... |
| 3 Ministry of Interior | ... | ... | ... | ... |
| 4. Ministry of Education | | | | |
| 5. Ministry of Defense | ... | ... | ... | ... |
| 6. Ministry of University Affairs | ... | ... | ... | ... |
| 7. Ministry of Justice | ... | ... | ... | ... |
| 8. Ministry of Finance | ... | ... | ... | ... |
| 9. Ministry of Industry | ... | ... | ... | ... |
| 10. Ministry of Transport and Communications | ... | ... | ... | ... |
| 11. Ministy of Commerce | ... | ... | ... | ... |
| 12. Ministy of Science and Tech. and Energy | ... | ... | ... | ... |
| 13. Ministry of Foreign Affairs | ... | ... | ... | ... |
| 14. Minisly of Agriculture and Co-operative | ... | ... | ... | ... |
| 15. State Enterprises | ... | ... | ... | ... |
| 16. Non-Government Non-Profit Agencies | ... | ... | ... | ... |
| 17. Business Sector | ... | ... | ... | ... |
| Total | 17 | 9 | 17 | 17 |

Notes: ... Most Involvement .. Moderate Involvement . Some Involvement

*Informal Co-ordination Mechanism.* In addition to the formal co-ordination mechanism and structure that exists, there are a number of informal processes going on which include a non-governmental consortium against AIDS in Bangkok, a northern Thailand non-governmental consortium, donors and United Nations agencies which all meet once a month, on a voluntary basis to be briefed and up-dated on the national AIDS policies, plans and situation in Thailand. These forums serve as an informal channel for groups to co-ordinate, share and exchange information on activities and resources. In addition, there is inter-communication and intra-communication, often through individual contacts with government, between ministries, non-governmental organizations, donors and United Nations agencies.

In the private sector, there is currently co-operation between businesses involved in the sex industry, the Ministry of Interior and the Ministry of Public Health in implementing the programme on 100 per cent - condom use policy. A more recent initiative is the Thailand Business Coalition on AIDS which was launched in September 1993 to educate and disseminate information about AIDS and to encourage businesses to adopt AIDS in the workplace policies for their staff.

*Lessons Learnt.* Strong political commitment by the Government is needed in order to mobilize all sectors to prevent and control HIV/AIDS. Substantial financial resources need to be set aside by the Government each year to sustain the momentum of efforts being carried out by public and private, non-governmental organizations as well as international agencies. Inter-collaboration and intra-collaboration/co-ordination among sectors and groups need to be strengthened and expanded.

The National AIDS Plan should be articulated within the framework of the National Economic and Social Development Plan. It provides the framework for long-term country-level co-ordination. The National AIDS Plan should be open for revisions and adjustments to address rapidly changing circumstances. As the epidemic expands, the plan leas naturally become broader and more inclusive of a diversity of groups which are playing increasingly active roles in AIDS prevention and control efforts in Thailand.

Financial contribution from multilateral and bilateral agencies to the National AIDS Programme tend to focus on their own priorities and interests. This may result in an unequal distribution of the assistance in certain geographical and programme areas. Financial commitments by multilateral and bilateral agencies are often of one-year duration creating short-term unsustainable activities for what is a long-term problem.

The Government of Thailand has made it a national policy to support the work of nongovernmental organizations by ensuring that a certain allocation of the national AIDS budget is made available to non-governmental organizations.

In conclusion, there are no blueprints for multi-sectoral co-ordination of the vast number of participating parties involved in AIDS efforts in Thailand. The country has recently embarked on a multi-sectoral planning process in order to formulate a revised National AIDS Plan for 1995-96, the fruits of which remain to be seen yet. however, experience has shown that in order to ensure maximum participation and co-operation by all groups, co-ordination must be done carefully and sensitively, and should be flexible and open to different views expressed by the various groups involved in the participatory planning processes.

## 5.2 National AIDS Programme Management: A Training Course

In order to enhance programme management at the national level, WHO has developed a training course which, like EPI, CDD and few other programmes. consists of modules. Each module addresses a major aspect of AIDS-programme development and contains exercises for the participant to practise what is leant. The titles of the 12 modules are:

1. Introduction
2. HIV/AIDS Problem, Control Activities and Target Populatioins for Preventicn
3. Interventions and Policies
4. Programme Prevention Priorities and Targets
5. Promoting Safer Sexual Behaviours
6. Condom Procurement and Distribution
7. Provision of STD Care
8. Prevention of HIV Transmission through Blood
9. Prevention of HIV Transmission through Injecting Drug Use
10. HIV/AIDS Care and Social Support
11. The National Plan
12. Monitoring and Evaluation.

On completion of this course, participants are expected to be able to plan, manage and evaluate a comprehensive national AIDS programme more effectively and efficicntly. The Global Programme on AIDS has a supply of training modules for inter-country training. SEARO will be supporting such courses in 1994-1995. If countries are interested in conducting training they should approach the WHO Regional Office. WHO can supply sets of the modules and offer the assistance of trained facilitators/course directors at no cost to the country.

## 5.3 Evaluation of National Programmes and Prevention Indicators

Over the past decade, pressure for speedy and visible action against AIDS has often led national AIDS programmes to neglect evaluation. While evaluation may appear to be a luxury at first sight, it soon becomes clear that it provides a crucial resource for planning and implementing successful programme activities. Unless plans are made early enough for evaluation, programmes run the risk of facing unfulfilled expectations, frustration and disillusionment for lack of feedback on the effects of the hard work already carried out. Carefully conducted periodic surveys provide reliable information for long-term trends to determine the progress and future direction of the programme.

An evaluation package has been developed by WHO for use by national AIDS programmes. The package is designed in the form of a loose-leaf notebook in orer to allow for individual use and update of each section as needed. National AIDS programmes are assessed in a number of ways: first, through reviews of their implementation. Programme reviews provide a broad assessment of the national AIDS progrmme particularly of its management capacity. Second, to complement information provided by national programme reviews, a set of indicators describing the progress of activities has been developed in order to strengthen the capacity of AIDS programmes to conduct their own evaluation. The periodic assessment of these indicators is expected to yield information on the achievement of national targets. The information collected through the various instruments in the "methods package" will assist managers of national AIDS programmes in planning and reprogramming effective interventions.

**Table 42.5. Methods for the Measurement of PIs**

| Methods | Population Survey/ Outlet visit | Health Facility Survey | Records | Sero-survey |
|---|---|---|---|---|
| PI 1. Knowledge of preventive practices | x | | | |
| PI 2. Condom availability (central level) | | | x | |
| PI3. Condom availability (peripheral level) | x | | | |
| PI 4. Reported non-regular sexual partners | x | | | |
| PI 5. Reported condom use with non-regular sex partner | x | | | |
| PI 6. & Pl 7. STD case management | | x | | |
| PI 8. STD prevalence, women | | | | x |
| PI 9. Reported STD incidence, men | x | | | |
| PI 10. HIV prevalence, women | | | | x |

A core set of indicators in the areas of prevention, care and support and reduction of socio-economic impact are needed to measure the progress of national AIDS programmes. As a first step, ten prevention indicators have been selected for their usefulness in monitoring the overall progress of the programme, their potential usefulness in the design of interventions and their relative ease of measurement. The areas covered by the prevention indicators are: knowledge of preventive practices, sexual behaviour, case management of STD, condom availability and use, and STD/HIV prevalence. The prevention indicators and their methods of data collection are shown in the list of prevention indicators in the table 42.5.

## 5.4 Budget and Financial Guidelines: Do's and Don'ts

Funds for AIDS programme activities are received from headquarters in instalments. Therefore, allotments actually received should be the guiding factor in implementation. WR's office while establishing obligations locally or sending request to the Regional Office (e.g. supplies and equipment etc.), should study the reports sent every month to ascertain whether adequate funds are available in the allotment concerned. If it is an approved activity *and* funds are available in the relevant allotment, it can be implemented locally or through the Regional Office (e.g. supplies and equipment). For the sake of convenience, funds are alloted by WHO Headquarters in BL 834—'All Local Costs'. However, the implementation should be done as per the workplan, and the funds can be reprogrammed by GPA/SEARO. Each activity or a group of related activities falling under one allotment should be assigned a separate sticker.

In the AFI system one sticker can be obligated under one allotment only. Obligation document quoting two allotments are received but with one sticker. Correct allotment reference should be mentioned on the transmittal letters. In many cases, the allotment reference given is GPA 001. In case of UNDP funded projects even the sublines should be mentioned. The amount obligated for programme support cost is not available for use. The Allotment Report (ACE 055) and the Obligation Report (ACE 026) being sent every month should be reviewed regularly. Timely review of unliquidated obligations would release funds for other activities. Feedback from countries is very important.

## GPA Country Allotment Structure 1994-1995—vis-a-vis 1992-1993 (Comparison)

1. Allotment '200' (i.e., Staff Cost) and '290' (i.e. Liquida-

tion of previous year's obligations) will continue as in 1992-1993.

2. Instead of the present four allotments per country, i.e.

   210—Programme Management

   220—Health Education

   230—Surveillance and Control

   240—Laboratory Support

There will be only one allotment i.e., '250' with six categories in it.

1. All activities in the workplan are to be given an ARC (Activity Reference Code). Similarly, all obligations (except those under allotments '200' and '290' series) whether under DP, FX or RB funds will also have to be coded. Any clarification in identifying the appropriate Activity Reference Code can be obtained from TL/GPA's office/SEARO.
2. Existing flexibility provisions are being reviewed by WHO Headquarters and will be comunicated later.

## GUIDELINES ON FINANCIAL MATTERS

1. Overall WHO/GPA Funds Controlled At HQ
2. IPF and Workplands for each country
3. Allotments
   - Receipt from WHO HQ
   - Availability of funds under different lines/components
   - Inter-line Transfers and Flexibility
   - SEARO
   - WHO HQ
4. Level of authority from implementation
   - Country Level
   - LCS/834
   - CSA
   - Short-term general service staff
   - Supplies and equipment (With delegation of authority)
   - Regional office
   - Supplies and Equipment
   - Short-term Consultant
   - Long-term staff
   - Group educational activities Etc.
5. Obligation
   - Government request
   - Conforming to workplan
   - Details of activity, budgetary breakdown and schedule of

payment

— Approval by the WR

— Approval by technical unit if not included in the approved workplan

6. Sticker

   Obligations (One sticker per activity) Transmittal every week (BFO's memo sea/bud/92/015 dated 30 January 1992 to WRs refers)

7. Payment for LCS

   As per schedule or up to use 50,000. (Advance over this amount to be approved by regional office)

   Sticker number and allotment to be quoted on the voucher cheque should not be in the name of an individual.

8. Submission of reports/accounts

   No further advance under LCS should be approved for same activity if accounts for previous advance have not been submitted.

## HOW TO IMPLEMENT LOCAL COST SUBSIDY?

## LOCAL COST SUBSIDY

| IF INCLUDED IN THE WORK PLAN (A) | IF NOT INCLUDED IN THE WORK PLAN (B) |
|---|---|
| | 1. WR should request GPA/SEARO for technical approval<br>2. Should also indicate the activities which will be replaced to make funds avail able.<br>3. The procedure stated as in case (A) to be followed. |

ACTIVITIES

## WITHIN DELEGATION OF AUTHORITY NOT WITHIN DELEGATION OF AUTHORITY

| | |
|---|---|
| If required funds are available in budget-line | Request GPA/SEARO for technical the approval/release of funds. Obligation to be established on Approval from technical unit |
| Obligations can be established locally, sticker assigned and funds released. | If Required funds are not available in the budget-line but are available in the Allotment. Suggest interline transfer while obligating documents if a part of the IPF remains to be received from HQ obligation can be established. Copies of allot. Notif. are sent to wR and monthly reports sent by bfo also indicate the sta tus of allotment received from HQ. |

## STICKER DOCUMENTS TO BE SENT TO BFO/SEARO ON WEEKLY BASIS THROUGH THE TRANSMISSION OF OBLIGATIONS

## OTHER POINTS

I. Each obligation document/activity (Request for LCS) should be assigned a separate sticker. One sticker can be obligated under one allotment only.

2. The sticker and the allotment should be clearly stated on the obligation document/ Transmittal letter. In case of UNDP funded projects, even the sublines should be mentioned.

3. Obligations should be established and funds released closer to the dates of activity as per the time frame in the approved work plan.

4. Flexibility limits- 100 per cent within the allotment 20 per cent between allotments. 1994-95- Existing flexibility Y provisions are being reviewed by WHO HQ and will be communicated later.

5. Savings under "290" are not available for use.

6. Reports sent by BFO every month to the WRs should be reviewed carefully and observations thereon should be communicated to BFO promptly.

7. Any increase in allocation/budget for a country. Request should be sent to TL/GPA/ SERVO WHO will in turn take it up with GPA/HQ. Only on receipt of allotment notification funds can be obligated/release.

8. Amount obligated for programme support cost (PSC) is not available for use.

9. In 1994- 1995

   (a) The present four allotments per country i.e. 210,220, 230 and 240 will be replaced by one single allotment i.e., "250".

   (b) All activities in the workplan and all obligations (Except those under allotments "200" and "290" series) whether under DP. FX or RB Funds to be assigned an activity reference code (ARC).

## 6. CONSENSUS STATEMENT AND RECOMMENDATIONS

The assembled National AIDS Programme Managers, expressing grave concern regarding the continuing rapid progress of the HIV/AIDS epidemic in the Region, reaffirmed their commitment to the important goals of HIV/AIDS/STD prevention and control and reiterated the need to strengthen programme management, strengthen evaluation and monitoring mechanisms and using surveillance as an indicator for the progression of the epidemic. After reviewing the status of activities in each country and exchanging international, regional and national programme advances, the participants proposed the following recommendations for future national and regional action.

## HIV/STD PREVENTION

Given the current status of the epidemic in this region, prevention programmes should remain the major focus of national programme activities:

1. Additional efforts need to be made in all countries to develop effective targetted interventions among high risk behaviour groups (injecting drug users, commercial sex workers and their clients, street children, etc.) including information, education, comunications, integrated STD service delivery and condom promotion and provision, utilizing community outreach approaches. Involvement of nongovernmental organizations and the private sector, particularly at the community level, are crucial in these efforts.
2. In the coming year ministries of health's ministries of education and other appropriate ministries should work co-operatively towards the integration of sex/lifeskill education into all levels of education (primary and secondary schools, universities, etc.), either as a part of the curriculum or co-curricular activity or both as appropriate, in collaboration with parent, teacher and student organizations.
3. Concentrated efforts need to be undertaken by the appropriate governmental and non-governmental organizations to develop effective education and intervention programmes targeted at youths out-of-school.
4. Comprehensive STD services, based upon the syndromic approach and including provision of effective, where possible, single-dose treatment, individual health education and counselling on risk reduction, treatment compliance, partner notification and condom use, and condom provision need to be integrated into existing health services, including primary health care services, MCH/FP clinics and non-governmental organizations/private health care services as a matter of priority.
5. National programmes should ensure that comprehensive condom programming strategies that address demand, supply and support functions are integrated into national prevention efforts, i.e., that plans and activities concerning research, IEC, appropriate distribution systems, logistics and training be co-ordinated to achieve national condom-related prevention goals. Condom social marketing programmes for disease control and family planning need to be developed and supported urgently.

6. Member countries should develop and adopt national policies for blood transfusion services, including voluntary donor recruitment and selection and the rational use of blood and blood products, in order to ensure a safe national blood supply.

## CARE AND SOCIAL SUPPORT

(7) Member States should begin to plan for comprehensive programmes on HIV/AIDS care by establishing linkages within the government health and social welfare structures and between government and community based care programmes to ensure a continuum of culturally appropriate care from the hospital to tile holne for those suffering from HIV/AIDS. This should include developing collaboration with traditional health care systems.

8. Member countries should ensure a national policy against any form of mandatory testing (testing without informed consent), while undertaking to make anonymous voluntary testing witil counselling services available to the community.

9. Member countries should be encouraged to examine any legislation or regulations which discriminate stigmatize or infringe on the basic human rights of persons suffering with HIV/AIDS. Special policy guidelines to deal with the care and social support of marginalized populations suffering from HIV/AIDS such as sex workers, injecting drug users should be developed.

## PROGRAMME MANAGEMENT AND CO-ORDINATION

10. All Member countries should develop, in an open participatory planning process involving all sectors, a national strategic HIV/AIDS plan as an integral part of the national health plan/development plan.

11. Member countries should ensure sustained political and financial commitment and support to the national AIDS programme through ongoing advocacy with opinion leaders, policy planners, politicians, the private sector and international and bilateral agencies.

12. Effective inter-sectoral and intra-sectoral collaboration should be ensured through the development of effective co-ordination mechanisms involving a broad-based multisectoral representation. This should include the private sector, nongovernmental organizations, religious

organizations and structures, local government structures, and international and bilateral agencies.

13. National AIDS programmes should strength their capacities to plan, implement, monitor and evaluate STD/AIDS programme activities through programme management training, including logistics management and training.

# 43

# HIV/AIDS and STD Surveillance Data Management and Use

(Report of an Intercountry Meeting, Bangkok, 6-9 December 1995)

## 1. INTRODUCTION

The AIDS pandemic, which was first reported in 1981, has started making an impact in Asia. The region has recently witnessed the most alarming increase in the level of HIV transmission: there has been a three-fold increase in HIV prevalence since the end of 1993. As of mid-1995, 3.5 million people in Asia were estimated to be infected. In Thailand, 22,000 cases of AIDS have been reported so far, of whom more than 80 per cent have been reported since 1993, while India has witnessed an increase of 100 per cent in the number of AIDS cases reported between 1993 and 1994. Some countries still have a low prevalence; however, this situation could change rapidly.

Although the understanding of the virology, immunology and modes of transmission of the disease have increased significantly over the last 15 years, there is still substantial uncertainty about the actual extent and eventual impact of the HIV/AIDS pandemic in many countries of the South-East Asia Region. More complete descriptive data on HIV infection rates and sexual behaviours of people are of immense value in improving understanding of the dynamics and changing patterns of the pandemic. Continued efforts to collect surveillance data and use it to update estimates and projections are needed for mobilizing national response and sustained support against HIV/AIDS within individual countries. Such estimates are useful for advocacy and for planning impact alleviation programmes, including care of and social support for individuals and families affected by HIV/AIDS.

To discuss HIV/AIDS and STD surveillance, data management and use, an intercountry workshop was organized by WHO which was held in Bangkok from 6 to 9 December 1995. The objectives were:

(1) To review the progress in establishing and sustaining HIV/AIDS and STD surveillance systems in the countries of the South-East Asian Region, including the use of computer based information system such as EPI Info, EPI Model and EPI Map;

(2) To exchange experiences on the methods that could be used for making estimations and short-term projections on HIV/AIDS and STD using available data, and

(3) To make recommendation for further strengthening HIV/AIDS and STD surveillance in the countries of the South-East Asia Region.

The workshop, which consisted of plenaries, group work and practical exercises using computers was attended by focal points at country level of communicable disease surveillance programmes and of HIV/AIDS and STD surveillance as well as from WHO.

The participants were welcomed at the opening session by Dr. Jai P. Narain, Team Leader, Global Programme on AIDS, WHO/SEARO. The Regional Director, WHO/SEARO, in a message ready by Dr. M.J. Wysocki, Regional Adviser, Health Statistics, WHO/SEARO, emphasized on WHO technical support to countries, especially in the area of HIV/AIDS epidemiology and surveillance. In 1992, WHO/SEARO had conducted a workshop in Bali, Indonesia, on HIV surveillance which addressed the technical aspects of sentinel surveillance and recommended that all countries must have sentinel surveillance programmes to monitor the trends of the AIDS pandemic. It was now timely that the progress made in this direction was reviewed with a view to identifying areas requiring further strengthening. This workshop will, therefore, not only help in reviewing and improving the functioning of the existing HIV/AIDS programmes but will also provide a forum for participants to use computer based information and data management system, particularly for the purpose of making countryspecific estimations and projections, based on available epidemiological data.

## 2. AN OVERVIEW OF HIV/AIDS AND STD SURVEILLANCE

Public health surveillance is defined as the systematic collection, analysis and dissemination of data on the occurrence of a disease or condition in order to guide decisions towards its prevention and/or management. With regard to HIV/AIDS, it involves surveillance of HIV infection, of AIDS cases, and of other sexually transmitted diseases.

The main objectives of HIV/AIDS surveillance can be summarized as follows:

— to detect and describe the geographic, demographic and risk-factor distribution of HIV infection;
— to monitor the progression of the HIV/AIDS epidemic;
— to plan prevention activities and health and social services for persons with AIDS and HIV infection;
— to evaluate the impact of specific elements of national AIDS programmes.
— to estimate present and future impact of the pandemic;
— to provide comparative data on the global and regional scope of the epidemic; and
— to increase public and political awareness of the disease.

While AIDS case reporting reflects the transmission of the infection 5-10 years in the past and the current burden of serious HIV-related morbidity, HIV surveillance, i.e., the study of the prevalence of HIV antibody, permits monitoring of the current prevalence of the HIV infection. These two surveillance approaches are complementary and, therefore, indispensable components of the public health surveillance of the epidemic.

AIDS case reports, when complete, can provide information on the demographic and geographic characteristics of the populations affected by the epidemic and on the relative importance of the various exposure risks (important for prevention); they can measure the extent of serious morbidity associated with HIV infection (important for short-term planning of health care at national and local levels). Furthermore, AIDS case reports can be used to calculate earlier HIV infection patterns and tuture short-term projections of AIDS cases. Reporting AIDS cases also raises public awareness of the impact of the epidemic. Finally, international comparisons of AIDS case rate may be possible, provided case definitions and surveillance systems are reasonably compatible.

In the mid-1980s, after an antibody test for HIV became available, seroprevalence studies were undertaken in population groups with varying degrees of risk for HIV infection. At the same time, some countries attempted random surveys of the general population in order to evaluate the current HIV prevalence. It became clear soon after that general population surveys were costly and could give an inaccurate impression of HIV prevalence due to participation and selection bias, and the fact that groups at high risk for HIV infection are not randomly distributed in the general population. HIV serosurveillance in sentinel populations (sentinel HIV surveillance) is now routinely undertaken in most countries of the South-East Asia Region. This is the systematic cross-sectional surveying of the prevalence of HIV antibodies in selected populations which may be repeated at intervals over time. It is recommended by WHO as the principal method of data collection for detecting the presence of HIV infection and its geographic, demographic and temporal distribution and trends over time.

Populations particularly suitable for sentinel HIV serosurveillance are persons attending antenatal and sexually transmitted disease clinics, drug treatment centres, and other groups at high risk of HIV infection who have blood drawn for other purposes (e.g. syphilis serology). Clinic or health facility based sentinel HIV serosurveillance, which allows HIV testing by the unlinked anonymous technique is generally recommended. Unlinked anonymous testing refers to HIV antibody testing, after the removal of all potential identifiers, of sera previously obtained for other purposes. By this approach participation bias can be minimized.

Sentinel HIV serosurveillance does not involve randomized selection of sites, and therefore data from different sentinel sites should generally not be aggregated. While sentinel HIV serosurveillance can be used to monitor the HIV epidemic, it can, to certain extent, also be useful for estimating the present and future impact of HIV, or be used to evaluate the impact of a national AIDS programme.

The meeting concluded that assessment of the epidemic in any country depended on data from all available surveillance sources. Although AIDS case surveillance and HIV serosurveillance were essential elements of national AIDS programmes, additional sources of data, particularly on STDs when available, were extremely important when monitoring the epidemic and directing prevention and control programmes. Although not discussed further in this document, these data sources could include:

- the accumulated statistics on HIV infections resulting from diagnostic evaluation, counselling and testing services, and other public health activities;
- tuberculosis and mortality statistics;
- behavioural studies of risk factors for HIV infection;
- estimations of the sizes of populations at increased risk;
- special studies to determine the prevalence of AIDS or HIV-related illness he hospitals; and
- special studies to measure AIDS-related mortality.

## 3. ISSUES AND CONCERNS RELATED TO AIDS/HIV AND STD SURVEILLANCE IN SOUTH-EAST ASIA

### 3.1 Improving AIDS Case Reporting

The factors which influence the accuracy of AIDS surveillance system include the sensitivity and specificity of an AIDS surveillance case definition, completeness of reporting, and reporting delays. Therefore, every effort should be made to enhance AIDS case reporting through training of health care workers assigning responsibilities to individuals, putting in place standard operating procedures, and developing diagnostic and reporting guidelines, including use of uniform case definition for reporting purposes. Even in countries such as Thailand, completeness of AIDS case reporting is not more than 30 per cent.

The desired attributes of an AIDS surveillance case definition include ability to identify severe HIV-associated disease; high sensitivity and specificity; simplicity; and suitability for national and international comparisons. HIV diagnostic testing and other laboratory studies, including CD4+ cell counts, will strengthen some of these attributes (such as the ability to identify severe HIV-associated disease, the specificity and the sensitivity). However, they are not a requisite for AIDS case surveillance. AIDS case surveillance can be and is carried out successfully without HIV antibody or immunologic testing, and without complex laboratory procedure to diagnose opportunistic infection.

The WHO AIDS surveillance case definition formerly called provisional WHO Clinical Case Definition for AIDS, or "Bangui" definition, was developed in 1985 and is based on clinical criteria only. This was modified in 1992 by the WHO Consultation to Review the Priorities for Surveillance of HIV/AIDS and AIDS Surveillance Case Definitions. The new case definition does not require HIV antibody testing. Although some studies have shown that it may lack sensitivity, it is reasonably specific and widely used in countries with limited health infrastructure and limited clinical and HIV diagnostic capabilities. This case definition is feasible, inexpensive and has high predictive value in areas of high HIV prevalence. Limitations, however, include low sensitivity, lower specificity than other definitions which incorporate HIV testing, positive predictive value is very low where HIV infection prevalence is low and lack of accuracy related to tuberculosis. (Tuberculosis patients without HIV infection could be counted as AIDS cases because of similarity of symptoms and signs.)

It can, therefore, be recommended that in countries where HIV infection exists but HIV serology and other diagnostic facilities are not routinely available, should continue to use the WHO clinical case definition for AIDS surveillance. For reporting cases to WHO, the amount of data required should be kept as minimum as possible. These should include information on age, sex, transmission category and geographic location. Reporting should be made in the format provided by WHO South-East Asia Regional Office.

### 3.2 Adhering to HIV Sentinel Surveillance Methodology

Sentinel surveillance for HIV is developed primarily to monitor trends for HIV prevalence in selected populations, determine the geographical spread of HIV infection, and provide information for estimation and projection of all levels of HIV infection. While implementing HIV sentinel surveillance, the following methodological considerations should be adhered to by national AIDS programmes. (These are described in some detail in the WHO/SEARO publication "Carrying Out HIV Sentinel Surveillance —a Guide to Programme Managers").

— *Sentinel Site*: Selection of population groups or sites that are easily accessible. Implementation of sentinel surveillance does not require a random sampling of sites or groups but rather attempts to identify groups or sites from which good data may be consistently collected over a period of time.

— *Sentinel Populations:* Groups or sub-populations in which HIV prevalence will be monitored must be clearly identified. For example, pregnant women seeking antenatal care and military recruits are most likely to be representative of the generally sexually active population. If hemogram or syphilis screening is routinely performed, blood drawn for this purpose may also be tested for HIV antibodies. In low prevalence areas, HIV screening for surveillance purposes may be limited to sub-populations that engage in a behaviour that places them at high risk of HIV transmission. Common "higher-risk" populations include Injecting Drug Users (IDUs), Commercial Sex Workers (CSWs) and STD clinic attendees. In countries where blood donated for transfusion is routinely screened, these data are a convenient source of information. However, HIV prevalence information from blood donors may be biased in two ways. In settings where blood donors are paid, HIV prevalence levels are usually higher than in the general population. In situations where donations are voluntary and donor selection programmes have been implemented, HIV prevalence rates are frequently lower than in the general population. Because of the large sample size and the continuous nature of screening activities, with appropriate interpretation, HIV prevalence rates among blood donors provide convenient and valuable information on the progression of the HIV epidemic.

— *Sampling Duration:* To obtain the most valid measure of HIV prevalence, blood samples for HIV sentinel surveillance should be taken in less than a two-month period. In an epidemic period the calculation of HIV prevalence rates based on sampling periods of longer than two months may result in an artificially low rate.

— *Sample Size:* To obtain an acceptable level of precision of the calculated prevalence rate, WHO recommends a minimum sample size of 250 for "higher risk" and 400 for "lower risk" population groups.

— *Sampling Method:* To facilitate implementation, WHO recommends that consecutive sampling be used and that each individual be included until the desired sample size is reached. In some settings convenience sampling may be necessary.

— *Sampling Frequency:* Except in situations where transmission is thought to be explosive, WHO recommends that rounds of sentinel surveillance be carried out once every year (same months).

— *Testing Methodology:* To minimize participation bias, WHO recommends that, whenever possible, unlinked anonymous testing be used. In settings where unlinked anonymous testing is not possible (usually among certain "higher risk" population groups), testing should be voluntary, confidential and accompanied by both pre- and post-test counselling.

Implementation of sentinel surveillance is an intensive effort that requires training, support, supervision and co-ordination. Experiences from other countries in the Region show that implementation should begin with a few sites and easily accessible populations and, based on experience gained, the programme should be expanded to include other sites and sub-populations. Close supervision and monitoring is essential for implementation of a successful HIV sentinel surveilllance programme. Data from HIV surveillance should always be presented in the form of rates rather than absolute number of persons detected with HIV.

## 3.3 Choosing an Optimal Surveillance Strategy

Each of the two surveillance methods previously discussed, "AIDS case reporting" and "HIV Sentinel serosurveillance", is important. For example, in areas where HIV infection is unrecognized or has been recently introduced, the main objective of surveillance may be to identify the areas or groups into which the infection is spreading so as to target prevention. In this situation, sentinel HIV surveillance of high-risk groups should take priority. Where HIV infection is already present and levels of prevalence are higher, the main objectives of surveillance should be to monitor the epidemic, to target prevention initiatives, and to plan health services. Sentinel HIV surveillance should be expanded to cover geographic areas and groups in which there is a risk of the infection spreading. In both situations (e.g. HIV infection recently introduced, or HIV infection at higher prevalence levels), AIDS case reporting should be undertaken and the choice of an AIDS surveillance case definition should be selected, based on resources and the level of clinical and laboratory diagnostic capability. Where resources are limited, the AIDS clinical case definition without HIV antibody testing may appropriately meet the surveillance goals. In countries where resources are less restricted, use of a more sophisticated AIDS surveillance case definition may be more appropriate.

It was stressed that other data sources on sexually transmitted diseases, sexual and injecting behaviour, socio-economic aspects, etc., should be used to supplement the information available from AIDS case reporting and sentinel HIV surveillance.

## 3.4 Initiating STD Surveillance

Surveillance of STD in the South-East Asia Region remains weak; there is a lack of reliable and accurate data on the prevalence and incidence of common sexually transmitted diseases in most countries. As a result, the magnitude of STDs and the trends cannot be quantified with any degree of confidence. The situation is further compounded by the lack of consensus on the approaches to be used to measure the disease burden and due to the inadequate laboratory diagnostic facilities available in most countries.

There is, however, a broad acceptance that collection and dissemination of surveillance data on STDs are essential to identify groups at high risk, establish realistic disease control objectives and evaluate the overall effectiveness of STD syndromic management and of HIV/AIDS primary prevention measures, as a good surrogate marker. Based on country reports, it is clear that the incidence and prevalence of STDs and complication rates are high in most countries of the Region. In Thailand, however, the incidence of STDs has been declining over the years.

The priority for the Region now is to establish a reliable but simple and practical STD surveillance programme using a standardized approach and format. In this regard, draft STD surveillance guidelines prepared by the American Regional Office of WHO were discussed with a view to adapting the same for South-East Asia. Consistent availability of reasonably accurate data on STDs will guide and assist STD/AIDS control programmes in evaluating the impact of control strategies, e.g., based on syndromic management of STDs and on IEC interventions targeted at individuals with high risk behaviour and in rationally planning for future strategies.

To assess baseline information, it would be useful to collate all available published and unpublished data and analyse them. Standard guidelines are needed to facilitate establishment of STD surveillance in countries, preferably based on and linked to the existing case reporting system. In men, surveillance should include reporting of grintal ulcers and uretheral discharge as syndromes from selected sites, while among women, STD surveillance should include report of VDRL/TPHA among antenatal clinic attendees and gonococcal cultures, where such facilities exist. *Monitoring of gonococcal antimicrobial susceptibility patterns should also form an integral part of STD surveillance.*

### 3.5 Using a Uniform Reporting Format

Uniform simple reporting forms should be used for reporting HIV, AIDS and STD data from periphery to control level within the country. For reporting of data to WHO, the amount of data required should be kept to the minimum possible. For example, AIDS case reporting should include information on age, sex, transmission category and geographic location. Format developed by the WHO Regional Office and provided to all national AIDS programmes should be used for reporting to WHO.

## 4. COMPUTERIZED DATA MANAGEMENT SYSTEMS

### 4.1 Analysis of AIDS Cases and Forecasting

The computerized data management system was introduced to the participants. It was emphasized that using computer systems for AIDS surveillance include the ability to enter, retrieve, delete and update data records using *Epi info* and an edit function to ensure data has been correctly entered and both summary and detailed analysis can be performed. The; summary analysis for reported AIDS cases should include cases by year and geographic area, and by age and sex. Information can be obtained in the form of line listing, histograms and pie charts. Detailed analysis of AIDS cases can include details on the clinical presentation and the modes of transmission. For HIV, the summary analysis should include the number tested for HIV, the number positive, the date of the sampling period, the geographic area or site, and the group tested.

Feedback should be presented to facilitate checking of data entered by data providers. Analysis and feedback should contain a comparison of information submitted by different providers. A report for communicating surveillance data to the WHO Regional Office should be generated and sent each quarter. (A prototype system illustrating the above was demonstrated and the participants practised entering data and producing reports.)

*Epi Model,* a microcomputer programme for making short-term forecasts of AIDS cases, was presented during the meeting. The three epidemiological assumptions necessary for a reliable forecast were discussed: the year widespread transmission began; the reference prevalence estimate, and the position on the epidemic curve. The year of widespread transmission is not necessarily the year the first AIDS case or HIV infection was detected, but rather the year when indigenous transmission reached the threshold necessary for continued local transmission. The reference prevalence level refers to the estimated number of adult HIV infections and not to the reported infections. The position on the epidemic curve is determined by taking into account the age of the epidemic, the likely peak prevalence level, and the annual distribution of observed AIDS cases and HIV prevalence levels.

## 4.2 HIV Estimation and Projection Methods

Because detection of HIV infection is limited by the sub-clinical nature of the infection and differential access to health care and HIV testing facilities, an estimation of the number of HIV infections is necessary to present a true picture of the extent of the epidemic. It is useful to set up a working group in each country which will be responsible for estimating HIV infections in the country. These estimates could be updated once a year based on available epidemiological data and using scientific methodology. Several methods of estimation were discussed in the meeting:

— *Enumeration:* Attempts have been made by some to use enumerated or detected HIV infections to estimate HIV prevalence. However, this leads to a gross underestimation of the level of HIV infections in a population. Individuals infected with HIV will develop symptoms and present for care only at the end-stage of the infection. Enumerated or detected HIV infections represent only the bare minimum. of the actual number of individuals infected with HIV; this also depends on the number of people and types of populations tested for HIV infection.

— *Population-based probability sampling:* A more reliable estimate of HIV prevalence could be obtained by probability sampling of the population. In many countries the prevalence is low and would require an extremely large sample. Because blood must be drawn, consent must be obtained and may lead to severe participation bias. If HIV is limited to "high risk" populations, access to these populations may be difficult. For ethical, logistical, financial and methodological reasons, WHO does not recommend that population-based sampling be undertaken.

— *Modelling:* If accurate information on transmission rates and behaviours that influence transmission are available, epidemiological models may be used to provide an insight into the dynamics of HIV epidemic. However, direct measures of HIV prevalence are frequently more reliable than estimates of the occurrence and distribution of behaviours influencing HIV transmission and are more easily implemented. The use of modelling to determine current estimates of HIV prevalence should be applied with care.

— *Expert judgement*—Delphi methods: in situations where data on HIV/AIDS levels, trends and distributions are limited, expert judgement can often provide a rough guess as to the likely range of prevalence. Knowledge of local situations and of infectious disease process (especially sexually transmitted diseases and epidemic theory) are an essential pre-requisite for involving experts.

— *Back calculation:* The number of incidents of HIV infection may be estimated using statistical back calculation. However, this method requires relatively complete AIDS case reporting over a period of time and is not able to estimate recent levels of HIV infection.

— *Extrapolation:* If a reliable estimate of HIV prevalence has been previously made, this estimate may be used to anchor future estimates for 1-3 years, assuming that there are no sudden changes in the populations effected. Long-term extrapolation should not be made and direct estimates from seroprevalence surveys should be frequently used to re-anchor the estimate.

— *Sero-surveys of sentinel populations* is often the most popular method of estimating the burden of HIV. It is well accepted that in many cases the most reliable estimate of HIV prevalence can be obtained based on seroprevalence studies of different sub-populations representing populations at different levels of risk. The HIV prevalence rate observed in different groups may then be applied to the population which the study group represents. For example, in epidemics where heterosexual transmission is predominant, HIV prevalence rates observed in pregnant women are generally applied to the sexually active population (usually aged between 15-49). in many countries, because HIV is not uniformly distributed throughout the population, separate studies for urban and rural areas may be necessary and the observed prevalence rates applied to urban and rural populations. If the epidemic appears to be confined to "high risk" populations, an estimate of the size of these groups is necessary. In general, such estimates may be made by applying the following formula:

$v = \Sigma \ (pi/ti)(Ri)$, where

v is the total estimate

p is the number positive in the group tested

t is the number tested in the group

R is the estimated size of the population for which the p/t may be applied. Care should be taken that the groups do not overlap. The meeting participants practised the use of above-mentioned methods with the help of computerized data management system, employing their own country specific surveillance data.

## 4.3 STD Estimates

STD estimates are important for programme development, management and evaluation. These are useful also to estimate the requirement of drugs and other resources as well as for general advocacy purposes. The first step in making specific prevalence estimates at country level is to determine the STD prevalence rates for syphilis, gonorrhoea, chlamydia and trichomoniasis, through a modified Delphi approach and after discussion with relevant experts in the country. Additional related information made possible through review of STD literature, library search and data from all available recent studies in the country supplemented by already available official STD prevalence figures can be shared with experts to obtain the best estimates of prevalence rates. Such data could include prevalence of positive serological test for syphilis among pregnant women or of gonorrhoea among women between 15-49 years.

By applying the estimated prevalence for each of the specific STDs to the mid-year population estimate of adults 15-49 year, it is possible to get prevalence or the number of STDs existing at any point of time that year.

The STD incidence can be estimated by discussing the estimated prevalence by average duration of infection. The latter, in terms of years, can be obtained roughly through discussions with experts and review of literature in each country. It needs information on the proportion of STDs that are symptomatic or asymptomatic, those who are treated and those who remain untreated, by sex. The exact methodology for estimating the duration seems complicated and is being refined.

## 5. RECOMMENDATIONS

The meeting made the following recommendations:

### For Governments

1. Additional efforts need to be made in the countries of the South-East Asia Region to adopt and implement the standard protocol for HIV surveillance according to the guidelines given in the WHO/SEARO publication "Carrying out HIV Sentinel Surveillance".
2. The need for unlinked anonymous testing and the fact that initiating HIV surveillance in low-risk groups may be relatively unproductive unless a critical level of HIV prevalence among those with high-risk behaviour has been reached, should be kept in mind. In countries with mature epidemic, it would be useful to include military recruits also as a sentinel group to monitor HIV trends in the general population.
3. The HIV sentinel surveillance may be supplemented with elements of behavioural surveillance whenever possible and feasible.
4. The results of HIV surveillance in a country should be regularly reported to WHO/SEARO with the use of the format included in the publication "Carrying out HIV Sentinel Surveillance". WHO/SEARO, on the other hand, should provide countries with regular feedback.
5. Estimates of HIV prevalence, based on the results of HIV sentinel surveillance, should be made annually by a working group at national level. Wherever possible, computers should be used for data management and for estimation of HIV infections.
6. Countries should continue efforts to develop, in cooperation with WHO/SEARO, the standard AIDS case

definition and adopt the same while reporting AIDS in a standard reporting form. Every attempt should be made to promote reporting of AIDS cases and deaths to the National AIDS Programme, and to

7. When carrying out AIDS reporting for surveillance, all efforts should be made to ensure confidentiality at all costs.
8. Standard guidelines on surveillance of STDs should be developed in the Region, which could then be adopted for use by Member Countries. The work on the preparation of regional guidelines should be one of the areas of co-operation between national experts and WHO during 1996-1997.
9. In order to monitor STD trends, reporting should be based on syndromes; for example, among men, genital ulcer disease and urethral discharge should be reported, preferably from selected sites both in the public as well as private sectors. Among women, VDRL/STS routinely carried out at antenatal clinics should be monitored. In addition, at sites where facilities exist, data on gonococcal cultures should also be used for surveillance purposes.
10. These selected STDs should be reported on a monthly basis within countries, and to WHO on a quarterly basis. The WHO quarterly reporting form should be modified to include data on STD surveillance as well.

## For WHO

1. WHO should continue to provide technical support to countries in capability building on HIV/AIDS and STD surveillance, particularly in the area of training.
2. WHO should draft guidelines on STD surveillance for use by Member Countries and finalize it in consultation with national experts.
3. WHO should provide feedback to countries on HIV/AIDS and STD surveillance on a regular basis.

# 44

# Development and the HIV Epidemic

(A forward-looking evaluation of the approach of the UNDP HIV and Development Programme)

Bruce Parnell, Gro Lie, Juan Jacobo Hernandez, Cindy Robins

## 1. INTRODUCTION: THE UNDP HIV AND DEVELOPMENT PROGRAMME AND THE SPECIAL PROGRAMME RESOURCES

UNDP's HIV and Development Programme is engaged in responding to the HIV epidemic using approaches consistent with the adoption of the development paradigm of sustainable human development (Banuri *et al.* 1994, p. 21)*. It aims to build the capacity of people, communities and nations: building capacity to understand the ways in which the epidemic evolves through its interaction with human development, and the ways in which people can act in response to its causes and consequences.

During the fifth UNDP programming cycle (1992-96), Special Programme Resources (SPR) were made available to enhance the relevance, impact and effectiveness of UNDP's technical co-operation programmes. These resources were to be used to improve current procedures for, and approaches to, programme and

** The term 'sustainable human development' is used here because it summarises the purpose and approaches of the new development paradigm which is emerging as a result of dissatisfaction with traditional methods of technical co-operation. Sustainable human development has been defined in UNDP discussion papers as, "the enlargement of people's choices and capabilities through the formation of social capital so as to meet as equitably as possible the needs of current generations without compromising the needs of future ones"* (Banuri et al, 1994, p.2 1).

** SPR allocations 'INT/92/400 - Minimising the impact of HIV on development', and 'INT/93/401 Partnership programme to enhance national capacity to analyse and respond to the psychological, social and economic determinants and consequences of the HIV epidemic': these two allocations were evaluated simultaneously, and for the rest of this report are referred to as the singular, "SPR".*

project design, implementation and evaluation; and for exploring new catalytic and innovative approaches to development. The HIV and Development Programme (HDP) was allocated $5m for the cycle, subsequently reduced to $3.5m*.

The HIV and Development Programme was established in January 1992 to provide policy guidance to the organisation on HIV-related personnel and substantive issues, to co-ordinate all activities undertaken by UNDP in this area and to provide programme support to UNDP country offices and other units.

The establishment of the Programme was funded from UNDP's inter-regional programming resources, complemented by extra-budgetary support from the Netherlands, Australia and Norway. Since SPR funds could not be used for staff costs, the Programme has used extrabudgetary support, received in recent years from the United States of America and from Australia, for core costs: staff, communication, travel, translation and publications. The SPR was used to finance the activities undertaken and managed by this staff. This has been a constructive use of both sources of funding. The work of the Programme depends essentially on both sources of funds: without the capacity created by other sources of support, the Programme could not have used the SPR in the way it did. Therefore, although the stimulus for the evaluation came from the need to evaluate the use made of the SPR, the evaluation is of the approach of the Programme as a whole.

The HDP used the SPR to explore and enhance understanding of the ways in which the principles and approaches of sustainable human development can be applied towards developing understanding of, and effective responses to, the HIV epidemic. Its approach was based on a set of related understandings about the nature of human development, the nature of the HIV epidemic and the role of UNDP.

Based on these understandings, the HIV and Development Programme recognised that the HIV epidemic demands an urgent and effective response. However, the Programme recognised also that this response must take place in a context in which governments, development professionals and other agents of change find themselves facing new and highly complex phenomena. New knowledge and programming approaches are needed to develop effective responses to the multidimensional aspects of the epidemic. It was therefore decided to use the SPR resources to explore the possibilities of such knowledge and programming approaches.

This was done through a series of interrelated activities which addressed key areas of focus using improved methods of development practice, working in collaboration with the people whose lives are affected, and the organisations which support them, and with other individuals and agencies, including UN agencies, interested in developing sustainable responses to the HIV epidemic.

The approach used by the HDP recognised that the most effective responses would grow out of people's action within their own contexts: their own communities and their own countries. The approach was therefore based on capacity building, with an emphasis on the development of effective partnerships with those responding, in order to ground responses in people's shared experiences of the realities of the epidemic. The approach involved constant reflection based on the lives, dreams and hopes of those people struggling to respond.

Within the framework of this approach, based on the principles of sustainable human development and recognising the collaborative role of UNDP, a central question which was constantly explored through the HDP in relationship with its partners was, "How can we, together, move forward?

## 2. THE EVALUATION PROCESS

### 2.1 The Nature and Purpose of the Evaluation

The purpose of the evaluation was to review the use by the HIV and Development Programme of Special Programme Resources (SPR) at global, regional and national levels during the fifth UNDP programming cycle (1992-1996), and to consider what UNDP should be doing during the sixth programming cycle*. The evaluation was intended to be forward-looking, starting with consideration of what has been learnt through the HDP to date, but *aiming to generate further and deeper understanding of the practices* of sustainable human development as applied to the HIV epidemic, its causes and consequences.

Evaluation is a process inextricably linked to a sense of purpose, and there is no such thing as an all-purpose evaluation (Weiss, 1972). Evaluation processes should therefore relate to the needs and interests of the *users* of the evaluation. In this case, the people for whom the outcome may be of value and interest will not be limited to those defined in many evaluation texts as "key stakeholders". Along with UNDP, the *users of this evaluation* will include a range of people and organisations interested in learning more about how sustainable human development may work in their own and others' contexts: the partners, direct and indirect, of the HDP initiatives, staff of national HIV/AIDS programmes. UN agencies, NGOs, communities, consultants, academics and others

---

*[3]The draft terms of reference for the evaluation are available on request from the HIV and Development Programme. The evaluation process was developmental in nature, designed collaboratively by evaluation team members and programme staff: the terms of reference were a starting point for this process.*

affected by the epidemic. The evaluation process was therefore designed to elucidate lessons learnt through the approach of the HDP in ways which would also be of value to these users of the evaluation.

The evaluation was also designed to fit within a framework outlined in a UNDP discussion paper on guiding principles for evaluation (Benbouali, 1995). In relation to programmes of this nature, the paper notes that, "The development objectives are finally the results of strategic effects of many programmes/projects and efforts" (Benbouali, 1995, p. 2). A suggested means of enhancing understanding of such strategic effects is to concentrate on issues of *relevance* and *sustainability.* This makes such evaluation distinct from auditing and assessment, which focus on managerial and financial issues, and on measures of programme activities and performance as predetermined in initial decisions about programme objectives.

An emphasis on strategic effects is also central to the suggestion, outlined in a recent UNDP discussion paper on sustainable human development, that one of the indicators of sustainable human development is the extent to which social learning has taken place, as indicated by "... the emergence of new habits and routines (as) a critical indicator of social change" (Banuri, et a., 1994, p. 28). The evaluation explored the extent to which the HDP activities had enhanced such social learning, and hence capacity development, by exploring a broader range of critical indicators, more accurately described as the emergence of new *understanding* and *approaches,* as the concepts of *habits* and *routines* were considered too static to describe either the activities of the Programme or the Programme's intended strategic effects.

In line with the forward-looking purpose of the evaluation, and acknowledging the need for sustainable human development to grow out of people's lived experiences, the central issue of the evaluation process, reflecting the central question of the Programme itself, was "How can we, together, move forward?" In this case, the question was asked in relation to how we can use evaluation processes to generate a deeper understanding of the newer approaches to development practice.

## 2.2 The Evaluation Framework

It was important that the evaluation be conducted in a manner consistent with the dynamic, and even opportunistic, nature of the Programme. The world keeps changing, the determinants and consequences of the HIV epidemic keep changing, and the opportunities available to a low-budget programme operating globally also keep changing. So does understanding of what works best to promote sustainable human development. Therefore, it was important that the evaluation avoid a result of "locking" the Programme into a fixed *modus operandi.* For example, an evaluation with a linear logic which simply considered inputs, outputs, or immediate impact would have been inappropriate. Such an approach would require some sense of "fixing" the Programme as a static entity, clarifying what were the precise goals and objectives and measuring the outputs at just one point of time and in one context: the world as it was at one point in time.

Understanding the approach of the Programme as being based on a set of principles, from which arise methodologies and approaches, was therefore considered more accurate than attempts to define the Programme based on assumptions about clearly defined inputs and outputs. Early in the evaluation process, in July 1995, Programme staff developed a list of some of the concepts which the Programme was then using to describe its work and some of the concepts it was not then using.

The evaluation process was *interactive* and *iterative.* The *interactive* process involved working with the partners of the Programme, and others who use similar approaches in their own work, to develop together a deeper understanding of how the approaches work. The starting point was the Programme, but the evaluation enabled people to explore such issues with reference to their own lived experiences. This is consistent with the principle that, "The perspectives of and experiences of those persons who are served by applied programmes must be grasped, interpreted, and understood if solid, effective, applied programmes are to be put in place" (Denzin, 1989, p.105). The evaluation process was *iterative* in that it started with shared reflection about the nature of the Programme, went back into the field to explore how this understanding relates to people's lives, then returned to shared discussion about that, and so on.

The process was, in these ways, based on the qualitative research method of *interpretive interactionism* (Denzin, 1989). This method emphasises the need to *interpret* real-life phenomena in order to reduce complex reality to understandable and debatable notions. It suggests doing this in an *interactive* way, because deeper understanding about the meanings and significance of experiences and relationships arises when people reflect and engage in dialogue with each other.

Such an evaluation process meets two important requirements for the use of qualitative methodology:

1. The need to combine the collection of data with a rigorous interpretation of the significance ofthat data, as outlined by Patton (Patton, 1990, p. 423):

> ... we must be constantly moving back and forth between the phenomenon of the programme and our abstractions of that programme, between the descriptions of what has occurred and our interpretations of those descriptions, between the complexity of reality and our simplifications of those complexities, between the circularities and interdependencies of human activity and our need for linear, ordered statements of cause and effect.

2. The need to ensure that the people who conduct such interpretive analysis are those for whom the analysis is most important, as outlined by Denzin (Denzin, 1989, p. 25):

> Interpretive interactionism asserts that meaningful interpretations of human experience can only come from those persons who have thoroughly immersed themselves in the phenomenon they wish to interpret and understand.

## 2.3 The Evaluation Process: What was Done

*Stage 1. Selection of evaluation team members*

The evaluation team consisted of four people who are themselves affected by the epidemic. They are all engaged in responding to the epidemic in their own contexts, and have all been involved in promoting sustainable human development as participants in international networks, as consultants, or as long-term staff in development projects. In response to the second evaluation requirement above, the team members have all been partners of the Programme. They reflect a diversity of experiences of the epidemic and come from different global regions. Directly including more people from developing countries in the evaluation team was planned but was, ultimately, not possible. The nature of the evaluation process ensured, however, that many people from developing countries had direct input in both provision of information and interpretation of results. The evaluation team members were Bruce Parnell (team leader, from Australia), Juan Jacobo Hernandez (Mexico), Gro Lie (Norway) and Cindy Robins (Canada).

*Stage 2. Selection of further participants in the evaluation process*

Decisions were made about countries to which field visits would be made and criteria for selection of participants in interactive discussions and in workshops. These decisions were based on the qualitative research method known as purposeful sampling, as defined by Patton (Patton, 1990, p.169):

> The purpose of purposeful sampling is to select information-rich cases whose study will illuminate the questions under study. ... The logic and power of purposeful sampling lies in selecting information-rich cases for study in depth. Information-rich cases are those from which one can learn a great deal about issues of central importance to the purpose of the research, thus the term purposeful sampling.

The selection of evaluation participants was therefore based on determining which people were most likely to provide significant knowledge and insights which would contribute to a better understanding of how the approaches used work in practice.

The Programme had used a variety of new and innovative programmatic and organisational approaches to assist governments, communities and organisations, and the selection of evaluation participants had to reflect these approaches. Criteria for selecting participants were that they represented groups with whom the Programme worked in partnerships, people who were involved in networks responding to the epidemic, people who had participated in SPR activities, and people who were identified by Programme partners or other participants as being people who work in ways that are compatible with the approaches used.

The Programmers analysis had indicated that every facet of human, social and economic life can be affected by HIV and development, and that national responses must include collaboration between individuals, families, communities and governments. This mix was also reflected in the selection of evaluation participants, so that they included people from the governmental sector, non-government organisations, community groups, and grassroots movements as well as from the international community.

The three countries visited were Zambia, the Philippines and Mexico. These reflect a diversity of regions, countries with different experience of the HIV epidemic and its impacts, and countries in which the SPR has had varying levels of contact. A fourth country, Senegal, was visited by the evaluation team leader for the purpose of conducting a limited number of interactive discussions. This choice was made because, although the Programme has worked in Senegal, availability of partners at the required time meant that it was not possible to conduct the full range of evaluation processes in Senegal.

*Stage 3. Interactive interpretation of the Programme's approach*

The evaluation team leader worked with HDP staff in July 1995 to collate information about SPR activities and sustainable human development; to collectively reflect on the purpose, nature and approach of the Programme; to consider evaluation options; and to design a relevant evaluation process. A paper outlining the conceptual framework for the evaluation was prepared and distributed widely for comment amongst partners of the Programme and others interested in evaluation. It was developed as part of the evaluation process and was written with input from a number of people familiar with the work of HDP and evaluation methodologies to clarify the understanding of both Programme staff and evaluation team members.

*Stage 4. Developing further understanding of the approach of the Programme*

A planning workshop was held in Zambia in October 1995 for the evaluation team members, two members of the HIV and Development Programme staff and the UNDP HIV and Development national professional officer in Zambia, Margaret Mutambo. At this workshop, further consideration was given to the conceptual nature and approach of the HDP, with reference to selected publications on development practice, social change and evaluation which were tabled by workshop participants. The outline of the development practice framework for the HDP which is included in Section 4 of this report is based on the results of this period of the process.

The process of interpretive interactionism was applied to exploration of workshop participants' own experiences of development, the HIV epidemic, and the Programme. This ensured that all evaluation team members were familiar with the concepts and methodologies of the evaluation process. It also ensured that the evaluation team commenced development of a collective understanding of the nature and significance of the approach of the Programme and a shared understanding of issues to be considered during the country field visits.

*Stage 5. Country field visits: interactive discussions*

Interactive discussions were held with selected participants from each visited country. This dialogue differed from a usual interview format, in that those interviewed were able to talk freely about what mattered to them, but the interviewers from the evaluation tearn were also free to pursue issues they considered important; hence, use of the description, "interactive discussions", rather than "interviews".

The interactive discussions aimed to explore evaluation

participants' own experiences of HIV and development and any involvement they had with the Programme, and to engage with them in discussion about what approaches they find useful, regardless of whether or not their experience of those approaches was within SPR initiatives. The discussions explored issues through eliciting "thick description", as defined by Denzin (Denzin, 1989, p. 83):

> A thick description does more than record what a person is doing. It goes beyond mere fact and surface appearances. It presents detail, context, emotion, and the webs of social relationships that join persons to one another. Thick description evokes emotionality self-feelings. It inserts history into experience. It establishes the significance of an experience, or the sequence of events, for the person or persons in question. In thick description, the voices, feelings, actions, and meanings of interacting individuals are heard.

*Stage 6. Country field visits. interpretive workshops*

Interpretive workshops were held in each of the three primary countries visited in order to:

— provide a chance for people from each country to interact with each other in interpreting understanding of how various approaches work within their countries;
— provide a chance for larger numbers of people to participate in the evaluation process; and
— ensure that interpretations made by evaluation team members were able to be further considered by the people whose perceptions of relevance and sustainability were being considered.

*Stage 7. Country field visits. review workshops*

People responding to the HIV epidemic and development in each country usually do so working with National HIV/AIDS Committees, UN agencies and international donor agencies. To further ensure that the findings of the evaluation process were based in reality, and to ascertain the extent to which new approaches in sustainable human development are understood and supported (or not) by these agencies in each country, a short review workshop was also held in each country, and these agencies were invited.

At least some members of national HIV/AIDS committees in each country had been included in Stages 5 and 6 of the evaluation process. For this reason, very few also attended the first reporting back workshop review in Zambia, as this would have required yet further time commitment. Accepting this likely scenario, and in order to reduce the workload on those who had voluntarily offered to make the arrangements, it was decided that members of these committees should not be invited to attend the workshops in the Philippines or Mexico.

Many staff of UN agencies and international donor agencies attended the review workshops in each of the three primary countries. The workshops had a simple format, in which the nature of the Programme and the evaluation process was explained, the lists of concepts currently used and not used by UNDP were presented and initial interpretation of data by evaluation team members was presented for further discussion.

These workshops generated much interest, and dialogue ensued. Many participants indicated a good understanding of issues which were relevant within their countries of work, and demonstrated a keen interest in developing understanding of the interrelationships between the HIV epidemic and sustainable human development.

*Stage 8. Commissioning of case studies*

To complement information collected through field visits and consideration of published information, two case studies were commissioned to further explain the way the Programme worked in practice.

The first of these, entitled "Enhancing National Capacity Through HIV Action Research", was written by Catherine Hankins, a partner of the HIV and Development Programme, and two members of the Programme staff. It summarises what occurred and some of the key lessons learnt through this component of the SPR. The initiative aimed to enhance the national ability of people to find out what they need to know and to incorporate what they find into policy and programme design. This case study is included to provide insight into the practical ways in which a specific project was developed within the framework of the SPR, to indicate some of the lessons learnt through these types of processes and, consequently, to provide an example of the way the Programme evolved over time in response to lessons learnt. This case study is included in the text of this report, after Section 5.

The second case study, entitled "The Partnership Between the Salvation Army and the HIV and Development Programme" was written by Alison Rader and Captain Doctor Ian Campbell of the Salvation Army. It summarises the conceptual understanding about the nature of effective practices in sustainable human development which evolved over a long period of partnership between the Programme and the Salvation Army, and partnership between the Salvation Army's International Headquarters and its own partners in many countries. This paper's focus on development of conceptual understanding is deliberate, for two reasons. First, Salvation Army personnel and HDP staff reported that gradually enhanced understanding of development practice was one of the primary benefits to all parties engaged in this partnership. Second, evaluation team members felt it was useful to highlight specific lessons learnt through one particular partnership, as a typical example of the richness of what was achieved through an approach based on partnership. This case study is also included in the text of this report, after Section 6.

*Stage 9. Interpretation of data*

Collected data included information arising from shared discussions: discussions within the evaluation team and with Programme staff in the first four stages of the evaluation process, and discussions held with individuals and within workshops in Stages 5 to 7. In line with the processes of interpretive interactionism, this data was then collated, analysed and interpreted by the members of the evaluation team through a final workshop in New York over five days in November 1995.

This workshop followed an open-ended format, enabling development as it progressed and input from evaluation team members and Programme staff. Once again reflecting the interactive nature of the evaluation process, participation of others in this workshop was encouraged. At various stages, the workshop was attended by all HDP staff, by Gary Engelberg (a partner of the programme based in Senegal) and by Alison Rader of the Salvation Army.

During this workshop, the evaluation team identified the key concepts about which the evaluation process had led to deeper understanding, and shared information about what had been learnt about these concepts through the country field visits. The summary of understanding of how the Programme approach works in practice, which appears in Sections 5, 6 and 7 of this report, is based on this final workshop.

*Stage 10. Report writing*

The report was written following the final workshop. A brief report such as this cannot capture all that was learnt either through data collection or through the interpretive discussions. It is expected that further information about what has been learnt will be disseminated through the work and lives of the many people who participated in this process.

Selected notes made by evaluation team members during the data collection process are available on request from the HIV and Development Programme. These provide summaries of interactive discussions with evaluation participants, and thus enable richer insights into the ways in which the approaches of the Programme have worked in practice. Statements made in confidence are not available for distribution, but these constitute only a small proportion of the data collected.

## 3. THE SPR-FUNDED ACTIVITIES

### 3.1 Overview

The work of the HIV and Development Programme was guided by a set of related understandings about the nature of the HIV epidemic, the nature of development and the role of UNDP in the response to the epidemic. It took place in a context in which there was rapid and continuing spread of the HIV virus, no cure, and a potential for the HIV epidemic to impact on all aspects of human development.

The issues to be addressed were complex and various: moral, social, cultural, religious, psychological, legal, political, strategic and economic factors had to be considered. The programming responses had to be sustainable for perhaps many years to come, resulting in development of the capacity of individuals, communities and nations to adapt to the changing circumstances which may arise through interaction between the epidemic and the ongoing challenges of human development.

The HIV epidemic impacts on the broad range of human endeavour including social and economic development, welfare, education and training, employment, defence and law enforcement. The causes and consequences of the epidemic are closely associated with other challenges to development including poverty, unemployment, civil unrest, indebtedness and rural-urban movements. For example, HIV-related illness and death creates new poverty, deepens existing poverty and increases family and national indebtedness.

This interaction between the epidemic and development demands a multi-sectoral and interdisciplinary response, with collaboration between many partners: governments, international agencies, community based groups, NGOs, research institutes, private sector groups and, most importantly, the people directly affected.

The development of the Programme was based on a

recognition that UNDP's role is to assist developing countries to accelerate the process of capacity building within both governments and nations, through support for human resources development, institution building, strategic planning and management, good governance, and the promotion of sustainable human development. Thes development and dissemination of models and guidelines was considered of limited effectiveness. New knowledge and skills needed to be developed collaboratively, and new issues needed to be addressed as they were identified.

The Programme aimed:

- to deepen understanding of the nature of effective responses to the epidemic, to determine what works and how, and what does not, and to take the best practices of development and apply them in this field; and
- to increase UNDP's capacity to programme its resources more effectively and in this way to strengthen national capacity to develop an effective multi-dimensional response.

The elements of the approach adopted by the Programme were:

- a continually deepening and changing *understanding* of the epidemic drawn from extensive and diverse experience in the response to the epidemic and in development practice;
- an approach based on *capacity building:* the Programme tries to bring its expertise into processes of interaction which strengthen those values, processes, skills and behaviours which make it possible to establish an effective response.
- an approach based on *partnerships:* the relation of partnership recognizes and respects the commitment and expertise that each partner brings to the work, accepts the importance of building consensus and solving problems across differences, is based on a set of ethical guiding principles and requires trust and respect; and
- the continual *grounding* of understanding and of the approach, and the checking of these against the realities of the epidemic. In particular, this involves actively seeking and listening to the insights, reflections and experiences of the Programme's partners as well as following the developments in understanding and practice of individuals whom the Programme respects.

Such an approach requires extensive communication amongst all concerned and consultation with people in their own environment. The Programme found it was important that, wherever possible, the occasions and spaces made for discussion and learning should be where people themselves live and learn rather than in institutional settings.

The working principles of the Programme include the involvement of those directly affected by the epidemic in all activities and aspects of its work; gender sensitivity, representation and responsiveness; supportive partnerships with agents of change: individuals and community and non-governmental organisations; the strengthening of partnerships between the government sector and the community sector; sensitivity to ethical, legal and human rights issues; and the strengthening of partnerships across regional language groups.

The areas of focus of the Programme have arisen from these interactive processes. They include:

# exploration of methodologies and instruments which can be used in national planning to minimise the social and economic consequences of the epidemic,
# exploration of ways in which communities and nations can address complex and delicate ethical, legal and human rights issues,
# consideration of the strengths and limits of initiatives directed specifically towards women,
# developing understanding of how processes of social learning through research can be used in programme development,
# ascertaining how networks can be supported and developed into sustainable institutional forms with the flexibility to accommodate to changing needs and circumstances,
# exploring ways in which insights and lessons can be learnt and shared,
# reflection on the role of language, images and metaphors in determining the nature of understanding and responses, and
# consideration of ways in which fatalism and despair can give way to a sense of agency.

The HDP is thus clearly situated within the overall conceptual and operational framework of UNDP's work. It adopts approaches consistent with this framework and is based on concepts of sustainable human development, especially human survival; social capital formation; capacity building; social learning and partnership (see Banuri, et al. 1994); expertise (see Chambers, 1994); gender responsiveness; process consultation (see Joy and Bennett, 1994); strategic questioning (see Peavey, 1994); and governance.

Consistent with the principles of sustainable human development, the inclusion of the people whose lives are affected was considered essential and the Programme encouraged continual input from people directly affected by HIV and by development. This commenced with a workshop in New York in October 1992, in which a range of people directly affected by the epidemic worked with HDP staff, government officials, community workers, researchers and activists to develop general guidelines for the development of the Programme, including the identification of key issues to be addressed. The development of the Programme included ongoing interaction with these and other people, resulting in continual evolution of the Programme's approach, enhanced understanding of effective practices and the building of consensus on addressing a range of sensitive and complex issues.

The relationship between the approach of the Programme and recent advances in UNDP's understanding of the nature of sustainable human development was reviewed as part of the evaluation process, and is summarised in Section 4 of this report. The rest of this section (Section 3) provides a concise summary of the major types of activities which have been undertaken by the Programme. Although activities are described separately, the inter-connected nature of the factors which were addressed by the Programme means that these activities were not always discrete.

### 3.2 Minimising the Development Consequences of the Epidemic: Exploring Methods for Planning

With HIV prevalence amongst adults in some African countries now reaching 20 or 30 per cent of the adult population, there is intensified destruction of human and non-human capacity, and thus a new and critical need to find ways of addressing the consequences, not just measuring them. The HDP has supported many innovative processes in Africa and other regions to strengthen the capacities of governments, families and communities to mitigate these effects.

The first step in this process was a consultative meeting in Vienna in 1992 attended by other UN agencies, academics and people directly involved in their national responses to the epidemic. This meeting mapped out the main direction for SPR activities around minimising the development consequences of the epidemic, and defining processes which would enhance effective responses. It was agreed that a shift in balance was required, away from describing the consequences and towards developing types of understanding which would lead to strategies to address those consequences. Many activities followed, and there is space here for only a few examples.

— In collaboration with the International Institute for Applied Systems Analysis in Vienna, new computer software has been developed and made available at low cost to users. This makes it possible to access in a user friendly way the HIV data of the US Bureau of the Census, the largest data set available, and also to play interactive "games" which enable users to explore processes of HIV transmission and develop better undertanding of the dynamics of the epidemic. The software has been offered to UNAIDS to be used in furthering communication objectives.

— An unsuccessful attempt was made to strengthen the regional planning capacity in the Kagera Region of Tanzania through the inclusion of activities which addressed the effects of the epidemic. This is an area where there is an existing UNDP planning project and where HIV prevalence is very high. Important lessons were learnt from this experience about the processes required for gaining commitment to programme development, together with improved knowledge of the constraints which affect what is possible under conditions of widespread denial.

— Nicaragua is a country with low reported HIV prevalence in a region where other countries are already experiencing rapid spread of the epidemic, and where socioeconomic factors may enhance further rapid transmission of the virus. Attempting to induce more effective prevention by government and others, the HDP, in partnership with a national NGO, cosponsored a workshop and follow-up activities to enhance understanding of developmental aspects of the epidemic. This strengthened local capacity to undertake economic analysis, to measure the effects of the epidemic and to identify appropriate responses to the needs of those affected.

— A project was undertaken in several rural areas of Mexico, in collaboration with the National AIDS Programme and other partners including the NGO, Colectivo Sol. The project explored how to better use local structures and organisations, such as public libraries, to strengthen links between information providers and community-based service organisations such as health centres and women's groups. Important lessons were learnt about processes for building local trust as integral to and necessary for programmes relating to HIV prevention and care.

## 3.3 Capacity Development Through Research

An ongoing project explores how to strengthen national capacity to define, undertake and make use of research on the socio-economic causes and consequences of the epidemic. The project, in four African countries (Central African Republic, Kenya, Senegal and Zambia), has developed innovative processes to support national teams of researchers and others, working in partnership with National HIV/AIDS Programmes, affected individuals, researched communities and other potential users of data and analysis.

Research is now underway and important insights have been gained about how to best ensure that research is timely and relevant to programme needs. Activities which build on the lessons of the project are being developed in other countries and regions, including Myanmar and Nicaragua, with proposals also under consideration in Vietnam and Botswana.

This initiative is developing new approaches to technical co-operation, based on principles of process consultation which entail different relationships and use of new working methods between development partners. The SPR initiative has thrown light on how best to strengthen national research capacity through technical consortia; how to involve potential users throughout the research process; how to strengthen research skills and improve understanding of the ethical and development aspects of the epidemic; and how to ensure early discussion of, and improved methods for, the dissemination of research results and their effective use in programme development. *Case Study* 1 describes this project in further detail.

SPR funds are also being used to explore how the processes of research can be used to stimulate solutions as well as to increase understanding of problems. Research on families of children left without social and economic support after the death of their parents is being undertaken in a seriously affected area in the west of Kenya. The research methodology is designed to lead to processes of discussion and consultation within families and communities and with local government so that adequate support can be provided to these children. The findings are also contributing to national policy and programme development.

## 3.4 HIV and Development Workshops

Training materials and workshops have been developed focusing on the human, social and economic development dimensions of the epidemic. The workshops aim to increase awareness of the complex nature of the epidemic, to analyse approaches to strengthening community-coping responses and national responses, and to identify the policies and programmes required at all levels to respond to the epidemic. The belief that the epidemic can be overcome is central to the workshop.

The workshop is based on three principles:

— placing the psychological and socio-economic causes and consequences of the epidemic at the centre of the training: the analysis upon which the workshop is based focuses on identifying effective processes for reducing the impact of the epidemic on human, social and economic development and the impact of these factors on the spread of the virus;

— placing people at the centre of the analysis: people and their communities are central to discussions within the workshop, which focus on their expressed needs and concerns, their resources, their coping and survival strategies and their development aspirations; and

— placing hope at the centre of the response: people are changing their behaviour, families and communities are providing support and care for those affected, and communities, businesses and governments are developing strategies for preventing further infections and reinfection and for minimising the adverse impact of the epidemic.

The workshop is designed for senior government officials particularly from ministries of planning and finance, the productive sectors (agriculture, mining, industries, transport, etc.) and the social sectors, for senior United Nations officials and for the organisations of civil society. In addition to the workshop itself, shorter workshops on HIV and Development have taken place at national level for politicians, community organisations, NGOs, the private sector and others. National and inter-country workshops organised by UNDP include workshops in Australia, Austria, Benin, Botswana, Cameroon, Central African Republic, Chile, Cote d'Ivoire, Gabon, India, Jamaica, Kenya, Madagascar, Malaysia, Mexico, Morroco, Nicaragua, the Philippines, Poland, Senegal, Uganda, the Ukraine, the USA, Zaire, Zambia and Zimbabwe.

Many examples of flow-on effects from these workshops and the training materials used were reported during the evaluation process. Three training for trainers workshops have been held (Mombasa 1991, Agadir 1992, Kuala Lumpur 1994) and those trained have subsequently adapted and used the materials in many settings. The workshops have had an impact in enhancing people's understanding of what is needed and what is possible, on the development of effective strategies, in initiating the development of effective networks of people who may not otherwise have met, and in stimulating engagement amongst those who had previously not considered the epidemic relevant to themselves or their work.

In the Philippines, participants reported that they often use components of the workshop in their work in rural provinces, as they have found this an effective way to engage people's interest and understanding as a prelude to acting in response to the challenges of the epidemic. In two states in India, the training materials are being used by women sex workers working in red light districts to increase the understanding of their co-workers of the epidemic and of the need for a collective response. Already by 1993, over 500 groups of women sex workers had seen and discussed the module on The Unfolding of the HIV Epidemic. In rural Zimbabwe, the materials have been incorporated into village theatre productions aiming to increase awareness of, and a commitment to respond to, the epidemic. In Senegal, it was reported that the workshop had created an emotional as well as an intellectual engagement amongst many people who were already engaged in responding but who, as a result of the workshops, now did so more vigorously and with much greater personal conviction. Thus, the workshops have been able to address needs in new ways which people find directly relevant across international boundaries.

In many countries networks of NGOs have incorporated the development practice approaches and conceptual frameworks presented in the workshops into ongoing projects building local capacities to understand and respond to the epidemic.

### 3.5 Learning how to Learn from and with Others: Facilitated Study Tours

Exploration and testing out of new and innovative approaches to learning how to learn from and with others has been integral to the work of the Programme. One approach that has been developed, tested out and found to be effective is the facilitated study tour. This was first developed in response to a request from the National HIV/AIDS Programme in Djibouti for assistance in understanding and developing a community-based strategy to address the HIV epidemic. A multidisciplinary team from Djibouti, with participation from the Ministry of Health, counsellors, hospital administrators, the media, women's groups, community groups and lawyers, travelled first to Senegal. There the NGO, ENDA-Sante, ran a workshop to explore the lessons learnt to date about the centrality of the community response to the epidemic, including the importance of developing an appropriate legal and ethical framework to facilitate such a response. The workshop included visits to community groups and discussion with interested officials, researchers and activists in Senegal.

Following this workshop, the Djibouti team and the ENDA-Sante facilitators proceeded to Zambia and Uganda. They visited selected community groups and then spent an additional day in each country to reflect upon the relevance for their own country of what they had seen and learnt. The team prepared a paper summarising the lessons learnt and their applicability for effective programme design and development in Djibouti.

On their return to Djibouti, the team spent a week integrating their findings into the national HIV/AIDS plan and planning a pilot project to build national capacity to develop a community-oriented approach to the epidemic; to establish an appropriate legal, ethical and human rights framework for such an approach; to utilise existing resources for such an approach (including use of counsellors, local government structures and community leaders); to strengthen the trust between those individuals and families already affected by the epidemic and government and other community members; to delineate the roles and responsibilities of community organisations and government; and to develop participatory community-based monitoring and evaluation systems to capture the lessons and feed them into policy and programme development discussions.

The approaches used in the facilitated study tour resulted not only in stimulating the national authorities to rethink and redesign their HIV/AIDS strategies, but were supportive of building national capacity and fostering exchanges of experience and learning amongst many African countries.

Facilitated study tours were subsequently organised in response to requests from Swaziland, where the government wanted to explore and develop a national strategy for community- and family-based care and support, and from Vietnam, where the Vietnamese Armed Forces wished to strengthen their military HIV prevention programme and to develop stronger links between the military and civil society.

## 3.6 Ethical, Legal and Human Rights Networks

Networks of activists and professionals have been established and supported as a means of building capacity to address legal, ethical and human rights issues. These networks, in Africa, Asia and the Pacific and Latin and Central America and the Caribbean, draw their members from legal, governmental and academic institutions as well as from organisations of civil society. They are active in addressing the legal and ethical issues central to responses to the epidemic, and in the provision of services to those affected. Indirectly, they contribute to institutional capacity building and to human resource development.

These networks contribute to social capacity building through drawing together diverse groups of those interested or implicated to address issues of common interest. They broaden the base of discussion and contribute to consensus building within the community sector and amongst civil society, public and private sectors. They also advocate for law reform, changes in legal practices, the provision of appropriate services, policy and programme development, and they play a guardianship role in ascertaining the legal and ethical appropriateness of responses to the epidemic.

The value of the networking approach is evident in an example given by Attorney Manual (Manny) Goyena, a lawyer from the Filipino NGO, Alter Law. He talked in an interactive discussion with the evaluation team of how his organisation provided legal advice, but worked closely with other NGOs more able to be directly involved in social action. He had attended various regional meetings either in the law and human rights field, or as part of networking within the Asia-Pacific Council of AIDS Service Organisations (APCASO). He had been a participant at the first meeting organised by HDP for the Asia and Pacific region in Cebu, the Philippines, in 1993 and at the resource persons training workshop in Tarrytown, New York in April 1995.

Many people from the Philippines are now engaged as "overseas contract workers", working in other more wealthy countries usually for lower wages than local people. A recognised difficulty is their lack of rights within those other countries. Through the APCASO network, contact had been made between the Philippines AlterLaw group and lawyers in Malaysia. Together, the two groups are now planning proposals to address the rights of Filipinos working in Malaysia. Manny explained:

> We got [a lawyer] to meet with the Philippine NGOs working in Malaysia. So, we tried to define a model, file a test case. For example, the government now is just assisting people on the receiving end of complaints, but we're moving them to assist with initiating cases ... For example, with trafficking of women, ... because there are international syndicates, therefore responses have to be international.

Countries in which UNDP has supported networks and networking on ethics, law and HIV include, in Africa: Botswana, Burundi, Central African Republic, Cote d'Ivoire, Gambia, Ghana, Kenya, Rwanda, Senegal, South Africa, Uganda, Zaire and Zambia; in Asia and the Pacific: Bangladesh, Cambodia, China, Fiji, India, Indonesia, Malaysia, Myanmar, Nepal, Pakistan, Papua New Guinea, Philippines, Sri Lanka, Thailand and Vietnam; in Latin America and the Caribbean: Argentina, Barbados, Brazil, Mexico, Nicaragua, Paraguay and Venezuela; and in Europe and the Commonwealth of Independent States: Poland, Russia and the Ukraine.

In response to requests from NGO partners for capacity building and skills development in this area, a legal and ethical resource persons workshop was held in Tarrytown, New York, in April 1995. The focus of this workshop was on the use of process facilitation and strategic questioning skills in network building. Participants came from all regions previously involved in legal and ethical networking. A manual of the workshop materials is being produced on the use of process facilitation for network building to address legal, ethical and human rights issues.

### 3.7 Networking: Creating Spaces for Discussion, Support and Action

In a similar way, networks of people living with HIV and AIDS assist in both building capacity for representation and participation in policy and programme development, and in ensuring that expertise and commitment contribute to the strengthening of local and national responses. Such networks are important vehicles for protecting the rights of those affected and for providing protection and sanctuary. They enable those affected to enter into partnerships and provide the possibility of continuing organisational effectiveness even when illness and death affect individuals' ability to continue.

The Programme has provided a range of support to people living with HIV in their efforts to create national, regional and global networks, in advocacy of the principles of recognition and involvement, in the recognition of the particular expertise that living within the epidemic creates, and through involving them as partners in all its work.

It worked with the UNDP Regional Project on HIV and Development for Africa to assist with the creation of the Network of African People Living with HIV and AIDS (NAP+). It has been active in the formulation and implementation of the UN Personnel Policy on HIV and AIDS. Assistance has been provided to the Global Network of People Living With HIV/AIDS (GNP+) through provision of training in strategic planning and programme development. Support has also been provided to the International Community of Women Living With HIV and AIDS (ICW) to report on the lessons learnt during a pre-conference meeting held prior to the VIIth International Conference for People Living With HIV/AIDS, in Capetown, South Africa in March 1995.

In preparation for the Capetown Conference of People Living with HIV and AIDS, the Programme funded two GNP+ Board members to visit and work with groups of people living with HIV in Zimbabwe, Zambia, South Africa and Namibia.

The Programme has also worked closely with networks and organizations providing care and support to those affected. In particular, it has strong and continuing partnerships with ICASO, especially through its regional councils. It has also worked with the International HIV/AIDS Alliance and its national linking organizations.

## 3.8 Understanding Gender and HIV

The work of HDP addressing issues of particular relevance to women has focussed in two main areas: creating a greater awareness and understanding of the gender dimensions of the epidemic and developing more effective strategies to assist women.

From its start, the Programme has adopted the principles of gender sensitivity, representation and responsiveness to guide its work. It has sought an equitable participation of women in all its work and has played an important early role, especially through its publications and presentations, in drawing global and national attention to issues such as the epidemiology of infection amongst women, the susceptibility of young women to infection, the need for methods of protection that women can use in their socio-economic settings, the relationship between cultural and medical practices and infection rates amongst women, and the inequitable burden of care that communities and nations place on women.

Analysis of the way in which social and economic policies and institutions increase the effect of the epidemic on women led the Programme to an understanding of the causes of men's vulnerability to HIV infection and of their critical role in any strategies for women. A number of publications and presentations have addressed this issue.

There is now greater awareness of HIV infection rates amongst women and of the other ways in which the epidemic affects their daily lives but much more work is needed to develop effective approaches and practices to address these issues. The complexity of the analysis militates against narrowly focussed or single item responses.

The Programme has worked closely with women, and with organisations working with women, to increase understanding of how initiatives directed specifically towards women can help. It has also considered areas in which approaches directed towards men, or towards the contexts in which male-female relationships occur, are needed in order to better assist women and those they care about and for.

## 3.9 Civil-military Issues and HIV

It is estimated that HIV prevalence in military populations in a number of countries may be as high as 50 per cent. Reliable information on infection rates is scarce because of the enormous sensitivity surrounding the topic. This has strategic, political, social, economic and security implications at both national and global levels. In some countries security forces have begun to take action by working with national HIV/AIDS programmes. However, HIV within the military will continue to pose very difficult policy dilemmas both in branches of the military and in national contexts. Issues of concern include the effect on civilian populations, the ethics of mandatory testing, civil-military collaboration for prevention and care, and implications for peacekeeping operations.

Over the past few years, the HDP has been working in partnership with interested governments and institutions to explore civil-military issues around HIV. One outcome of these efforts has been the establishment of an international organisation, the Civil-Military Alliance to Combat HIV and AIDS, which now receives support from a number of UN organisations including UNAIDS and the World Bank, as well as from bi-lateral agencies including USAID.

Within this context, the HDP has been providing technical support and guidance to countries through facilitated study tours, missions and consultations. It has participated in meetings and training workshops of the Civil-Military Alliance and is represented on the Board of that Alliance. In December 1995, at the request of the Vietnamese Armed Forces, the Programme organised a facilitated study tour to enable them to discuss policy and programme issues with neighbouring Armed Forces and to explore ways for civil organisations and the military to work together. A group of senior military and civilian officials from Vietnam visited Thailand and the Philippines. The study tour was facilitated by a senior military doctor from the Papua New Guinea National HIV/AIDS Programme, a partner of HDP.

## 3.10 Learning, Advocating and Disseminating: Promoting more Complex Understanding and Action

The HIV epidemic is challenging accepted ways of understanding health and human development in our societies and demanding new forms of expertise and more integrated responses. It is raising conceptual, ethical and programmatic issues, many of which still need to be named, all of which need to be raised for discussion and exploration. The aim of the HDP publications and presentations has been to raise new or neglected issues, to encourage people to consider old issues in new ways, and to articulate the questions many of these issues raise about accepted ways of doing things.

The publications policy has been to keep papers brief, simply written and limited to issues not addressed, or not addressed from the same perspective, elsewhere. Authors are asked not to outline solutions but rather to stimulate the reflection and discussion essential for well-informed processes of change to arise within their own contexts. Publications have included issues and working papers, research studies, posters, statements of principles, training materials and a book.

Declarations drawn up at consultations and conferences organised by either the HDP or by UNDP's regional HIV and Development projects have been distributed in poster format, encouraging policy makers and practitioners to display them on walls of government offices, resource centres, clinics and other places used by people responding to the epidemic. These included the *Statement of belief on behaviour change as a central issue in responding to the HIV epidemic,* drawn up at an informal consultation hosted by the HDP in Senegal in December 1991, and the *Dakar Declaration of the African Network on Ethics, Law and HIV.* These short statements were widely distributed, both promoting and summarising new forms of discourse arising through sustainable human development responses to the HIV epidemic.

Many other issues were covered in papers which examined the multisectoral nature of the epidemic's socio-economic causes and consequences, and the development of effective, sustainable and compassionate responses. These papers cover themes relating to all the areas of the HDP, and titles include: *The HIV epidemic and development: the unfolding of the epidemic; The economic impact of the HIV epidemic; People living with HIV: the law, ethics and discrimination; Sharing the challenge of the epidemic: building partnerships; Young women: silence, susceptibility and the HIV epidemic; Children in families affected by the HIV epidemic: a strategic approach; The HIV epidemic in Uganda: a programme approach; The socio-economic impact of HIV and AIDS on rural families in Uganda.*

In order to diversify the voices of the HIV epidemic and to disseminate the lessons learnt thus far in developing countries, the HIV and Development Programme published a book entitled, *HIV and AIDS: The Global Inter-Connection* (Kumarian Press, 1995).

In order to ensure that the issues are accessible, the HDP has worked in a number of collaborative ways to ensure that its publications are available in a number of languages. It is working with Spanish-speaking and French-speaking HIV support organizations to strengthen their capacity to translate and distribute relevant HIV materials. The partner organization chooses material considered to be of relevance to the region and sets priorities for translation. It also identifies material for translation into English and other languages. The book, *HIV and AIDS: The Global Inter-Connection,* has been translated into Bahasa Indonesian, Bengali, Sinhala, Thai, Urdu and Vietnamese through a partnership programme with local publishing houses. It is presently under discussion for translation into French, Spanish, Japanese, and into Swahili by a consortium of people living with HIV or AIDS and government officials in Kenya and Tanzania. HDP materials have also been translated into Arabic, Russian, Chinese and Portuguese.

HDP materials are considered as public domain materials and it is made clear that they can be reproduced in whole or in part by any person wishing to understand and explore these issues further. HDP asks only for some acknowledgement and for suggestions for further papers and for comments on the series.

The HDP distribution policy is to distribute materials free of charge within UNDP programme countries, whenever interest is shown in receiving them. The materials have been widely distributed, in and outside of urban areas, to government and non-government organisations, to libraries and academic institutions. They have also been handed on from person to person.

The value of these publications in catalysing the responses to the epidemic of people in their own contexts was highlighted in comments made by Eduardo Nierras, an evaluation participant in the Philippines:

> My interest grew from my apprehension about the way HIV issues are gender and development issues. This leads to all sorts of understandings that people were, or are, trying to move towards, ... these papers showed me that other people were also thinking about these issues ...

## 4. UNDERSTANDING THE APPROACH IN THE CONTEXT OF EVOLVING NEW DEVELOPMENT PARADIGMS AND PRACTICES

The time is ripe for a thorough rethinking of development theory and practice. The costly mistakes based on the conventional modernisation paradigm and a top-down approach to development have to be rectified, and the right lessons must be learnt.

Perhaps the key lesson is that development starts with the people, and with their knowledge, culture and traditions as assets rather than liabilities. Unless this is taken as the point of departure, insensitive or impatient governments—and foreign donors— may easily destroy valuable social capital in the name of growth and "modernization."

Stefan de Vylder, development economist and practitioner (de Vylder, 1995, p.57)

These pleas for revision, made as concluding remarks to a recent UNDP discussion paper, provide a useful starting point for considering the association between the new approach to development and the HIV epidemic. The HIV and Development Programme explored the relevance of new development practices to the response to the HIV epidemic and, in turn, contributed to a better understanding of development practices generally, and specifically of UNDP's evolving approach to human development.

## 4.1 Key Lessons Learnt

This section is based on a review of selected literature on development practice and the nature of social change, and on interactive discussions which were held between evaluation team members and staff of the HIV and Development Programme. Consideration of what is now known about sustainable human development, capacity building and the role of UNDP led to deeper understanding about the way in which the approach of the HDP fits within the evolving framework of development practice and, in turn, has been able to contribute to development of this framework.

Discussions were informed by publications on the need for reappraisal of traditional approaches of technical co-operation in development, along with a recognition of the nature of the HIV epidemic. The HIV epidemic epitomises the need for new approaches to development practice because of the close association between the epidemic and human development, the continually changing nature of the causes and impacts of the epidemic in specific local settings, the fact that traditional approaches have mostly failed to reduce either the spread of the epidemic or to minimise its impact and, most importantly, because no one can claim to have expert understanding of what will work in all contexts to address the challenges of HIV and development.

The evaluation found that the work of the HDP is clearly situated within the conceptual and operational framework of UNDP's work, and that its approach is consistent with concepts used by UNDP. The Programme is contributing to the development of understanding of UNDP's evolving approach through learning more about what works in practice.

In particular, the Programme has put into practice the challenges of working in a way which catalyzes analysis and action by the people whose lives are affected. It has explored the implications of working to develop capacity through approaches based on partnership rather than dissemination of pre-conceived knowledge, it has learnt how to act as an agency which mobilizes people, and it has learnt how to be self-critical and self-evaluating.

The Programme's approach is situated within theoretical frameworks which help to guide these new approaches, and draws on understanding of social learning, strategic questioning and process consultation. Each of these frameworks emphasises the central role of transformation: transformation of individuals' perceptions and sense of personal empowerment, transformation of institutional approaches, and transformation of the roles of development practitioners. In these ways, the Programme has contributed to understanding of how sustainable human development works in practice, and of how such practice can contribute to more effective responses to the HIV epidemic.

## 4.2 Recognising the Need for New Approaches to Development and to the HIV Epidemic

Many development agencies, including UNDP, are re-considering what types of development practice may be effective in the context of current crises in meeting development needs (Banuri, *et al.* 1994). The imperative for change arises from a recognition that traditional forms of technical co-operation have been less than effective in meeting their objectives.

The report of a recent High-Level Seminar of the OECD's Development Assistance Committee, UNDP and the World Bank notes some current problems with technical co-operation (OECD/UNDP/World Bank, 1994). Though referring to development in general, some of these problems apply also to the field of HIV and development:

> Technical co-operation is donor driven ... Any single donor may be marginal, but in the aggregate, donors exert a powerful distorting influence on national processes of priority setting and resource mobilization and allocation.
>
> Technical co-operation has supported the monopolization of resources and power by governments ... (which) has not been compatible with social and economic progress.
>
> Within donor agencies there are short time horizons and pressure to deliver resources.

In facilitating responses to the HIV epidemic, top-down approaches based on what has been learnt in a few wealthy countries, and based on the need to be seen to produce quick results, are often the norm in developing countries.

Many programmes are funded by donors in a manner which assumes that people in various contexts simply need to be told "the truth" about the HIV epidemic; that the only sensible responses are use of condoms and treatment of those who are ill using expensive modern drugs which do not in fact save lives; that measuring the numbers of people infected is possible and is an essential component of an adequate response (at no matter what cost); and that tradition, especially religious beliefs and traditional medicine, is a hindrance in dealing with such a new phenomenon as the HIV epidemic.

The net result of such programmes, as widely acknowledged, is that responses to the HIV epidemic in many countries are ineffective in slowing down transmission rates, in reducing stigma and discrimination against those infected and those close to them, and in generating effective responses to the challenges the epidemic presents to human development.

The inadequacy of the application of classical approaches to technical co-operation to the HIV epidemic is further highlighted because so many of the problems which need to be solved are not yet fully understood by anyone, no matter how expertise is defined. For example:

— the epidemic in one country may be very different to that in another;
— the problems at one stage of the epidemic may be different to those at a later stage;
— the way the epidemic spreads is influenced by different development strategies, economic systems, and political situations;
— the possible range of responses to the epidemic depends just as much on personal and community-wide commitment to their resolution as on what may be externally viewed as necessary; and
— there are no obvious technical solutions, or even models of programme design, which are either entirely effective or readily transferable from one context to another.

How, then, can this be changed? What is required to generate effective responses to the challenges presented by the HIV epidemic in the context of development, or to the challenges of development in the context of the HIV epidemic?

## 4.3 Possibilities for Reform, and Implications for Addressing the HIV Epidemic

Partial answers to these questions may be found more readily in recent discussions about the nature of development than in discourse about the HIV epidemic. The OECD/UNDP/World Bank seminar suggested the following as part of an "Agenda for reform":

> On the donor side, there would need to be ... a commitment to provide support over longer periods with realistic time frames ... a different approach to the design of technical co-operation, with longer periods taken for a thorough analysis of problems and more extensive discussion of possible solutions, including the establishment of mechanisms for participation in decision making at each stage, and without donor pressure to regard technical co-operation as a necessary part of the solution to problems identified...On the recipient side, ... a strategic vision of the role of the public sector, governance, and the elements of an enabling environment for development.
>
> (OECD/UNDP/World Bank, 1994; see also OECD, 1991)

UNDP has responded to the challenges of this "Agenda for reform" through the development of more complex perspectives on human development:

> Sustainable human development is the enlargement of people's choices and capabilities through the formation of social capital so as to meet as equitably as possible the needs of current generations without compromising the needs of future ones.
>
> (Banuri, *et al.* 1994, p. 21)

The UNDP discussion paper in which this definition first appeared suggests that sustainable human development will result from new approaches within what it describes as "a new development paradigm". The HIV and Development Programme has explored approaches consistent with these suggestions.

Working within the framework of sustainable human development, the Programme has been based on a commitment to ensuring that solutions to the problems of HIV and development arise from:

— an enhanced capacity of individuals, communities and nations to understand the nature of the epidemic in their own contexts; and

— an enhanced capacity of individuals, communities and nations to find effective means to address those problems; which in turn depends on

— an enhanced capacity for people and organisations in all sectors (government, NGOs, the private sector, health and development agencies, religious organizations, and others) to work co-operatively and communicate with each other about problem definition as well as resolution.

No amount of technical co-operation can, on its own, enhance these capacities but it can facilitate necessary social change:

- — change in people's perception of their own roles and capacities in enhancing human development;
- — changes in the ways individuals and institutions relate to one another;
- — changes in the focus of analysis (from virus to people and their inter-relationships);
- — changes in the nature of what needs to be done, who needs to do it and where and how the impetus begins.

For these changes to be sustained, there needs to be a strong and widespread willingness to respond to the epidemic, and an external environment which enables such responses: an environment which encompasses cultural, policy-making, political and legal factors which influence people's abilities to understand and to act.

What, then, is the most useful role for an international development agency? How can effective development practice be applied within the HIV epidemic? Such questions cannot be explored independently of advances in understanding of development practice, nor of advances in understanding of the epidemic. The UNDP HIV and Development Programme complements the roles of many other UN, bilateral and NGO donor agencies working in development and in response to the HIV epidemic. The HDP therefore deliberately focuses on exploration of the association between HIV and development, and how more effective development practice can generate more effective responses.

The Programme is thus situated within the overall conceptual and operational framework of UNDP's work. Its approach is consistent with concepts used by UNDP, especially the concepts of sustainable human development, capacity building, social learning and partnership (Banuri, *et al.* 1994). Discussion about the new paradigm of sustainable human development has led to suggested guidelines, or starting points, for practice within this paradigm. The Programme contributes to this new discourse through having learnt more about what works in practice.

## 4.4 Learning to Move Forward, Along an Ever-Changing Path

A central question being constantly explored through the SPR is, "How can we, together, move forward?" Answering this questions leads to choices in the types of processes used, with the ultimate goal of assisting social change. Interim processes include identifying people and organisations who are social change agents, working with them and supporting them through partnership, and the facilitation of their networking with each other.

A useful framework to inform the nature of such social change processes can be found in a seminal work by Schon, *Beyond the Stable State* (Schon, 1971). Although written in response to crises in the welfare states of wealthy countries in the 1970s, the theoretical frameworks outlined by Schon have relevance for human development now.

Schon explores the nature of social change. He notes that the dominant model for diffusion of new ideas is based on the concept that, "A communicates to B what B does not know but A does". Like classical technical co-operation in development, which is based on the same model, this is inadequate to facilitate the range of innovations which are required to meet the complex realities of modern societies.

In what could now be seen as a forerunner to recent discussions on crises in development and in the international organisation of societies and nations, Schon notes that,

> Over time, we shift our perceptions on the problems that need solving. But institutions have an internal life of their own; consequently there are always mismatches between the institutional map and the problems thought worth solving.
>
> (Schon, 1971, p. 182)

The complex problems caused and/or highlighted by the HIV epidemic provide good examples of a proliferation of such problems. Just as the problems of human development are not solved just by the creation of good banking systems, so the problems of an epidemic driven by complex and dynamic social and behavioural systems are not solved by the improvement of medical or educational systems alone.

Schon's central thesis is that as such mismatches between problems and institutions becomes endemic, so do all sorts of responses, which vary in effectiveness and can in turn create their own problems. The net result is the loss of "the stable state". The challenge, then, is to find productive ways to deal with the consequences of the loss of the stable state.

The answers, Schon suggests, arise through processes of "social learning": a concept central to the newly defined human development paradigm. An imperative for effective change is the application of social learning to changing the nature of the state in general, rather than focussing on independent institutions. Failure to do so will result in endemic crises, as have now been identified in current discussions on development (Banuri, *et al.* 1994, pp.9-11; de Vylder, 1995, pp. 8-1 l).

Social learning requires an emphasis on process rather than

forseen outcomes, and on the generation of autonomous yet networked responses akin to the characteristics of social movements, rather than on the restructuring of individual institutions:

> The importance of this movement is not that it permits once-and-for-all redesign of institutions, but that it permits continual redesign of organisational elements within the framework of broad functional systems. Hence, the need for an internal organisation which can be continually redesigned without flying apart at the seams. Within the system, the foreground condition is not stability but change. Attention focuses on the process of transforming one structure into another rather than on the resulting structure.
>
> (Schon, 1971, p.184)

This is entirely consistent with the recent suggestion that, "UNDP must see itself as: (1) a catalyst and an advocate for social change; (2) an agency which mobilizes stakeholders in sustainable human development; (3) a supporter of potential partners; (4) a self-critical and self evaluating body; and (5) a promoter of institutions that enhance accountability and responsibility of all partners" (Banuri, *et al.* 1994, p. 7). It is also consistent with the approach of the HDP in that the Programme works in these transformational ways, is process-defined, and consciously works with, and promotes co-operation between, governments, NGOs, communities and individuals affected by HIV and by development.

Practical suggestions on how to bring about the required changes can be found in three critical components of the new approach to development which have all been drawn upon to directly inform the work of the programme: the need to start with people's own perceptions of their realities and to promote more actively the role of expertise which arises from lived experiences (Chambers, 1994); the use of "strategic questioning" (Peavey, 1994); and the culmination of a range of new approaches in a method of facilitation developed by Management Development and Governance Programme of UNDP and called, "Process Consultation" (Joy and Bennett, 1994).

## 4.5 Who Defines what is Real, and what is Needed?

The first of these was suggested in a paper prepared as an overview for a recent UNDP roundtable discussion (Chambers, 1994). Under the title, "Poverty and livelihoods: whose reality counts?", the author draws attention to the vast differences between the perceptions of poverty held by professionals and the perceptions experienced by the people who actually live in poverty. He suggests that the most valuable expertise in both understanding reality and knowing what changes are needed is the expertise which arises from lived experience. This understanding of expertise presents major challenges to those working in development and requires major changes in approach: "If poor people's realities are to come first, development professionals have to be sensitive, to decentralism and to empower, enabling poor people to conduct their own analysis and express their own multiple priorities" (Chambers, 1994, p.16).

The author notes that these challenges are not simple:

> The challenges are paradigmatic: to reverse the normal view, to upend perspectives, to see things the other way around, to soften and flatten hierarchy, to adopt downward accountability, to change behaviour, attitudes, and beliefs, and to identify and implement a new agenda; in sum, to define and embrace a new professionalism. (Chambers, 1994, p. 20)

Again referring to the need for a new agenda in development, this author suggests four pillars for a poverty agenda:

— analysis and action by local people, and putting first the priorities of the poor;

— the promotion of sustainable livelihoods (rather than simply economic growth);

— decentralization, democracy and diversity; and

— professional and personal change.

Such changes, he suggests, demand, "... altruism, insight, vision and guts" (Chambers, 1994, p. 28).

The scope of the changes required in development practice as a result of starting with people's own realities should not be underestimated. People's realities include not just perceptions of the world as it is, but also understandings of the ways it can be changed. These can lead to entirely new ways of defining and reaching programme goals.

## 4.6 Asking Useful Questions to the Right People

A second component of enhancing understanding of people's realities is the use of "strategic questioning" (Peavey, 1994). Strategic questioning is a process in which the person investigating and the person investigated become equal partners in a process of learning. One can find power in approaching a problem with the feeling of, "I don't know", or in allowing doubt into what is already known. Such attitudes open doors to new possibilities, through which both the listener and the person being questioned can realise change.

Strategic questioning is the skill of asking questions which will make a difference. It is characterized by six key features. In summary, strategic questions:

— are dynamic and create motion (for example, by asking, "How can we, together, move forward?");
— create options;
— can be a lever to reveal in-depth information;
— do not lead to "yes" or "no" answers;
— empower the person being questioned; and
— sometimes include "unaskable" questions which challenge assumptions and values.

## 4.7 The Central Role of Process in Building Capacity

Finally, a set of processes which have been adopted by the HIV and Development Programme is suggested in the guide, "UNDP Process Consultation: Systemic Improvement of Public Sector Management" (Joy and Bennett, 1994). This guide was developed to assist countries to face the challenges of building capacity for systemic public sector change and reform. It suggests that UNDP's role is to support that process by contributing resources and by, "... facilitating the sharing of experiences and insights in different areas of development" (Joy and Bennett, 1994, p. iii). In essence, the role of the external agency is to suggest issues to consider and processes which might be used to consider them, not to explain "realities" or to provide "answers".

Suggesting issues and processes is exactly what the Programme did, for example, with work in the legal, ethical and human rights fields. It would have been inappropriate and ineffective for the Programme to determine exactly what changes should be made to the legal and ethical environment in each country, because each country is different, as highlighted in the UNDP guide to process consultation:

> Client systems are not all in the same state of change-readiness or need: technical co-operation must start where the change programme is and support what the change programme needs next ... UNDP has a role in maintaining momentum not in providing direction. ... Action plans evolve with commitment; the client context is constantly changing and the UNDP programme needs to be responsive to and patient with this. ... Different forms of technical co-operation will be needed at different stages of a reform programme.
>
> (Joy and Bennett, 1994, pp. 3-5)

Consistent with the general approach of sustainable human development, the guide suggests a strong emphasis on working with processes rather than endpoints. It suggests that a further aspect of the approach required now, as used by the Programme, should be to explore the nature of the new development paradigm through simultaneous practice and reflection, rather than through desk-top programme planning followed by action: "New roles, and the new relationships they imply, are worked out and learnt by discussion and interaction" (Joy and Bennett, 1994, p. 37).

Importantly, the guide to process consultation also recognises the importance of the view of reality of an agency such as the HIV and Development Programme, recognising that there is room for outsiders to bring their own perspectives to problems, so long as those perspectives are offered in dialogue, not as "solutions" to which funding is tied. Such an approach was typical of the Programme's work in capacity building for undertaking research which would contribute to better policy and programming responses to the epidemic (see Case Study 1). The Programme's central role in this project was to ensure that an adequate range of people was involved in determining both research needs and methods, rather than a role of indicating what should be investigated through research.

## 4.8 Transformation as an Essential Component of Development

The UNDP process consultation guide affirms that "transformation" plays a central role in the new development paradigm. The central concern of the guide is with transformation of structures and processes, whereas the HDP staff are more critically aware of the need to enhance the understanding and practice of social change agents as a means of working towards this.

There is consistency between the guide and the Programme's approach in seeing transformation as something which will not happen overnight, in using processes which lead towards transformation rather than specifying the outcomes of that transformation, in recognising the central importance of developing relationships, and in continually grounding the programme in people's lived realities:

> There should be no attempt to specify all activities in detail, no pressure to complete every step within the timeframe stated or to hold inflexibly to what at first seemed the best sequence of activities. Expectations should be modified based on feedback from actual experience.
>
> (Joy and Bennett, 1994, p. 21)

## 4.9 The Evolving Nature of Sustainable Human Development

It is in this context that the Programme has worked, through developing, implementing and constantly evaluating new approaches through partnership with people in their own contexts. Indeed, the evaluation has been merely one more form of gaining the "feedback from actual experience" suggested in the above paragraph.

Most importantly, both the Programme and the evaluation are elements of a necessarily ongoing process of experimentation and learning. While much has been learnt to date, the path ahead is by no means certain, and there is a need for continual questioning in the context of ongoing partnerships with those whose lives are directly affected by the challenges of HIV and of development. The promotion of better understanding and more effective action in response to the HIV epidemic and development is at a stage which is typical of the field of sustainable human development in general:

> It is still too early to attempt a synthesis of the new theory of growth and development which appears to be emerging. The trend is clear, however: a more multi-disciplinary approach to development is gaining ground, signifying, among other things, more emphasis on people, ideas and institutions, and less on money and factories.
>
> (de Vylder S. 1995, p. 11)

The Programme has incorporated the need for continual learning with the need for urgent practice. In so doing, it has enhanced understanding of what is needed and has demonstrated that it is both possible and desirable to continue questioning the value of approaches as they are being implemented.

A final lesson, along the lines of what is now called "international best practice", may never be reached. This is because each country and each context within countries is different; the epidemic is evolving, and sustainable human development is itself a process, not an outcome. In the words of an evaluation participant from the Philippines, "International best practice is about starting a process." The most useful role for outsiders, then, may well be to help people to find their own effective processes. The development which results would then be relevant, sustainable and centred on people's most crucial needs.

# 5. DEEPENING UNDERSTANDING OF PRACTICAL IMPLICATIONS OF A SUSTAINABLE HUMAN DEVELOPMENT APPROACH

## 5.1 Key Lessons Learnt

This section is based on the results of interactive discussions held in the field between evaluation team members, partners of the Programme and others who have been involved in using similar approaches. It reports on issues of central concern to the evaluation.

It is one thing to say that new approaches are needed in development practice. It's another thing to build capacity in situations, like the HIV epidemic, in which no-one knows what will work, in which inappropriate development practices have sometimes already stifled the creation of effective local understanding and action, and in which the people whose lives are affected are often marginalised through poverty, cultural factors and lack of involvement in community and national decision-making processes.

In developing better understanding of what does work, it was therefore considered important that the evaluators go out into the field to engage in dialogue with the people whose lives are affected, and to not limit discussion specifially to the approach of just this one Programme. People were able to explain and discuss, with the evaluation team and with each other, what has worked to develop their own capacities, what has led to their own sense of creative engagement with the challenges of HIV and development, and what has resulted from these approaches.

Participants talked of their own experiences of capacity development. They often mentioned the need for the new approaches to proceed slowly at first, reporting that their own engagement and empowerment had arisen not from being told what to do, but through working in partnership with others who respected and encouraged gradual development of their own understanding, skills and actions.

Central to these processes was the concept of partnership. The evaluation process generated deeper understanding of what sorts of partnerships lead to capacity development. Key themes which arose through interactive dialogue are summarised here and explained in further detail in the text.

Many key findings centre on the nature of partnerships which build capacity:

— If development and maintenance of partnerships is genuine, then they will follow the usual patterns of human relationships

— Effective partnerships take time to establish and essentially involve two-way dialogue and development
— Effective partnerships are not always initiated or controlled by donor agencies or by central government authorities
— Effective partnerships allow all partners to make choices
— Effective partnerships acknowledge the contributions of all parties involved
— Effective partnerships are not always easy.

Others indicated some immediate effects of such partnerships:

— Inclusion of the people whose lives are affected in developing understanding and responses
— The development of 'safe spaces' which enable those included to discuss issues of central importance to them.
— The reflection and sharing of experiences, thus leading to understanding which would not normally be generated

Finally, a set of key findings indicated the longer-term results of the partnership approach to capacity building:

— Validation of people's own experiences and perceptions
— Development of empathy and deep understanding amongst the people whose lives are affected and thus amongst the people most likely to be able to work together to find effective solutions
— Experiences of solidarity which enable people to act together
— Empowerment and the releasing of energy, particularly amongst people who previously had felt disempowered and unable to either fully understand their own situations or act to bring about useful change
— Ultimately, effective and sustainable outcomes which result in long term and adaptable social change which addresses the challenges of HIV and development.

Following description of these key themes, a case study is presented which outlines the way approaches based on capacity development worked in practice in an ongoing project of the Programme to enhance national capacity through HIV action research. This case study demonstrates, from the perspective of the Programme, how the approach evolved, what was learnt about what works, what difficulties have been experienced through this practical experience, and thus what suggestions can be made for ongoing work by the Programme and others.

## 5.2 The Process of Capacity Building within the HIV Epidemic

The following sections highlight some of what has been learnt through the use of SPR about how the new development paradigm can be realised in practice. They are based directly on the data collected through personal interaction during the evaluation process: dialogues with individuals in the four countries visited, and interactive workshops.

Much information was collected in the form of narrative and "thick description". Of necessity, this section includes only the most significant findings, collated and summarised by the evaluation team after further dialogue and shared reflection ("interpretive interactionism". One important finding that is almost impossible to convey through a written report was the depth of feeling expressed by many evaluation participants about their involvement in responding to the epidemic. These included feelings associated with grief, loss and pain, but also included equally intense feelings of hope and confidence that they were, indeed, engaged in effective responses to the epidemic which are leading to worthwhile and positive changes. Many participants responded enthusiastically to the very idea of discussing processes which work, noting that such processes are often overlooked in attempts made to understand the global response to the epidemic.

Although grouped into sections in order to make the information more accessible, in reality there was much overlap between people's understanding of various concepts. The information is presented here as a further contribution to the discourse about the new development paradigm and its interaction with the HIV epidemic.

Central to discussion on sustainable human development, and to the work of the Programme, is the concept of capacity building. This was included in the list of "Concepts UNDP is currently using," which was used to generate discussion during Stage 5 of the evaluation process. The HDP aims to build capacity not just of individuals and organisations but of whole nations. Reflecting the need to commence with building capacity to understand, not just to act, the programme uses partnership and processes of shared problem solving, rather than skills transition, to develop capacity.

A crucial aspect of capacity building is that it builds on what is already there, even when existing capacity is not recognised by those who have it, as explained by John Musanje, from Zambia: "We need to mobilise the indigenous potential." The resulting enthusiasm expressed by evaluation participants who had been involved with the Programme is typified in the comment of David Chipanta, also from Zambia, that, "They (HDP) helped me see capacities that are dormant, such as the capability to listen, to change and to adapt."

What are the features of capacity building which generate understanding and more effective responses to the HIV epidemic? The next few sub-sections explain processes which people have found helpful in developing their own and their nations' capacities. Before these, the report addresses some more general aspects about the nature of capacity building within the context of the HIV epidemic.

## 5.3 Building Capacity to Respond in Different and Changing Contexts

A central feature identified by evaluation participants is that people and nations now require capacity to quickly understand and respond to changing contexts, not just to familiar or repeated situations. While some people noted that each stage of the epidemic presents different challenges, many noted also the evolving nature of their understanding of what is occurring and what is now required. Consider this quote from Roland Msiska, the former National HIV/AIDS Programme Manager in Zambia, reflecting on both his personal development of capacity and the way his programme now has to work:

> So, none of these deaths is the same. Each death raises different questions, different challenges. Each time you change, you become less dogmatic, more one who asks questions. ... Each death gives a different dimension to the epidemic. Yet we may have been dealing with the epidemic as if it's a single epidemic. There are different epidemics, moving around; they are constantly dynamic.

The changing nature of the epidemic and of emotional and cultural responses is not widely acknowledged, yet is an important feature of people's own perceptions of reality, and therefore affects their requirements in capacity building.

A corollary of the complex and dynamic nature of such capacity building is that capacity must be developed across institutional and state/community boundaries. This requires working with a range of institutions, as is reflected in the Programme's commitment to bringing together governments with NGOs, military with civil organisations, and researchers with users of research. In order that this work be effective, it simultaneously requires an emphasis on working with individuals, as noted by Carlos del Rio, the National AIDS Programme Manager in Mexico:

> Deep cultural changes have to occur, you need a societal response. Children must learn. Social realities must change ...

we need a deep effort ... But I have learnt that responses are personal not institutional.

The challenge of catalysing social change which grows from individual commitment can be met, in part, through working with individuals who act as social change agents. This can sometimes mean identifying people who already play that role, and sometimes mean drawing out the capacity of individuals to act as social change agents. This concept was well understood by many evaluation participants: individuals can catalyse sustainable human development within their own communities, through using processes similar to the concept of process consultations, as highlighted in a comment from Teresita Bagasao from the Philippines, who said that, "Being a social change agent is about asking questions."

The need for identifying and working with individuals who are potential social change agents was identified early in the Programme's development. The value of doing this was also a central theme in evaluation participants' comments about both their own and others' responses to the epidemic. The importance of individuals' commitment was highlighted in comments made by the National AIDS Programme Managers interviewed; from Zambia, the Philippines and Mexico. All three talked of the complexity of their jobs and the need to work across institutional and professional boundaries, of occasional or regular tiredness, but also of a strong commitment to their work; they had also noted varying levels of engagement and commitment from those with whom they work.

Another central requirement of capacity building is that of honesty, especially the honesty of being able to admit when simple solutions are not available or appropriate. Due to the complex and dynamic nature of the epidemic, it is not possible for any one individual or organisation to know how to deal with every problem that arises. During interactive discussions, for example, evaluation participants often responded very positively to being told that the Programme is questioning the nature of expertise. The general feeling was that so many of the problems which people now face are so new, so complex and so different to problems which can be addressed by one professional discipline or another, that there can no longer be "experts" in the traditional sense of the word. However, the nature of honesty and expertise is also relevant in a strategic sense: "Even saying, 'I don't have the answers', you have an answer", was a typical comment (again from Roland Msiska in Zambia). It expressed that working together with people to find answers can build capacity much more quickly than claiming that your own expertise is universally applicable.

Rather than focusing on skills transition, the Programme has found that capacity building arises from the development of shared learning through working in partnerships, as explained by Teresita Bagasao with reference to her own interaction with the Programme and the flow-on effects within her own work with NGOs in the Philippines:

> How do you consider agents of change? They can be experts and manipulate things. Or they can be experienced people but know that they're entering a different set of circumstances, so merge one's knowledge and experience with the country they're entering. That's the essence of partnership.

## 5.4 Characteristics of Partnerships which Develop Capacity

Consistent with the general approach of promoting sustainable human development, the role of the outsider in identifying social change agents is, to a large extent, indirect. The aim is not to go into other people's contexts (countries, communities) and identify individuals as social change agents but, rather, to establish partnerships which facilitate communities identifying and working with their own social change agents. A primary means of doing this is through bringing people together in groups and networks.

Thus, the first consultative meeting to discuss directions for the SPR, in October 1992, determined that a key element of the Programme should be, "To identify and to characterize the necessary and sufficient conditions for the development and maintenance of group and social cohesion". A primary reason for this was that, "The functional group—family, village, community, society—is the ultimate resource for behaviour change, for care and support, and for coping with the impact of the epidemic."

One method used to explore what is needed for development and maintenance of group cohesion was the development and maintenance of partnerships, commencing but not limited to partnerships between the Programme and those affected by the epidemic. Many comments were made by evaluation participants about the nature of those partnerships which develop capacity. Some of the recurring themes in these comments are summarised in the following points.

*If development and maintenance of partnerships is genuine, then they will follow the usual patterns of human relationships.* Sometimes partnerships will succeed without effort, sometimes enormous emphasis will have to be placed on maintaining the relationships, and sometimes they will fail. Ultimately, when partnerships work, they result in growth and changes amongst all partners concerned. These sorts of comments were made with reference to the Programme's relationships with its direct partners, to those partners' relationships with others in their own countries and in international networks, and to other partnerships which were identified by evaluation participants as examples of effective capacity building.

*Effective partnerships take time to establish and essentially involve two-way dialogue and development.* Capacity building does not work through patronising relationships, such as when donors have all the ideas and claimed expertise and involve local partners only in programme implementation. An example of this way of operating and the long term result was given by Peter Resurreccion, who works constantly across government/NGO boundaries in the Philippines, as he talked of earlier experience in the Department of Health:

> In the early years, foreign donor agencies came in and just did what they wanted. This led to me feeling like an admin person. I was just there to answer what they need ... and when they left, it all stopped.

In contrast to this, effective partnerships involve all partners being able to constantly question and challenge themselves and each other. Many participants reported that the HDP, and UNDP in general, often allowed this to occur. For example, Assistant Secretary Antonio Dujua, from the Department of Justice in the Philippines, noted that,

> UNDP doesn't foist things upon us ... they give hints, but don't say, "This is the way." And that gives us a sense of independence, with more room for creativity and productivity ... At the [UNDP] workshop on ethics, law and HIV there were people from many Asian countries. Each country has different legal systems and approaches, but the main objectives of the people at the workshop were the same. For example, trying to ensure that there would be no mandatory testing ... There were spaces where we could express ourselves, across cultures ... Some countries already had legislation. I came back here thinking that I could be able to push legislation.

The way effective dialogue can flow on from Programme partners to others was highlighted in comments made by staff of two Filipino NGO agencies which work to build the capacity of others in the Philippines through ongoing partnerships based on approaches identical to that of the Programme. These two people, from Kabalikat and Phansup (Philippine AIDS NGO Support Network) each noted that their own work reflects the way that Programme staff spend time "up front" in identifying potential Programme partners and in working to establish mutual understanding of roles and expectations before rushing into long-term partnerships. Such time consuming work does not always result in effective partnerships, but was reported to be an essential component of those which are effective. The results of such work are not always measurable using traditional measures of cost-effectiveness or project outputs, especially when time spent early on leads to decisions to discontinue potential, but in practice ineffective, partnerships.

*Effective partnerships are not always initiated or controlled by donor agencies or by central government authorities.* Participants in Senegal, Zambia, Mexico and the Philippines noted that many successful initiatives in response to the epidemic had commenced through voluntary activity, often starting with no clear idea of where their initiatives were heading, and receiving external funding only after difficult project development phases were complete. A few NGOs in the Philippines noted initial distrust of government involvement, claimed that successful initiatives almost always commenced with NGOs, and noted that when partnerships between government and NGOs work it is often because, in the words of one workshop participant, "NGOs have taken the pains to involve government." Hearteningly, some government workers in the Philippines also drew attention to this aspect of their partnership with NGOs.

*Effective partnerships allow all partners to make choices.* In provision of external assistance, there must be an ability for recipient partners to choose which aspects of that assistance they want, and what aspects of the external agent's experience they find useful. Partners of the Programme, especially those who had attended HDP workshops, reported that this was most often the case. Outsiders also need to be free to choose which partners they want to work with, but this may be complicated by the requirements of ongoing political challenges as, for example, when international agencies want to work with NGOs which are not close to their own countries' governments.

An important element of the importance of choice within partnerships was also noted by a participant from Senegal, when he talked about the importance of involving people with HIV but doing this in ways which enable them to choose when, where and to whom they come out:

> Yes, it's important to involve people with HIV in your projects, but also to look after them, not to leave them with a mess in their lives because you made them go public.

*Effective partnerships acknowledge the contributions of all parties involved.* Some participants reported that donors often assume that direction should be by them because they provide the funding, forgetting that the donation of time and expertise is a large expense for people living in poverty: "Donors and the community are both investing", said one participant, drawing attention to the need for both parties to determine the desired long-term outcomes of that investment. In contrast, effective partnerships engender mutual respect for the dignity and contribution of all involved.

Likewise, effective partnerships do not remain in the control of those who initiate them. This was highlighted, again, by Teresita Bagasao from the NGO, Kabalikat, in the Philippines:

There is a role for encouraging networks. We have 100 groups doing their own thing. We still respond to individual organisations but we encourage links. Our vision is that we will just be one of those organizations, not the central one. Not necessarily running the show.

*Effective partnerships are not always easy.* Some partners of the Programme reported that on some occasions they felt they were being presented with rigid views of the epidemic and development, or that their own expertise was not always recognised. This reflects that processes to build consensus on shared senses of purpose, and mutually beneficial learning, must also be ongoing. Others reported difficulties in their ongoing relationships with each other, as when members of networks noted that it was not always easy or productive for NGOs and governments to work together, or even for NGOs from different countries to respect and work with each other. A few participants in the Latin American and Caribbean Council of AIDS Service Organisations (LACCASO) noted that this network had experienced difficulties but had overcome them over time.

## 5.5 Some Immediate Effects of Partnerships which Build Capacity

Partnerships are important not only for their own sakes, but because of what they achieve. Throughout all stages of the evaluation process, much was said about how working through partnership achieves relevant and sustainable responses to HIV and development. Comments of participants can be grouped in various themes, and these in turn can be grouped into themes about the immediate effects of successful partnerships and what people experience through these processes, leading to more powerful and sustained effects. Amongst the immediate effects are concepts of inclusion, the creation of space, reflection and sharing of experiences. The way people experience these processes is addressed in the next sub-sections.

### Inclusion

Evaluation participants indicated the value of learning through interactive processes. However, such learning does not happen automatically whenever people meet together. An essential prerequisite to mutual learning is that all participants feel included.

Notions of expertise are important to this. In brief, if people feel that their own experience is valued by others, they will be more likely to talk about it and to share both what they have learnt and what they still have doubts about. This leads to others doing the same, and reflective dialogue helps in the development of solutions to newly identified problems.

The use of a wide range of available group processes, simulation games and other methods drawn from the fields of adult education and community development is important in these inclusive processes. While often used in local projects, the HDP has demonstrated their usefulness also in international networks and workshops.

It is important to include in sustainable development programmes the people whose lives are directly affected by the epidemic, to ensure that their experiences are valued, and to ensure that they feel able to contribute. A classic example is the inclusion of people with HIV in programme and policy planning. Promotion of this has been a feature of the UNDP HIV and Development Programme's work since the beginning. Recognition of its importance is now common on national HIV/AIDS committees and in many (but not all) international forums. However, this inclusion has often been tokenistic, resulting in people with HIV sitting in on committee meetings to which they have been invited at the last minute, not adequately informed of what is going on, and not included as equal partners in problem-solving within those meetings.

The HDP has explored ways to improve this situation, by promoting networks within countries, regions and worldwide so that people with HIV could share their experiences with each other before participating in wider networks, by inviting people with HIV to participate in all workshops and meetings held by the Programme, and by exploring within workshops various means of involving people with HIV in ways which enable them to participate and discuss their HIV status as and when they feel appropriate. The value of these types of initiatives was often mentioned by people with HIV who were involved in the evaluation process.

The issue of inclusion of people with HIV in workshops has led to much discussion amongst people with HIV, people involved in NGOs working in development, and other partners of the Programme. Gradually, it was reported, people are building up trust and understanding of how to make this work, by acknowledging that the answers are not simple but that they can be found through interactive processes.

Likewise, the Programme has promoted the involvement of others affected by the epidemic based on principles of including people affected and recognising expertise which arises from lived experience. Again, evaluation participants often acknowledged the importance of this.

The HDP evaluation process itself ensured inclusion of people whose lives are affected by the HIV epidemic, often to the surprise of those people themselves, because they are so often excluded. Reflecting a common experience of internalising lack of power, some participants in Mexico asked, "Why me? Why do you want to interview me?" One woman identified by HDP partners as being an active social change agent said her organisation was ".. just a grassroots organization", and asked, "Why don't you go to the big ones?" Constant experiences of exclusion result in a lowering of expectations about inclusion. The result is that the experiences of some of the people engaged in the most effective responses to the epidemic are often excluded from policy and programme development unless conscious efforts are made to invite their inclusion.

The lack of inclusion, or even active exclusion, of some people in many responses to the epidemic was also noted by many participants. Exclusion can be a damaging process which crushes hope and stifles the development of effective responses. Consider, for example, this statement by Eduardo San Miguel from Mexico:

> If NGOs do not revise or review their own approach to tolerance of opinions that are not their own, very little can be advanced. For example, the voice of those who are in the first circle around those with AIDS has to be listened to ... A female relative (of someone with HIV) at the national consultation had been talked down because someone said that the only people who are important are those with AIDS. That comment pleased the public, and left the woman discredited.

Another group not often included is the next generation. This is often reflected in countries in which it is believed HIV has a low prevalance: for example, when almost all HIV resources are spent on surveillance and education, with little interest in planning for future needs in care and support of people who are ill and the living dependants of those who have died. In contrast, a group of women in Zambia who are caring for the children of those who have died, a group called Kwasha Mukwenu, meaning "Help your friend who is in need", told evaluators that they are now teaching the older children how to care for the younger ones, in the conscious hope that their work will be continued in the years to come when they themselves are unable to continue providing care.

## The Importance of Space in Enabling Inclusion

One immediate impact of effective partnerships is the creation of space in which people can think, feel, say and thus share things that are not always possible in the spaces of their everyday lives. The concept of space was recognised as an important component of inclusion. Again, simply being in one spot does not lead to people feeling included, or to them bringing to the sharing the things which may matter most to them. Two considerations are important here: first, having a space where people are free to talk undisturbed, and where time to reflect is deliberately allocated; second, creating a type of emotional space, in which people feel free to discuss some things they do not normally discuss. The requirements of such space, and the range of issues this enables people to address, are summarised in this quote from As Sy, the Executive Director of the African Council of AIDS Service Organizations (AFRICASO):

> Physical, geographical, places to meet ... but ... without being accused, discounted, excluded, assaulted; ideological space ... where you can feel safe to talk about sex, serostatus and human rights.

The use of space, like many other processes of inclusion, needs to be valued and cherished if it is to be effective. An example of this was learnt directly by the SPR evaluation team in Zambia. A workshop which had led to the telling of many important stories and the sharing of many emotions was joined after lunch by a few people who had not been there in the morning, and who held senior positions in government. The trust and the sense of sharing the same space which had been developed throughout the morning and continued during the lunch break suddenly disappeared, and discussion reverted to common bureaucratic and planning language, with little allowance for the importance of emotion or cultural insight. In retrospect, it would have been important to insist that participants attend for the whole day, or just for the morning, but that they could not arrive mid-way through the workshop.

Participants reported that one of the most effective uses of space is to allow people to bring their emotions into discussions: in the words of one participant from Senegal, allowing "... permission to feel." Despite the overwhelming significance of human emotions in enabling people to come to terms with and respond to the effects of the HIV epidemic, this is often not allowed, especially in international meetings. The assumption is, too often, that effective responses arise from scientific insight alone, and that emotions get in the way of good programming.

Likewise, discussion about religious beliefs is often excluded in policy making, on the basis that religion somehow interferes with rational responses to the epidemic. Thus, participants in Zambia and the Philippines reported that many outsiders had told them either to make special efforts to "get the church on our side" or, conversely, to make sure the church was not involved because it would interfere with the promotion of condoms. In both countries, efforts to include the church have proved of value.

Indeed, both communities and people's religious and spiritual beliefs were central to many of the evaluation participants' own experiences with the epidemic. What is often forgotten is that a faith community in many communities is the only institution which brings people together in groups. If group sharing is an essential component of developing capacity, then the involvement of faith communities is also essential. If action arises from understanding, then no action will arise if key components of understanding are denied: these include religious belief and spirituality, which are often intricately entwined with feelings of hope, empowerment and solidarity.

The importance of, and methods for, creation of space in which people can reflect on and share their innermost feelings and beliefs in relation to the epidemic was highlighted in an evaluation workshop in the Philippines. Discussion at one stage addressed the question of the extent to which Filipinos feel able to talk about sex. The experience of many participants was that Filipinos find this difficult, but this was challenged by a Catholic nun, who said that she had found that Filipinos like to talk about sex. Only when asked to explain how she enabled them to do this did she recount that such talk usually occurred, "... at the end of the second day of closed workshops." Thus, the evaluation workshop itself had created space for Filipinos to talk about the circumstances in which they could talk about sex. The result was that all participants learnt how to create space for this, by hearing from someone who regularly does so but perhaps did not realise how rare this is.

## Reflection and Sharing of Experiences

Reflection, on one's own and others' experiences, was another immediate effect of working in partnerships which was reported by many participants. This was noted by Margaret Mutambo, from Zambia, as having obviously occurred amongst staff of the HDP:

> I don't think anybody can write what she (Elizabeth Reid, Director of the Programme) writes without reflection. The epidemic itself is something that makes you sit down and just think of things that are important.

The importance of reflection, and the types of insights to which it leads which are different from those which can simply be passed on as knowledge from one person to another, was also highlighted by Sr Marie-Luc, from Senegal:

> We don't have the answers, so we have to share. ... It's the entire being that's touched. People called upon to work in (the epidemic) ... have to feel all the implications of what it means. If all you do is campaigns and condoms, then you're missing the point. It becomes mechanical ... it is more multifaceted and profound ... it touches the individual in the most profound aspect of her being.

Like inclusion, reflection does not happen automatically, but can be invoked. Learning this through having participated in workshops which encouraged reflection was, in itself, an important lesson for Margaret Mutambo, from Zambia:

> Just bringing people together and giving them the chance to share, of course, with guidance. That is something that made me think, "I can apply that." People sharing, not something they have back in the office.

## 5.6 What People Experience as a Result of these Processes

It is the more powerful and sustainable effects of partnerships which lead directly to the types of understanding and action which are required for sustainable, adaptable and effective responses to the HIV epidemic in the context of human development. These include validation, the creation of social learning, solidarity, empowerment and the releasing of energy and, ultimately, sustainable and continuing social change.

### Validation

One of the important effects of inclusion and sharing is the sense of validation that people attain and can give to each other. Validation is about making sure that people are not only included, but also that the value of their experience is acknowledged and affirmed.

Validation is important in any work which is attempting to redefine the nature of expertise. Expertise which arises from experience is not always valued, and people whose expertise arises from experience rather than formal education often internalise feelings of inadequacy and lack of expertise. The required validation need not come from external "experts" in a patronising way, but may more often come from people learning to value each others' experience. In Senegal, a number of workshops had been held based on the Programme's workshop in HIV and Development. Evaluation participants reported that within these workshops they had listened to one another and shared their understanding of what might work to bring about change. These processes had been very useful in validating not just their individual expertise, but also the power of sharing and developing that expertise together.

One seemingly ironic aspect of validation is the benefit some participants reported could arise from validating uncertainty. Sometimes, coming together with others to share understanding about the epidemic results in sharing doubts, uncertainties and even a sense of despair about what is occurring and what might be done. Rather than stifling responses, participants reported that finding that their own uncertainties were also being experienced by others was empowering, because it enabled people to see that the problems did not just rest in their own individual lack of power or insight. The sharing of uncertainty often leads to identifying ways to move beyond that uncertainty.

## Developing Empathy and Deep Understanding

Many participants spoke about the importance to them of having developed the capacity for social, or community, learning through having first developed a deeper capacity for understanding the complex realities of the epidemic and its effects. Eduardo San Miguel, from Mexico, similarly talked about the nature of understanding which is effective in producing action:

> I've been trying to understand the epidemic in my own way. This has happened gradually. When you interact and you start listening to what people want to know, you have to think a lot, because when you ask questions around HIV and AIDS, you become vulnerable. To really understand, you have to ask concrete things, refer to specific experiences.

An important aspect of this was the acknowledgement that people must become engaged in understanding emotional aspects of the epidemic.

## Solidarity

The sharing of experiences, amongst people within similar contexts, can result in important developments in people's ability to learn about and understand locally-situated realities in ways which may not always be understood, and certainly cannot be predetermined, by outsiders. The concept of solidarity which arises from sharing, and supporting each other through, difficult experiences was noted as important by many participants.

Solidarity was not always seen as solidarity in action; often, it referred to solidarity in hope. For example, Sr Marie-Luc, from Senegal, noted that she gained an important sense of encouragement in her work from people in France:

> Solidarity means you are not an isolated person, you can't stay in your corner, what touches our brothers touches us. A solidarity in sharing the misfortunes of others, individuals and nations. When I went to France last year and spoke about what we're doing here in Senegal, I told them you have to express solidarity with countries worse touched than France, and with less means than you have. Then, France sent me messages, documents, magazines, and the exchanges I have with those people ... we are carrying this together, it's not just one person. Solidarity means helping and giving of yourself ... to feel compassion for the problems that the other person is living.

Mary Kanene, from Zambia, noted that the evaluation process itself had provided her with a sense of solidarity, simply through allowing interactive discussion:

> It was a blessing ... through talking (with Cindy) I realised how much I really was doing ... I know that in my small things I can be of value. You don't have to stand alone on a hilltop to be able to access others who are in need.

Solidarity is not something which arises through transfer of skills, but it can be catalysed through programming approaches which promote the sharing of personal experiences. A powerful example of this was provided by Roberto Castro, a member of a research team in Mexico:

> We are studying coping strategies, but we also have to learn to cope with our own reactions to our findings. We are overwhelmed, sometimes it is too much ... Sometimes what we find touches some very, very personal experience. One person we interviewed told us about being abandoned by the family. ... When we discussed this, we moved from the interview experience to the experience of one of our team members. He had polio as a child. At the age of five he was attending a rehabilitation centre to train his movements. The children were picked up by a bus every morning and brought back at the end of the day. Once there was one child who was not met by his parents or anybody else. He had to be brought back to the rehabilitation centre. Later they found out that the family had simply moved, leaving the handicapped child behind. When our team member understood, he told his mother what had happened and the mother cried and cried. He realised he was so lucky to have a caring family. When my team member shared this story with me it changed my perspective. I used to think I was luckier than him since I had no polio, but his polio story had shown him that he was lucky to have a caring family.

The richness of understanding and empathetic feelings experienced by all members of that research team, as a result of the telling of this story, has helped them to develop a much better understanding of the way the epidemic has affected the people with whom they interact through their research, as Roberto explained:

> We are somehow understanding the complexity. A world in which people have very little control of their own fate. This way of looking at the world is very rooted in their everyday life ... Changing is possible, but difficult, and involves slow processes ... I would like to see that the insight we have gained through our research will have practical implications.

## Empowerment, and the Releasing of Energy

Feeling that they are able to understand and respond to the challenges of the HIV epidemic and development was reported as centrally important to people's actual responses. Partnerships which lead to empowerment, which can sometimes be indicated by the presence of such feelings, are far more effective than those which build dependence. Anuar Luna, from Mexico, noted the close links between feelings of solidarity and feelings of empowerment: "The model is the tool, but the solidarity is the energy."

Programmes which work to build enabling environments, such as through changing attitudes and laws to make partnership between NGOs and governments easier, are therefore important. The means to develop enabling environments are many and complex, and require the interaction of numerous activities and the development of widespread understanding. Many participants reported that feelings of empowerment, feelings that they can act within their own environments, have come gradually and slowly developed through collective action.

Others reported that bursts of energy which enable them to respond to the epidemic are often associated with anger. Sara Longwe and Roy Clarke, from Zambia, were two such participants. They noted that a sense of anger at injustice and at patriarchal systems was an important motivating force, but that their anger at wider structural barriers was separate from the feelings they had working with people in their own lives. For example, Sara said that, "What gives me energy is to have one foot working in the NGOs and one foot in the grassroots." Roy acknowledged that he felt a sense of anger, "But at first when I felt anger it was a patriarchal anger: I am not having my wife treated like that! But later, I understood that the patriarchal reaction was a barrier to change."

A good example of how inclusive processes can be empowering was provided through a series of experiences related by Margaret Mutambo, the UNDP HIV and Development national professional of ficer in Zambia. She noted the value of processes of the Programme which enabled people within her own country to attend inter-country workshops in which they shared experiences with each other and with those from other African countries. The types of processes used within those meetings and workshops had resulted in her feeling able to act with strong commitment in response to the epidemic in Zambia. These processes, she said, were based on a recognition that everyone present had something to contribute, irrespective of levels of education or professional experience. Their very attendance indicated interest, and part of that interest was to learn. What the Programme had done, however, was to ensure that everyone also contributed to that learning, even in ways they had not expected themselves:

> Recognition of the person, not their skill. This leads to where you might not know you have something to offer until it comes out. Because there are some hidden skills that only another person can help you discover. They made clear that they thought I had something to offer. They did not know what that was, and I did not know what that was, but the workshop brought it out.

## 5.7 Sustainable Results: Responsive Social Change

The net result of partnerships, inclusion, solidarity and social learning is personal and social change which slows down the epidemic and minimises its negative impact. The importance of such change was often noted by HDP staff throughout the evaluation process, as was the interim step of change, or even transformation, of individuals and institutions.

The importance of transformation was also acknowledged by many evaluation participants. Transformation results in people feeling that they do understand enough to be able to act, that they want to take action, and that they are somehow "changed" as a result of that action. This was highlighted in comments by Anuar Luna, from Mexico:

> The [HDP] workshop gave me the capacity to see myself and others. This was my personal process: to discover the link between the personal and the global. The paper on strategic questioning also gave me a lot. In that workshop I felt the importance of meeting. I felt the global challenge and the importance for change, or deeply felt transition. The workshop was very, very important. ... We can influence many of the underlying problems of the epidemic. I think my life has changed in many ways. I have plans. I am enthusiastic. ... For me it was a long process to learn to think differently, to build a new way.

Evaluation participants reported various types of transformative processes which they found had been personally useful. Most often, these processes involved a combination of having lived through powerful experiences *and* having engaged in shared reflection about those experiences. As Roland Msiska, from

Zambia, said, "You go through these personal changes. Through a state of fear, to hope."

Thus, in workshops aiming to enhance understanding, processes which led to emotional responses had been very useful in generating commitment to responding to the epidemic. Likewise, people who said they had lived through traumatic experiences within the epidemic had found it useful to incorporate reflection on those experiences into general dialogue about policy and programme development. In turn, the involvement in policy and programme development had helped them to make more sense of their feelings of grief and loss.

Two particular components of the workshops on HIV and Development were mentioned by many participants, either as experiences which had led to changes for them, or as methods they use to help others understand various aspects of the epidemic. One is the simulation game, *Wilds fire,* originally developed for family planning situations by the Family Planning Association of New South Wales (Australia) and adapted for the Programme workshops. Another is an exercise called, *The Unfolding of the epidemic,* developed by HDP staff to enable people to understand the likely impact of the epidemic on individuals, families, communities and nations. Details of both exercises are available from the UNDP HIV and Development Programme. What is significant to this report is not those details, but a recognition that both of these exercises enable people to learn through shared reflection based on their own experiences, and both exercises enable learning at both an intellectual and an emotional level.

Some evaluation participants reported significant effects arising from a single interactive experience, such as a facilitated visit to a nearby country or participation in a single workshop. Transformation can result from single experiences which lead to feelings of, "Aha! Now I understand", or "Now I have changed." An example of this was the reaction of Santhi, from Senegal, to the exercise *Wilds fire:*

> You overcome your fear of AIDS. It's an adversary, but you've developed an idea of how it uses its tricks. So, it's no longer a fear of the unknown. It's transformation from not knowing, to being part of a network. I was the object of the transformation ... you suddenly realised anyone can get AIDS. ... You remember, "That bastard infected me!"

A participant reported in a final evaluation note of a workshop in Senegal that it had helped him to realise that:

> I thought I understood, but I didn't.
> I thought I was involved, but I wasn't.
> Things will be different from now on.

More often, participants reported that they had sensed changes in their own levels of understanding and commitment over time. This could come from continued involvement in a network, ongoing involvement in the development of training materials, or the repeated running of workshops for people in their own countries.

One person in Zambia reported the transformation he had experienced as a result of attending policy meetings on and off over a period of months during which a number of relatives and close friends died. The continual need to think about what should happen in national responses to the epidemic, interspersed with the intense personal experience of having people close to him dying, had resulted in an unshakable commitment to find better ways to help others respond to the epidemic. Similar experiences were reported by others working in UNDP, governments, NGOs or simply in their local communities.

Some government officials engaged in policy-making responses to the epidemic reported the importance of transformative experiences leading to changes in their perception of the significance of their work, and to a different type of engagement with their work in relation to HIV than what they had with other work. In helping to develop capacity, it is important to remember that government officials are also people who live in families and communities, and the importance of providing space for sharing of emotions and for validation of lived experience is as important for them as it is for others involved in responses to the epidemic.

The ultimate result of processes of capacity building is that people are able to further develop their own understanding and their own collective responses to the HIV epidemic and the challenges of human development. This was summed up well by Gary Engelberg, from Senegal:

> The virus is moving too quickly, so we need to involve people very quickly, ... I can't imagine knowing what's at stake and then not acting. ... That's the challenge, to get them to see what's at stake. Because it's dealing with procreation, love. Once people understand that, you just let them loose. You can create mutual support for those kinds of processes, follow up networks ... but what you have to create is a *mass movement* of people to stop the epidemic.

## CASE STUDY 1:

## ENHANCING NATIONAL CAPACITY THROUGH HIV ACTION RESEARCH

Although the economic determinants of vulnerability to HIV at both the individual and societal levels are increasingly being recognised and studied, most attention so far in the social sciences has been focused on the impact of HIV, primarily in the industrialised world. The socio-economic impact of HIV on developing societies has been less well studied and understood. The HIV epidemic threatens social and economic development because, in contrast to other life-threatening infections which attack primarily the young, the aged and the infirm, HIV affects people responsible for the support and care of children, the elderly and extended family members, and it affects adults in their economically and socially most active years. HIV-related illness and death have the potential to deplete the labour force, undermine public sector capacity to govern, and lead to social and civil unrest.

At the macro-economic level, selective erosion of slices of the economy occurs as people with critical capacities such as bank managers, teachers, engineers or nurses become ill. Reduction in productivity and workforce depletions in key formal sector industries such as mining, tourism or agriculture can affect gross domestic product, export earnings and public revenue generation. Countries may then experience investment reductions in education and training which, combined with the loss of skilled labour, can lead to decreased output, skills, experiences, and aspirations with resultant further decreased investment. These macro-economic effects compound those of structural adjustment programmes in many countries (Lurie et al., 1995).

At the household level, reductions in earning capacity, increases in health related expenditures, the opportunity cost of time spent caring for the sick, and extra burdens placed on women threaten to substantially reduce household resources. Coping mechanisms may include changes in household composition and the modification of roles and activities within the family. Children may be withdrawn from school to assist with household duties or to enter the job market (Ainsworth and Koda, 1993, 50), cash crops may be abandoned in favour of subsistence crops that require less attention (Barnett and Blaikie, 1992, 89), traditional knowledge systems may be irrevocably lost and customary mechanisms for the care and support of orphans may be overwhelmed. Conventionally determined direct and indirect costs will clearly underestimate the real psychosocial, interpersonal, emotional, and economic consequences and costs of the HIV epidemic at the individual, household, community and national levels.

This case study describes and discusses the generalisability of a programme, currently underway in four African countries, which is aimed at enhancing the capacity of nation states to understand the threat that the HIV epidemic poses to their economic, social and political development and to respond effectively.

## Extractive Research Approaches in Developing Countries

Research can provide information critical to formulating effective programming and policy initiatives that can increase the capacity of countries to meet the challenge of the HIV epidemic. To date, however, a good proportion of HIV-related research has not achieved these ends, which is not surprising given the long and notorious history of North-South research relationships. The approach used is the antithesis of local capacity building. Researchers from industrialized countries define a line of inquiry and then seek out local collaborators, both to ensure that the relevant approvals can be obtained and to provide on-the-ground assistance with the challenging logistics of data collection.

Following the operational phase, some data entry, verification and cleaning may be conducted locally but, more often than not, the information leaves the country with the industrialised country researchers never to be seen again. If and when the results are published, it is in the form of a scientific article, in a highly-rated journal priced beyond the resources of institutions such as the local university, let alone local collaborators. Local members of the research team are lucky to be included as co-authors, the standard gesture often being a simple acknowledgement of their help. Increasingly this approach is being rejected but it remains common.

## Local Research Processes and the Link to Programming and Policy

The charges levelled at foreign investigators can also apply to the way local researchers behave. Indigenous scientists trained in industrialized countries, or in similarly-styled regional learning institutions, now form the elite cadre in developing countries. Following traditional approaches, topics and methodology may often reflect the individual curiosity of the researcher. In other, perhaps more common cases, research priorities and methodologies may be determined by donors with little interest in what is needed for more effective responses to the epidemic. Indeed, even in those unfortunately rare circumstances where local priorities are taken into account there is very little evidence that research is effectively used in the formulation of policy and programmes. For example, among 73 studies profiled in a directory of social and behavioural research on HIV and AIDS compiled in Zimbabwe in 1994, fully 71 per cent gave no indication that the results were being used in the formulation of programmes and policies (Misihairabwi et al., 1994, 23). Many studies conducted in developing countries are never published in local journals or even in the form of a final report and only exceptionally are results disseminated to the communities which were researched or to service providers and decision makers. It is unsurprising that in the conditions which prevail in many countries, where the norm has research being largely externally funded and determined, that local policy and programme needs are low on the agenda and that results are rarely translated into effective programmes or policy changes.

In addition to an evident opportunity cost to the *status quo,* ethical concerns are raised by issues of ownership of the data. At issue is whether research, particularly research addressing the cultural context and meaning of sexuality, will provide baseline data for programme development and evaluation or whether it will simply produce voyeuristic impressions and serve to increase the stigmatization of the community and its members.

Methodological concerns have been raised about the extractive research model and the tendency for quantitative questionnaire surveys to reflect the pervasive and tenacious assumptions of biomedicine about culture and behaviour (Schoepf, 1991). Ultimately, choice of methodologies, whether quantitative or qualitative, will depend on the nature of the research question being posed and should be based on whether the research findings generated by the chosen methodology will be informative and valid, and have the potential to significantly advance understanding and stimulate social change. Mobilising society will be essential for an effective response to the HIV epidemic and research which is capacity building is thus an important instrument in the process of strengthening social capital.

## Capacity Building Through Research

Responses to the complexity of the HIV epidemic must be timely and must act to slow down the spread of the virus and provide support and care to those affected within communities. Research will play a critical role if results contribute to the development of effective HIV programming and policy and if the research process itself is empowering for research participants and their communities.

If research is to support the development of effective HIV programming, it should fit within a locally articulated plan of research needs and priorities, be timely and be affordable.

Moreover, given the urgency of the problems to be addressed through policies and programmes there has to be a reasonable likelihood that research will in fact yield results which can be embodied in effective responses to the epidemic. Small-scale, multifaceted, multidisciplinary projects may be more cost-effective than expensive large-scale ones and may furnish results more rapidly. The best way to ensure that such findings are used by those responsible for HIV programme development is to involve decision makers, programme developers, community activists and representatives from National AIDS Programmes (NAPs) from the outset of research design and continuously throughout the research process. The latter are critical partners since NAP staff know what research is being undertaken, planned or has been completed, and are the point of contact at the national level for bilateral and multilateral donors.

Individuals affected by HIV are central to a complex understanding of the nature of the epidemic and to the utilisation of eventual findings, and should be fully integrated into research processes from the start. Effective action-oriented research will involve people living with HIV and affected by HIV in the setting of research priorities, in the choice of research questions, in evaluations of the relevance of proposed investigations, in the research design phase, and in study conduct, analysis and dissemination of results.

Development is now understood as sustainable if it empowers people to take charge of their own well-being, if it builds on the strengths of local knowledge and values, and if an enabling environment is created at national and international levels which fosters and supports local initiatives (Banuri et al., 1994). In development practice the role of experts or donor agencies is increasingly understood as involving facilitation of processes for creating norms, values and practices that enable people and their organizations to gain greater control over their lives. In this paradigm, development is constituted by local sources of experimentation, of innovation, and of diversity fostered within a supportive macro-level institutional, policy and legislative environment.

At the heart of this new form of development practice is the recognition that sources of learning must be local in part so as to enable people to engage with "the global" on their own and better terms (Appadurai, 1990). For ideas and programmes to take root within communities, they must spring from within, they must be based on the realities of lived experiences, and they must be disseminated and defended from there. At the centre of this new development practice are concepts of consensus building, promotion of partnerships between the organizations of civil society and public institutions, human and social capacity building, ethical practice, and facilitation.

Participatory research initiatives can support and strengthen local processes of social learning and national capacities which transform social learning into policy and programmes. Community level responses empower participants, particularly infected individuals and communities, to identify their own needs and to ensure that chosen strategies can be implemented and maintained. It follows that researchers who are close to or part of affected communities are better placed than external teams to identify research themes and methodologies which are relevant and to ensure that their findings are of ultimate benefit to affected people, activists and organizations responding to the epidemic.

## Programme Development: The UNDP Research Capacity Building Initiative

Based on a development approach of social learning and capacity building, the UNDP partnership programme was created to assist selected communities, academic institutions and countries to create capacity to undertake action-oriented research into the extent and nature of the psychological, social and economic causes and consequences of the epidemic; to analyse the data and findings in ways that would be directly relevant to programme and policy development; and to assist community organizations, programme managers, activists and leaders to assess and redesign their policies and interventions in light of the research findings. This work is being undertaken in Senegal, Central African Republic, Zambia and Kenya (Hankins, 1994, 1995a, 1996) as well as Myanmar (Porter, 1995) and Nicaragua. This case study focuses on progress to date in the African component, and includes discussion of the difficulties encountered and lessons learnt to date.

Programme Implementation Phase I of this pilot programme began in April 1993 with the formation of Country Groups in four African countries. Research topics were chosen, infrastructural support was provided, an inter-country training seminar was held in Senegal, research protocols were elaborated, technical support missions conducted, and presentations made to donors. Phase II, which focuses on the translation of data into programming and policy, was launched in August 1995 with skills building workshops for Country Group representatives, NAP managers, technical support partners, donors and African academics.

### Phase I: From Research Needs to Raw Data

The four African countries evaluated for eventual participation in the Partnership Programme were chosen to represent both East and West Africa, francophone and anglophone cultures, and to provide a spectrum of HIV prevalence ranging from Senegal with the lowest rates at one per cent (Mbaye et al., 1993), Central African Republic at approximately ten per cent (Global Programme on AIDS, 1991), through to Zambia and Kenya in the ten to twenty per cent range for overall country HIV prevalence among adults (Hira et al., 1989; Kitabu et al., 1992; Mungai et al., 1992). Between April and June 1993, exploratory missions were conducted in each country, with NAP personnel, other pertinent government ministries, and key donors being consulted as to the relevance of such a programme. Their willingness to participate actively in the programme was assessed since neither the HIV and Development Programme in New York nor the HIV and Development Regional Project in Dakar would be directly funding any of the research projects developed within the initiative. Potential candidates for the multidisciplinary Country Groups were interviewed and asked to provide a written statement of why they wanted to participate. They were informed that the exchange being contemplated was one in which their time contribution would be balanced by new knowledge, skills and contacts. The Country Groups included a mix of senior and junior researchers, concerned community members, affected persons, institutional leaders and other users of research findings.

Country Group meetings were held to define priority areas for research and to draft initial proposals equivalent to letters of intention. A seminar attended by all Country Groups during September 1993 discussed principles, methodologies and ethical issues involved in psychosocial and economic research. It aimed to strengthen participants' awareness of the nature, determinants and consequences of the HIV epidemic and, in particular, to create a common conceptual framework for viewing HIV and development. The seminar paved the way for a collaborative effort among researchers from within and outside the region, and quantified the financial resources required to undertake designed studies and follow-up activities. Infrastructural support of $US5,000 was then provided to each team for research training, language courses and pre-pilot work.

In 1994, a technical assistance consortium of experienced researchers from within Africa, from other regions of the developing world and from elsewhere was established with the resultant diverse blend of researchers having both scientific expertise and experience working in partnerships of equals with others. Following this, technical support missions to Senegal, Central African Republic and Zambia focused on quantitative and qualitative research methodologies, economic theory and analysis, ethical issues, and presentation strategies. These assisted Country Groups to finalise their research objectives, determine appropriate research methodologies and study sample sizes, refine analysis plans, justify budgets, and prepare workplans. Fourteen proposals were prepared initially by the four teams. By early 1996 data collection had been completed in two projects and was underway in three others. Strong donor interest had been expressed in a further four projects and funding negotiations were proceeding. Research projects underway include evaluations of the management of HIV infection within the family, the socio-economic determinants of the HIV epidemic, the role of church groups in HIV/AIDS prevention and care, the socio-cultural factors associated with HIV prevalence, and the impact of AIDS in the business sector.

## Phase I: Lessons Learnt

The lessons learnt during this pilot project are as relevant to Asia, and other parts of the world, where the socio-economic impact of the HIV epidemic is also being felt (Panyarachun, 1995), as they are to Africa. How well each step of the programme was implemented had predictable consequences for subsequent steps. Countries and their National AIDS Programmes had varying levels of commitment to the programme, some research teams were not well-balanced with respect to experience and motivation, stakeholders did not participate fully in the defining of research priorities, infrastructural funds were not disbursed in a timely manner, some members of the technical assistance consortium lacked process facilitation skills, and several local donors were reticent to fund projects. Some suggestions for avoiding these and other problems are presented in the discussion which follows.

Countries chosen should be those most likely to implement the programme successfully, to attract funding for research activities, and where the NAP and local UNDP offices have expressed interest. Although the partnership process is UNDP's responsibility, particular attention should be paid to ensuring that key individuals in the NAP comprehend what is being attempted and are prepared to integrate research projects into the NAP.

Country Groups have a tripartite composition of researchers (intergenerational and interdisciplinary), data users (government, civil society, professional associations), and members of concerned communities and affected individuals. The mix of disciplines and perspectives within Country Groups can be maximised by ensuring that those interviewing and selecting members have a clear understanding of the implications of the capacity building objectives for the choice of participants. Medical doctors, epidemiologists, survey sociologists, economists and other quantitative researchers should be fully complemented by anthropologists, ethnographers and others with qualitative research and strong conceptual backgrounds. In each Country Group, it is essential to have at least two representatives from infected and affected communities and their support organisations so as to reduce the possibility that illness will interrupt community representation or that token representation will lead to reduced participation due to intimidation based on hierarchy and position.

To minimise the tendency for Country Groups to define areas of inquiry on their own without outside consultation, a workshop should be held within each country to create a common understanding of the HIV epidemic and of the objectives of the programme. This should occur after the creation of the Country Groups and prior to any definition of relevant research tasks. Such a workshop could initiate a process of consultation with key stakeholders, such as representatives of both governmental and non-governmental organisations, community-based groups, donors, individuals and communities affected by HIV and others. Incorporating brainstorming sessions concerning the range of possible research topics, the workshop would help create top-level commitment to the process, and engender in the researchers a moral engagement for ongoing consultation and follow-through with key stakeholders and in particular with users of the research including the NAP and the Ministry of Planning. Although responsiveness to the needs of civil society is critical if social capital and social change are to be created it is important to be inclusive because the focus of each country's response to the epidemic is its strategy for HIV in which the National AIDS Programme plays a pivotal role.

Team building activities should incorporate a team-driven self-assessment of individual capacities and complementarities as well as of overall team composition, allowing for the possibility of adjustments. Team cohesiveness depends on several factors including leadership, team composition, personality factors, previous relationships, individual commitment and strategic replacement of members who leave the team because of lack of interest, conflicts of interest or new job responsibilities. Criteria for selection and procedures for choosing replacement members should be defined by participants at the first country workshop. Since both the personality and vision of the leader were found to be critical to team functioning and progress, selection criteria could be suggested at the time of Country Group formation. This may reduce the possibility that pre existing local power relationships play the predominant role in the designation of team leaders. The underpinning philosophy is one of minimization of direction to the teams with emphasis on a process of technical co-operation which is based on principles of process consultation. This means providing guidance, challenging old ways of looking at things by raising new questions, offering expert information, analysis, and judgement while facilitating collective ownership in the design and implementation of new capacity building approaches to research, policy, and programme development (Joy & Bennett, 1994).

To avoid misunderstandings, it is important that the conditions of research participation be made clear from the outset. Team members are asked to make a personal commitment to exchange their time on a quid *pro quo* basis for capacity building without the possibility of either assured project funding or personal monetary recompense. Once a research project has been financed, direct payment of Country Group members or reimbursement to the employers of salaried individuals to cover time devoted to actual research work, such as the conducting of key informant interviews or participation as assistant moderators in focus groups, is justifiable.

The timing and objectives of a regional inter-country seminar should be carefully defined. The 1993 seminar succeeded in encouraging South-South collaboration and inter-country cooperation within the region and across language barriers but failed to meet some objectives, in part because often the definition of research needs had been carried out in isolation and, in part, because protocol development was well underway. Ideally, the initial inter-country seminar should follow country seminars and local processes of consultation for research question definition. Representatives of the Country Groups and of technical consortium members who have been involved in facilitating country workshops can usefully participate in the planning and programming of the inter-country one.

The establishment and maintenance of an appropriately skilled technical consortium were crucial to the success of the partnership initiative. In addition to specific technical back-up, more general support was provided for enhancing comprehension of the concepts of HIV and development and of the principles of research into the psychosocial and economic dimensions of HIV. Capacity to use research in programme design was strengthened by discussions identifying the linkages between research and policy and programme development. These in turn laid the groundwork for collaborative efforts among researchers, decision makers, affected communities, activists, and organisations responding to the epidemic. Down to earth advice on identifying and quantifying the financial resources required to undertake designed studies led naturally to the development of strategies for follow through at country level with donors and UNDP field offices.

Finding members for the technical assistance consortium with a broad understanding of both the HIV field and participatory development strategies, with appropriate scientific skills, and with personalities suited to a mutual learning process was challenging.

Constituting a technical support team composed of individuals who would complement each other in specifically addressing the needs of each country required consultation with numerous sources, evaluation of consultant capacity, performance appraisal of participants, and an element of luck concerning availability for specific missions. Facility in the language of the Country Group was obviously essential. The calibre of each technical support team had direct effects on the quality of the interactions between mission members and their country counterparts as well as on the overall benefits derived from technical visits, benefits which varied by country. Drawing on the specific expertise of members of the technical consortium, technical support missions provided assistance for three projects in Senegal, two in the Central African Republic, five in Zambia, and four in Kenya. Lack of time prevented assistance being given to most projects in the development of research instruments, codification manuals or interview guides as had been originally intended. Practically, Country Groups could choose two projects for external technical consultation which would provide the template for refinement by the research teams of any additional protocols.

The provision of supportive and facilitative technical assistance can tread a fine line between critique and criticism. Personality factors play a major role as does the experience of country counterparts and mission members in honest but affirming project review procedures. When most technical mission members come from industrialised countries and not all have training in process consultation principles and techniques, positive interactions may be hindered and traditional North-South one-way information transfer reinforced. Members of the technical assistance consortium must fully understand the implications of the programme's capacity building objectives for modes of interaction. The provision of specific training sessions designed to enhance the preparedness of consultants to participate effectively in the programme, combined with on-the-job training and performance appraisal, should be built into the programme. An emphasis on skill development with respect to process consultation (Joy and Bennett, 1994) and strategic questioning (Peavey, 1994) would help avoid inappropriate consultant behaviour during technical support missions.

To strengthen intra-regional ties, two of the three technical support missions included at least one member from a country within the region. As the programme matures two or more regional resource people should be used. As part of national capacity building, Country Groups should first assess whether technical assistance is available within the group and then if necessary seek assistance from other resources within the country. External technical support should be called upon only as a last resort although the provision of local assistance will also need to be facilitated to ensure that the programme's capacity building objectives are understood and respected. Technical support missions can reinforce the importance of qualitative research methodologies—such as focus groups, key informant interviews, and rapid appraisal techniques—in a synergistic blend with quantitative methodologies in the overall response to the epidemic. Technical support needs in the realm of qualitative research should be identified early so that technical mission composition reflects these needs.

As with all work undertaken by UNDP's HIV and Development Programme, the research capacity initiative is intended to be taken up and supported by UNDP country offices and other partners. Funding of specific protocols by UNDP was not an expected outcome of the programme since it would not have built local capacity to secure research funds. However, the local donor community often identified the research protocols as "UNDP projects" rather than acknowledging UNDP's role in a process of capacity building that led, *inter alia*, to the production of research protocols. Once such hurdles are overcome, donors who potentially may fund the actual research work should be involved early in the process to increase the likelihood that funds will be made available in a timely way. Expeditious financing of an initial project or of a pilot research activity, such as key informant interviews or questionnaire testing, significantly strengthens team cohesiveness and allows people to learn by doing.

The process of obtaining research funding commitments was facilitated by two factors. First, Country Group members who developed convincing formal presentations engendering donor confidence in the research teams' capacity found these to be effective in generating commitments from funders. Thus, an emphasis on refining funding presentation skills should form part of the technical support mission terms of reference. Second, Country Groups that created strong ties to the National AIDS Programme (NAP) and ensured that their work was perceived to be—and actually was—integral to the development of programmes and policies were more likely to obtain funding. The inter-relationships between NAPs and the Country Groups, and the priorities and interests of both parties should be the focus of formal and informal ongoing discussions throughout the programme.

## Phase II: From Data to Policy and Programming

The first Phase II workshops, held in August 1995, focused on skills for the transformation of collected raw data into findings useful for policy and programme development. Participants included members of the Country Groups, NAP managers, technical support partners, invited African academics, and multilateral and bilateral donors. Workshop formats were derived from notions of partnership and shared responsibility for programming. Specific sessions considered a spectrum of issues, including processes to ensure continuing ownership of research by the communities involved, appropriate dissemination of research findings, research as empowerment, and strengthening capacity to use research in programming and policy. Skills building focused on facilitation, process consultation, strategic questioning, and development of performance appraisal criteria. Communication was enhanced and links forged between NAP managers and respective partnership programme Country Groups. Short and medium-term plans for in-country activities were developed through collective problem solving. The workshops highlighted the implications that capacity building approaches to research—aimed at stimulating social learning, building local research capacity and meeting the needs of programme managers, activists, and decision makers—have for technical co-operation, bilateral donor procedures, current practices of peer review and academic publication, and development practice.

## Social Learning and Implications for the Provision of Technical Assistance

The UNDP partnership programme is based on the recognition that participatory research initiatives have the potential to support and create local processes of social learning which, when complemented by strengthened national capacities for thinking, reflection and analysis, lead to the transformation of social learning into policies and programmes (Banuri et al., 1994, 27). In addition to building local capacities for social learning, as this case study has shown, this UNDP initiative aims to create new approaches to the provision of supportive technical assistance. National teams and local communities take direct responsibility for establishment of research priorities and methodologies and for the development of ethical principles to govern the research. They set the conditions under which technical assistance is provided and determine the areas where their own research competence needs supplementation or strengthening. Technical assistance is then provided in a way that is both more complicated and yet more relevant and sustainable, with outside expertise fitted into local processes of social learning. The programme facilitates the drawing down of assistance from the best available external academic and development sources, national, regional and international. Currently this includes individuals from academic as well as national institutions in countries as diverse as Canada, France, the US, the

UK, South Africa, Zimbabwe, Senegal, Ivory Coast, Spain and Australia. The processes of learning and skills building occur within, facilitated from without.

The HIV epidemic provides the impetus for rethinking the role of outsiders, be they governments or others, in the creation of social change and in development practice. It poses a set of dilemmas for classical approaches to research and, since the issues it raises are the basic ones of development, research findings and processes will necessarily contribute to both development theory and practice. For research to play a critical role in the response to the HIV epidemic, communities, non-governmental organisations and community-based groups, as well as policy makers and programme planners, will have to come to view research as a useful tool for programming and forge mutually beneficial partnerships with researchers and donors. For the researcher, as for everyone, a new paradigm is required, one which Chambers (1994) describes as being people centred, participatory, empowering and sustainable. Much of the challenge is to give up power, to enjoy handing over the initiative to others so they can do more and in their own way, and to learn to value and enjoy these satisfactions.

## References


Ainsworth, A. and Koda, G., 1993, 'The impact of fatal adult illness on school enrolments and attendance'. in Ainsworth, M., Koda, G., and Lwihula, G. (Eds.), Report of a Workshop on the Economic Impact of Fatal Adult Illness in Sub-Saharan Africa, The World Bank and the University of Dar es Salaam: Bukoba, Tanzania, 50-6.

Appadurai, A., 1990, 'Disjuncture and difference in the global economy', Public Culture, 2(2): 1-24.

Banuri, T., Hyden, G., Juma, C. and Rivera, M., 1994, Sustainable Human Development. From Concept to Operation: A Guide for the Practitioner, United Nations Development Programme, New York.

Barnett, T. and Blaikie, P., 1992, AIDS in Africa: Its Present and Future Impact, Bellhaven Press, London.

Chambers, R., 1994, 'Poverty and livelihoods: whose reality counts?', Overview Paper II, United Nations Development Programme, Stockholm, Roundtable, Change: Social Conflict or Harmony?

Global Programme on AIDS, 1991, Weekly Epidemiological Record, 66 (35), 257-9.

Hankins, C. (ed.), December 1994, Partnership for Capacity Building (Newsletter), HIV and Development Programme, United Nations Development Programme, Montreal, pp. 6-7.

Hankins, C. (ed.), August 1995a, Partnership for Capacity Building (Newsletter), HIV and Development Programme, United Nations Development Programme, Montreal, pp. 3-5.

Hankins, C. (ed.), February 1996, Partnership for Capacity Building (Newsletter), HIV and Development Programme, United Nations Development Programme, Montreal, pp. 6-7.

Hira, S.K., Kamanga, J., Bhat, G.J., Mwale, C., Tembo, G., Luo, N. and Perine, P.L., 1989, 'Perinatal transmission of HIV- 1 in Lusaka, Zambia', British Medical Journal, 299, no. 6718, 1250-2.

Joy, L. and Bennett, S., 1994, Process Consultation, Systemic Improvement of Public Sector Management, Management Development Programme. United Nations Development Programme: New York, 33-56.

Kitabu, M. Z. Maitha, G. M., Mungai, J. N., Plummer, F. A., Ndinya- Achola, J. O., & Temmerman, M. 1992, Trends and seroprevalence of HIV amongst four population groups in Nairobi in the period 1989 to 1991, VIII International Conference on AIDS, Amsterdam, PoC-4018.

Lurie, P., Hintzen, P. and Lowe, R.A., 1995, 'Socio-economic obstacles to HIV prevention and treatment in developing countries: the roles of the International Monetary Fund and the World Bank', AIDS, 9 (6), 539-46.

Mbaye, N., Diouf, A., Kebe, F., Diadhiou, F., Sarr, M., Fall, M., Sarr, M.A. N.G., Ba, D.S., Tall, N.D., Ouangre, A., Gueye, A., Siby, T., Boye, C.S., Mboup, S. and Kanki, P., 1993, 'Histoire naturelle de la transmission verticale VIH 1 et VIH 2 Dakar', unpublished paper presented to VIII International Conference on AIDS in Africa, Marrakech, Morrocco, Abstract M.O.P.046.

Misihairabwi, P., McChaven, N., Ray, S. and Weiss, E., 1994, Fostering Collaboration Between Researchers and NGOs on Women and AIDS in Zimbabwe, Women and AIDS Support Network and International Center for Research on Women, Washington, D.C.

Mungai, J.N., Maitha, G.M., Kitabu, M.Z., Plummer, F.A., Ndinya- Achola, J.O., Bwayo, J.J and Temmerman, M., (1992), 'Prevalence of HIV and other STDs in three populations in Nairobi for year 1991', unpublished paper presented to VII International Conference on AIDS, Amsterdam, PoC-4714.

Panyarachun, A. 1995, AIDS and Social and Economic Progress in the Asian and Pacific Countries, [Plenary Address] Third International Conference on AIDS in Asia and the Pacific, Chiang Mai, Thailand.

Peavey, F., 1994, 'Strategic questioning, an approach to creating personal and social change', in Peavey, F., By Life's Grace, Musings on the Essence of Social Change, New Society Publishers, Philadelphia.

Porter, D., 1995, Wheeling and Dealing: HIV and Development on the Shan State Borders of Myanmar, Study Paper 3, HIV and Development Programme, United Nations Development Programme, New York.

Schoepf, B.G., 1991, 'Ethical, methodological and political issues of AIDS, research in Central Africa', Social Sciences and Medicine, 33, 749-65.

This Case Study was prepared by Catherine Hankins, MD, MSc, FRCPC, a founding member, Group for Research to Action, McGill AIDS Centre, Montreal; Elizabeth Reid, Director, HIV and Development Programme, United Nations Development Programme, New York; and Des Cohen, Chief Economist, HIV and Development Programme, United Nations Development Programme, New York.

**Acknowledgements**

Catherine Hankins, Elizabeth Reid and Des Cohen wish to thank Sylvie Gauthier, Fiona Percy, and Mina Mauerstein-Bail. Co-ordinated by the Centre for AIDS Studies of the Public Health Unit of the Montreal General Hospital, now known as the Group for Research to Action of the McGill AIDS Centre of McGill University.

## 6. GROUNDING RESPONSES IN PEOPLE'S REALITIES: LISTENING TO HOW PEOPLE TALK ABOUT THE EPIDEMIC

The way people communicate about their own lives and the epidemic is an integral part of their own understanding, which in turn is the basis of action they take. Consideration of the language people use is therefore important to supporting the development of understanding and action. An example of the importance of this was noted by Dr Evelyn Gacad, the National AIDS Programme Manager in the Philippines. She referred to the fact that the recently developed National HIV/AIDS Strategy was written by Filipinos and included use of "Filipino English". This, she said, meant that people reading the strategy would recognise that it had been written by Filipinos, not outsiders, and that this would result in more widespread commitment to understanding and working within the principles outlined in that strategy.

### 6.1 Key Lessons Learnt

This section is based on the results of interactive discussions held in the field between evaluation team members, partners of the Programme and others who have been involved in using similar approaches. It focuses on developing deeper understanding of the way in which the language people use helps them to understand and act in their own contexts, and the way in which the language used in development practice can either enhance or hinder such understanding and action.

If development is to commence with people's perceptions of their own realities, and continue in ways which are consistent with their views about what is desirable and how change comes about, then it is important that they be able to bring their own understanding into the process. If development practice continues to be described and implemented using only the languages of technology, power, medicine, colonialism and social engineering, then there is little chance that different perspectives can even be described, let alone incorporated into the process. Yet this is what often happens in the global response to the HIV epidemic. Programmes are almost always described using words like "targeting", "intervention", "inputs" and "outputs": words which fit clearly into an overriding metaphor of social engineering, and which are not consistent at all with the underlying purpose of most of those same programmed which is to empower people to respond to the epidemic in ways which make sense within their own cultures and social realities.

Two issues were therefore apparent for the evaluation team. First, the need to create space for people to talk using their own chosen words and metaphors, to enable them to describe how capacity is developed in ways which make sense to them. Second, to engage with people in shared reflection about they types of words and metaphors which they are already using. As a result, some alternative metaphor systems could be identified in various contexts: metaphors which are different to the dominant metaphor of social engineering, and which may help explain how capacity development comes about when attempts are made to come to terms with what it means to work in genuinely collaborative relationships.

In this section, further background information is provided to explain why the use of language is so important, and how the HDP has attempted to address some language issues. Then, the results of interpretive discussion about the language people are using in the response to the epidemic are summarised, with some tentative conclusions made about the types of metaphors which arise when people talk from the heart about their own experiences.

Following description of these key themes, a case study is presented which outlines and explains the way the development of appropriate language and useful concepts became central features of one series of partnerships, commencing with but moving beyond the partnership between the Salvation Army and the HDP.

## 6.2 The UNDP HIV-Related Language Policy

A crucial component of the approach of the HDP has been the promotion of widespread discussion about the use of language in discussions about responses to the HIV epidemic. One example of this is the production of a document entitled, "UNDP HIV-related language policy". This document has been used in UNDP workshops and circulated amongst partners of the programme. The document suggests the use of language which is inclusive and which does not create and reinforce a "Them/Us" mentality or approach; which is drawn from the vocabulary of peace and human development rather than from the vocabulary of war; which uses descriptive terms which are those preferred or chosen by persons described; which is gender sensitive; and which suggests that terms used need to be adequate and accurate.

A simple one-page document, this language policy has had far reaching impact, perhaps because its basic purpose and the issues it outlined made immediate sense to the many people who have read it. It has been used all over the world, and evaluation team members have all either seen the document or heard of its use in sparse and unrelated networks, including the HIV and Development Network of Australia, the Global Network of People Living with HIV, the Philippine National AIDS Council's committee on policy development, and networks of NGOs in rural areas of Senegal.

## 6.3 Noting the Emergence of New Forms of Discourse

The UNDP HIV and Development Programme has expressed concerns about the dominance of particular types of language in public discourse about HIV, drawing attention to the way in which some uses of language can limit understanding, but also noting the emergence of new forms of discourse which are more optimistic and empowering to those affected by the epidemic. These include use of, "... a language of processes rather than interventions, of people as responsible actors rather than as manipulable objects of interventions" (Reid, 1994). The approach of the HDP, using the inclusive and empowering processes outlined in Section 5, has enabled people to bring their own experience and understanding into programming responses. The language they use provides a good example of how such processes lead to deeper understanding. In planning the evaluation process, evaluation team members and Programme staff members identified language issues which the evaluation team decided to consider, centring around the use of metaphor in discussions about HIV and development.

## 6.4 Understanding the Role of Metaphor as a Means of Understanding Reality

The every day language of people, within many languages, is pervaded by the use of metaphors, to such an extent that these metaphors influence the way people understand the world. This has been documented and explained by Lakoff (Lakoff, 1992). An example provided by Lakoff is that metaphors such as, "Love is a journey" enable us to understand all sorts of complexities about love, which may otherwise remain an abstract concept which is very difficult to understand. Such metaphors may be primarily used in literature. However, there are more complex, more pervasive metaphors which are infused into our every day understanding.

Put together, these result in "systems" of metaphorical use which influence not just our understanding of single concepts, but also the relationships between many different concepts.

Use of metaphorical systems, rather than just single metaphors, is a feature of many discussions about HIV. The most dominant and obvious metaphorical system is the system of the metaphor of "social engineering".

## 6.5 The "Social Engineering" Metaphor

Within the metaphor system of social engineering, an example of a single metaphor is the use of the term, "expert". The idea is that an "expert", just like an engineer working with a mechanical system, can learn all there is to know about a particular situation, through observation, and then change that situation, through some sort of "intervention", to make the whole thing "work better". No one says that social systems are mechanical, but an unconscious implication of use of this metaphor is that the methods used to fix machines can, by and large, be transferred to the field of human development.

Such simple use of metaphors may appear harmless enough. However, when they are put together within an overall metaphorical framework, they come to dominate the ways people think about particular situations. Again, referring to programming responses to the HIV epidemic, consider the following terms, which appear again and again, and think about how they may influence the way people think about the epidemic:

input
output
analysing the situation
fine tuning of programmes
programming
measuring effectiveness
targeting
intervention
expert
control
testing

There would be no problem with use of these terms within a metaphorical system of "social engineering" if they enabled better understanding of different situations and if they led to more effective responses. The problem is that use of this particular metaphorical system has been so pervasive that it has led to exclusion of other ways of talking about the HIV epidemic. As one participant from Zambia noted, "They used these methods to deal with small-pox. Now they're trying to do the same with HIV. HIV is far more complex than smallpox, but the language they use does not acknowledge that". The result is that the use of this metaphorical system has limited the development of effective responses to the epidemic.

The way in which use of this metaphor has worked against the inclusion of many people's concerns within an epidemic intricately linked with culture and values was highlighted by Eduardo San Miguel, from Mexico:

> Social engineering does not refer to social relations. It seemed to be very technological, market oriented, reflective of state intervention versus participation in activity, with a high role for hierarchy. Authority without taking anybody into account.

Language consistent with this metaphor was most often used by participants responding to the list of "Concepts UNDP is not currently using". Common reactions to this list involved recognition that these types of terms were often used by funding agencies, and often led to forms of project proposal writing and reporting which conflicted with participants' own experiences in working with people in their own contexts. Some participants noted, for example, that they have to work with people in one way and report back to international agencies in another way.

## 6.6 How do People Talk about the Epidemic?

The evaluation team paid close attention to the way people are talking about the epidemic, in order to see if it was possible to identify aspects of emerging new types of discourse which are being used in people's everyday experience of responding to the epidemic. This process involved listening to the language people are using and considering whether there are some alternative metaphorical systems already in use. Through these sorts of listening processes, of which the evaluation was merely a simple example, a more comprehensive understanding of use of language may evolve, helping to connect the processes used in development assistance with the realities of people's lives.

Using interactive processes, the evaluation identified some recurring metaphors which seemed to form metaphorical systems, centering around concepts of "farming", "war", "building", and "family". Importantly, use of different types of metaphors seemed to vary between countries. This may reflect different cultures, but also may arise from different experiences of the epidemic.

## 6.7 The "Farming" Metaphor System

Many participants in Zambia used words and expressions that are often associated with farming. For example:

> We are planting the seed of love in these children so that they will grow up and be caring persons. We know that not all seeds will grow, but we have to put our faith in the future of these children. They will also be the ones to take care of our children when we die.
>
> *(Rose Mwitelela from Kwasha Mukwenu, a community based programme for care of children whose parents have died as a result of AIDS).*
>
> It is like growing something: it doesn't take a day. You must be prepared to wait. you need to nurture and care for the tree to yield fruits which you may never yourself get to see. *(Sister [Dr.] Auxillia Bupe Ponga, D.O.R., Director of Women and Development, National Commission for Development Planning).*

Farming in African societies is often done by women, and is connected to sustaining life through providing food for family members. It involves responsibility, care, patience, knowledge, attentiveness, and being sensitive to the surrounding environment (changing weather conditions, droughts, floods, access to water, etc.).

Farming in the African context means interaction with natural surroundings, and an understanding of interdependence. It also means that even if you have to put in a lot of work, the product of your work will not come immediately, but the product of your work may be essential for surviving. Farming is not linear: it is not a question of putting in the seed and waiting for the result. Conditions change and responses must change accordingly. Farming follows certain cycles and is process-oriented. Note the similarities with approaches in sustainable human development, and with the approaches of the Programme.

The responses to the HIV epidemic of the women quoted above centre around responsibility, care, flexibility, and the changing of responses after taking into account many different circumstances. The responses were future-oriented and illustrated hope in what many other people would see as the most grim of circumstances.

The Programme works with concepts that form an integral part of a farming metaphor, such as "nourishing", but it has not consciously used this metaphor. Many of its initiatives involve similar understandings of the importance of preparing the ground, planting seeds of hope, and following up with nurturing processes rather than use of control and reporting mechanisms.

## 6.8 The "War" Metaphor System

Some words used by evaluation participants can be used within several metaphors. This illustrates the importance of interactive exploration to identify patterns of meaning behind use of words. Words that are used within the metaphors of both social engineering and war include, "targets", "operations", "interventions" and "they". Some other words used in a metaphor system based on war are:

> fight, barriers, conflict, battle, resistance, shield, targets, power, power-imbalance, hostility, invasion, enemy, oppression, submission, victim, win.

Within the war metaphor the perception of the *enemy* varies. The enemy may be the virus. Often, however, the enemy is perceived to be the HIV-infected person, either as the one who destroys others or as one who is already infected, degraded, made unworthy, demoralized through being victimized and thus no longer one of 'us':

> ... the first time I opened up to those pastors' wives, I saw a judgemental spirit. ... There are words still being used that should be removed. "Victim!" ... so people put a label on you. *(from a Zambian HIV-positive woman who is active within the church and who works voluntarily in hospitals helping people with AIDS).*

Other people may also be seen as enemies:

> Don't come near me because I am going to get it from you (the homosexuality). The attitude of many of my colleagues is that homosexuality is "vampirism". ... Social images of sexuality as the unnameable and filthy are reinforced by prejudice and intolerance ...
> *(Eduardo San Miguel, the National Commission on Human Rights, Mexico).*

Amongst people engaged in effective and voluntary responses to the epidemic, the perception of the enemy is often very different to that in the above quotes:

> ... The conflict is really a struggle for dominance and a struggle for resisting dominance ... of course we meet resistance, but we soldier on ... AIDS is a crosscutting issue. This is really about fighting the patriarchal structure. And if this is not recognized in the response to the AIDS-epidemic we will have no movement forward!
> *(Sara Longwe and Roy Clarke, private development consultants, Zambia).*

There is a danger with the use of metaphors. Sometimes we use them firmly without reflecting on them. I realize I am always fighting. I am constantly talking about breaking the walls of the ghetto, about tearing down barriers. I am thinking and functioning within the war metaphor and this is the first time I have stopped to reflect on it. The NGO's in Mexico are also fighting between themselves. This discussion has been really valuable for me. I discover that I don't always need to fight, that actually a lot of the NGOs and others involved in responding to the epidemic can communicate and co-operate and have a lot in common in spite of the diversity.

*(Irma Rosado, ASPANE, participating in the workshop in Mexico).*

## 6.9 The "Building" Metaphor System

The metaphor of building was used in several ways amongst evaluation participants, and was particularly noticeable amongst evaluation participants in Mexico. It is used to illustrate construction and creation processes, as processes involving collective action and solidarity. The building is often seen as a home—providing sanctuary and protection. The metaphor of building was also used in the context of constructing barriers:

> If you are a caring person you get a lot of satisfaction seeing that people get out of distress. When facing a challenge you can see that you are one of the builders—that also gives you energy.
>
> *(John Musange, Family Health Trust, Children in Distress Project Manager, Zambia).*

In Mexico, exploration of the building metaphor revealed that building was associated with traditions of neighbours and friends helping each other in building homes. It evokes such associations as "solidarity", "reciprocity", "mutuality", and "belonging in a community".

When discussing people's decisions about when to discuss being infected, concepts like "coming out" and "out of the closet" were used in association with the concept of building. Interactive reflection in the workshop in Mexico revealed that coming out can make you vulnerable because it could put you in the open with no protection, with no shelter, with the risk of losing belonging. Use of the metaphor helps make clear some connections between the issue of "coming out" and the issue of "enabling environments".

## 6.10 The "Family" Metaphor System

Language centring around the concept associated with "the

family" was often used by participants in the Philippines. This was not observed during the workshops held in the Philippines, but was identified during later interactive processes when evaluation team members who had visited the Philippines reported back to others. Hence, use of the metaphor has not been discussed with participants in the Philippines, and its inclusion here is very tentative, aiming to provoke discussion rather than to draw conclusions.

Use of this metaphor was typified in discussion about the fact that many successful projects started with very humble beginnings, with no clear understanding of long term goals or even general directions. People simply, "... came together" to explore what they might do. People work together, support one another, and grow together, just as children grow within a family. There was a strong sense of nurturing new developments in a caring way in the Philippines. For example, many NGOs which have worked successfully on issues around the epidemic in Manila are now engaged in encouraging the development of NGO initiatives in other regions of the country. This work was often reported as using similar approaches to those used by the Programme. For example, the use of validation was important. One NGO worker drew attention, for example, to the importance of what she called,

> The principle of acknowledging small successes. For example, with kids learning to walk the one or two steps when they don't fall. So they glean some satisfaction when they start to move. Think maybe three or six months later what they'll be doing.

## 6.11 The Use of Inclusive Processes in Enabling People to Share their Understanding

This discussion on metaphors is included as an example of the way the inclusive processes explained in Section 5 create the opportunity for people to bring in their own understanding of reality, and to develop effective responses based on that understanding.

The language people use is but one indicator of their understanding. Inclusive processes enable the sharing of ideas using language which the people involved relate to and understand, and also the development of responses to which people feel committed because they are based on their own choices. Limiting the way people speak about the epidemic, even when this occurs unconsciously, will almost certainly hinder the development of effective and sustainable responses.

Active listening, the promotion of dialogue as a means of developing shared understanding, decision-making, and consensus are therefore important components of new programming practices in sustainable human development. Such processes are based on mobilizing the expertise of all involved rather than on the notion of "experts" coming in from outside and determining what responses should be developed within specific contexts.

## CASE STUDY 2:

## THE PARTNERSHIP BETWEEN THE SALVATION ARMY AND THE HIV AND DEVELOPMENT PROGRAMME

### "Sharing Experiences Means Extra Space for Mutual Growth"

### Introduction

Not all organisational interactions are healthy—those of the UN system and non-government organizations can bring to mind situations of awkwardness, tension, competition and exclusion.

Occasionally that is not so—the reflections of conversations, key events, key lessons learnt through organisational sharing of the UNDP HIV and Development Programme (New York) and the Salvation Army International Headquarters (IHQ) (through the IHQ technical assistance team) recall a healthy experience of mutual learning expressed through:

* Informal discussion.
* Regional and national co-operation with a focus on local programming.
* Participation of the Salvation Army in UNDP formal processes, e.g. SPR.
* Participation of UNDP in Salvation Army processes, e.g. International conference on HIV, Leysin, July 1991; participatory evaluation of the work of the international technical assistance team, Ottawa, Canada, September 1992.

The values that underscore co-operation need to be identified not only because they are crucial to organizational collaboration, but because mutual learning is essential for an effective response to the HIV epidemic. No longer do communities and organisations have the luxury of time to "play games", to be "territorial": the problem is too big for all of us combined, let alone any organisation trying to do it alone.

The values for effective co-operation include a willingness to share, to listen, to learn from the other, to be enabled in personal and organisational development because of the influence of the other, to be secure in sharing, to recognise the common foundation of sensitivity to the personal and community voice of suffering and of the search for hope, the need for a commitment to an ethic of care, and to a belief that change is possible. These values are expressed and developed in a context of belonging rather than separateness. They are the cement which holds together the foundations of programme development at local, regional and international levels. Complementing these values are the use of key concepts which include the link of care to prevention, and community involvement in social change.

*How have values been shared, concepts formed, and programmes developed in more effective ways because of the co-operation between the two international organizations?*

## 1. Zambia 1988

Picture the Chikankata AIDS team, frantically integrating daily work with evening planning and late night writing, entertaining, hosting, being hospitable to constant visitors, all of whom seemed to want to come at the weekends because that was when they had spare time!

Occasionally the visitor was not ordinary, but somehow communicated an insight.

Such a visitor was Elizabeth Reid (of UNDP). She came as an analyst, as a human being, as a person enmeshed in the emotions associated with the impact of the virus on a person and a family. She seemed to see something different, and what was so implicit to the implementing team was named by her.

She saw that the person with HIV had been placed fairly and squarely in the middle of circles of concern—that the person mattered and yet the person was in relationship with others.

She saw an attempt to articulate, at that stage, the link between the care of a person and the positive motivation towards protection and prevention by and in affected others.

The key values observed appeared to be:

1. Care is necessary for human dignity, encouragement and development.
2. Care links with motivation of affected others towards prevention and positive development through change.
3. Programme implementors don't have to be interventionists but can be participants.
4. Outside experts need to live the rhetoric—they need to sit with others, listen, absorb, sense, reflect, and learn.

These values were the basis of the Chikankata programme, characterised by the word "integration".

This concept of integration implied the interlinkage of many disciplines; the community voice was linked with the national voice in policy development; and, in a most basic sense, the integration of a care process with a prevention response came from within the motivation and initiative of people rather than relying primarily on external interventions (which were popular at the time).

## 2. London 1990

Ian Campbell, appointed by the Salvation Army to be Medical Adviser to the Salvation Army, finds his way to London and, within the first few days of arriving in February 1990, is in contact with "the network".

One early link was with UNDP New York, out of respect for relationship, as well as the felt need in Ian to find out what was going on internationally and to strengthen the process of international linkage of the Salvation Army.

*The values and concepts expressed by the Salvation Army* at that time with respect to AIDS had been more clearly articulated as "transferable concepts"—care linked to prevention; community related to belonging; change relating to attitudes, behaviours and environment; decentralised approaches embracing the notion of teamwork and linked to sustainability; the search for and discovery of hope; normalization meaning the realistic recognition of living with HIV/AIDS; and others.

A facilitator group had formed to develop programme and concept transfer internationally through the Salvation Army system.

Elizabeth Reid and Mina Mauerstein-Bail (of UNDP) together encouraged the identity that was being expressed by the Salvation Army. In a visit to the Salvation Army International Headquarters, including an interaction with the Commissioner, Bramwell Tillsley (second in command of the Salvation Army internationally), the statement was made by Elizabeth Reid that, "It is not our job to shape you in the UNDP image but to affirm you in your own identity, as the best way to help the international response to AIDS."

The values expressed by UNDP included the following:

* Unity in diversity—but a common belief that social change is possible.
* Respectful affirmation that religious belief is the key to effective living in many people's lives and in the identity of many faith organizations.

One *key concept was inter-organisational sharing as a means of strengthening identity and performance.* This has been the foundation for informal and formal interaction since 1990.

### 3. Leysin, Switzerland, July 1991

By agreement of the General, the first Salvation Army international conference on AIDS was held. This proved to be a catalytic event to a sequence of programme design, support and evaluation, and organisational sharing. This sharing is currently inclusive of 30 countries, with 50 community-based programmes still emerging, some of which can still be directly related to the Leysin conference.

A key feature of conference programme design, by the international technical assistance team, was the inclusion of other organisations to underscore the value of mutual learning.

The values expressed by the Salvation Army and by UNDP (represented by Mr. Wally N'Dow, then the UNDP Resident Representative from Central African Republic, subsequently in Tanzania, and now the Assistant Secretary-General of HABITAT, and Secretary-General for the HABITAT II Conference, June 1996) were that inclusiveness is valuable, and that inclusiveness is of direct benefit to work because of its influence on programme planning and development.

Wally N'Dow, a Muslim, was stimulated by the conference, and clearly felt that he belonged. An indicator was seen at the conclusion when he gathered everybody together, holding hands, and led the group in a song. He felt free to share his own faith background with another faithbased organization. The common ground was of response, in a spirit of service and facilitation, to the intrusion of HIV/AIDS. The common vision was the opportunity for community development, change, and hope.

### 4. Senegal, November 1991

Informal Consultation on Behavioural Change. Through a process of interlinkage between the UK NGO/AIDS Consortium, the Salvation Army, Save the Children (UK) and UNDP (New York), a reflection happened on the process of behaviour change. An influential and succinct statement on behaviour change emerged as the product of the work of 16 local programme teams, and of a facilitation process formed by inter-organisational sharing. This was in itself an indicator of successful sharing of values and concepts, and was ahead of its time because so many unusual boundaries were crossed.

The meeting in Senegal seemed to have that quality of reaching out into the future. A significant shift was felt in development of consensus about the concept of "*community*".

The Salvation Army view for some time had been that people are interconnected in relationships in community—people are "autonomous" and yet that does not mean that they work alone. Their decisions are influenced by others and the intricacy of the community process for seemingly simple actions should never be underestimated. Apart from a statement on the influences on behaviour change, this was another major outcome of the Senegal meeting, but it was subtle in that the connection between the person and community relationship had already been discerned mutually by UNDP and the Salvation Army. Perhaps it was more distinctively observed by Elizabeth (of UNDP) at the meeting, particularly through informal conversation in lunch hour times and after hours with people such as Roy Mwilu and Noerine Kaleeba. The meeting formed the environment for productive healthy mutual strengthening of learning, particularly the interconnection between community belonging and change.

## 5. Other Connections

In betwen these "major events", informal visits to New York, warm connections at regional and international meetings continued ...

## 6. Washington, June 1992

The US Congressional Forum on HIV/AIDS. An opportunity for influencing US policy on funding? A time for talking between people belonging to organizations? Politics?

Ian (of the Salvation Army) presented on "Care and traditional values in relation to responses to AIDS and HIV", with reference to the Chikankata Hospital experience of connecting care to prevention. Elizabeth spoke on "contracts" between people—using a different language but reinforcing the shared values and concepts contained in the former conversations and experiences. She spoke movingly of contracts between persons, men and women, communities and nations, linking this to development, positive change and hope.

The key value affirmed was that people develop through relationships, not by power and conflict. The key concept strengthened, which is crucial to effective programme development, was that people in the intimacy of their relationships need to respond as relational beings and as people in groups, as well as being persons functioning as individuals.

## 7. Berlin, July 1993

"HIV/AIDS and Military Populations", a UNDP supported

initiative, examined creatively the role of military populations in responding to and perpetuating the epidemic.

Another type of "military"—the "Salvation Army"—was creatively incorporated by Elizabeth Reid and Mina Mauerstein-Bail (of UNDP), probably as an effort on their part to increase the representation of values and concepts that go beyond the prevailing images associated with military populations.

Instead of seeing military populations as isolated units, the reality is that they connect to civilian populations in times of war and peace, through sexual activity, and through family and community life. The meeting did not ignore the accentuation of the risk environment provided by military populations in times of instability and civil war.

The key value shared indirectly and directly was that people in "groups" are actually not isolated in those groups— in this sense "targeted interventions" need to be very strategic and linked to the recognition that people in groups are also in other relationships.

The key concept underscored by this exploration of linkage to the wider community was that people who define themselves as being within a very select community or group are actually a subgroup of a wider community.

This is crucial to effective programme development because it is clear that through targeted interventions alone, marginalisation often increases for people who are commercial sex workers, truck drivers, youth, military people, religious people, etc. It is still commonly the case that targeted interventions are named as the only practical way forward. Even if other strategies are named, there is often a tendency to rely on targeted interventions as the priority, and in isolation from other relationships, because this appears to be easier.

## 8. Community Response

After Ian's visit to Zambia, Zimbabwe, Uganda and Kenya in May 1994, the emerging distress felt within families and communities impacted Ian (of the Salvation Army) with a sense of urgency that there needed to be a definitive reflection on processes of behaviour change. He wrote about this to Elizabeth (see letter).

Elizabeth responded to Ian's letter with her own letter—there was evidence of an instinctive perception of the real issue, beyond the words, of personal family and community impact that was way ahead of anyone's ability to name (see letter).

A key value being expressed was, "We do not know what we think we know." The epidemic teaches us that it is impossible to say that we have arrived, and that the best we can do is to share together, looking at relationship variables, real people, real experiences, real behaviours. This will give some opportunity to stretch out to touch the meanings associated with the epidemic, most of which are felt non-verbally and often missed by most people.

26 May 1994
London, UK

Dear Elizabeth,

I will be in New York for the afternoon of Wednesday, 8th June.

I hope it will be possible to see you even briefly. It will be important to share experiences gained through the mission just completed to the Congo, Zaire, Zambia, Kenya and Uganda.

The linkage of care in the home to change through and by the community is more clearly affirmed. At field level, systematic home visits by a team can be linked through 'confidential sharing' to community mobilisation for support and change.

Every household in the Chikankata catchment area is now listed, by the initiative of the community. Although it is not yet established, the view is emerging that every house can be visited on a systematic basis when there is someone who is sick and every house can be included now in a present and future plan for neighbour support and visitation. These two extra elements of neighbour to neighbour support and inclusion of a future need, expressed now, are two simple but very important elements of a workable approach to management at field level in high prevalence places.

Organisations like the Salvation Army are ready made for this sort of involvement but catalytic funding is needed in low, medium and high prevalence countries to normalise the process of home visits, community involvement and change. It seems to me that this can take anything from six months to several years, and that it can happen in low prevalence areas (e.g. Mizoram, India) as well as high prevalence areas (e.g. Chikankata, Tshelanyemba Hospital).

The team at Chikankata tried to describe both 'community pain' and 'hope'. The pain is reflected by serious disposition in people, lessening or disappearance of wailing when deaths happen, and adjustments to counselling processes that include, for example, recognition that though one person of a couple to be married might be sero-positive, they may still go ahead if they know what the future might hold because otherwise how can love be found and expressed? Also the recognition has dawned that the loss is accumulative and that it is only just beginning. The hope, as we said a year or so ago, is both concrete and mysterious—people can care for each other, but at the same time, the mystery of belonging energises people and motivates them to care, to love, and to be realistic.

Definition of hope is an important theme to spread around the world, because as people find capacity to cope, they can become disabled by the increasing accumulative loss and pain.

I know you know these things but I felt you should be the first to have a reflection letter on my return (today is the first day in the of five)..

We (Alison and I) look forward to seeing you and/or Mina, if possible.

Yours sincerely,
Ian D. Campbell
Captain
MEDICAL ADVISER
The Salvation Army

---

30 May 1994
Rosedale, Australia

Dear Ian,

It was such a pleasure to hear from you. Particularly since, as usual, we seem to be seeing and thinking the same things. I have recently had two brief trips to Zambia. How desolate that country will be one day. Unless... Both times I got out into the villages but the second trip I went down to Livingstone to see the work of three UN Volunteers working to strengthen community based responses to the epidemic.

One of the images that I will long carry with me was sitting in the courtyard of an urban health centre in one of the poorest compounds talking to the home-based care team that one of the volunteers was training and working with. When we arrived, it was the day of their normal weekly meeting, none of the women were yet there. We were told that they would be late since they had gone to a nearby compound to collect food for the work that they had been doing in a public works programme. This food, we were told, was all that many of them had to keep going. They were all volunteers from the surrounding compounds. They all had families of their own and each day was a struggle for survival. Yet they volunteered. And to do what must be one of the most depressing works of neighbourliness that exists: offering solace with little if anything in the way of physical support to the (mainly) AIDS dying.

The system was, usually, that when the neighbours heard that someone was sick, they told or sent a message to the Counsellor attached to the Health Centre. After she (almost invariably; in the home-based care team, one man had been trained but had not ever shown up after — this needs some reflection) had visited the house, she would add the family to the list for the care team. With a system such as this, the carers are not helping the HIV infected, but only the dying, the terminally ill. And usually those who are caught unawares by the dying, without preparation. The team told me that often they find the whole family starving, with no thought having been given to how those surviving the dying person will survive. The team has little to offer. Mostly they do not even have soap to wash the sick and themselves afterwards, no disinfectant, no food tor the starving or protein supplements for the weak, etc. (This lack of support needs to be addressed within the programme.

But what they do have is extraordinary. They have courage and compassion. By just turning up and crossing the threshhold, they challenge, and encourage, the rest ofthe community to do likewise. They ensure that the family is not humiliated and neglected but rather remains part of the community. They help start the essential process of changing attitudes towards the HIV infected and dying. Once inside, they bring concern and care. They are someone to talk things through with. For everyone, the sick and the well, the spouse with her or his fears and the children with their fears. They take over, for at least two short periods each week, the care of the sick, the cleaning up of the diarrhoca, the washing up, the making of the beds, etc.

Who are these women? What motivates them to do this? I do not know the answer to the latter question for that would have required more time to listen to and understand the answers than I had there. But I asked them who they were. Mothers all of them, as I recall. At least one recently widowed. All of them having trouble coping themselves, few of them with much education, all of them searching for ways to earn a little extra money. I wondered ifithe answer to the second question included an element of what you call a future need, an investment in the care of others now in the hope that there will be someone there to care for you when your turn (inevitably, one feels is the extent of the despair) comes. I talked about these women at the recent SWAA regional conference in Zambia.

Thus, even in this micro example, one sees the linkages from care to change through and by the community, to a network of concern and compassion that links present giving to the possibility of future needs, to a process of community mobilisation, that you talk about in your letter, an approach,that I too believe can be put in place in both low and high prevalence areas.

In many ways the UNV programme and the Salvation Army are similarly placed: at community level, where these processes of care and change must be set in place. At present, the Salvation Army has the critically important advantage of your team there to give them guidance on how to do it well. The UNVs need similar support if they are to do it effectively and sustainably. There are others also that we must identify.

The uniqueness of the Chikankata and similar programmes is that the person at the centre of this process is not always terminally ill, the condition with which they went to hospital may have been treatable, and so the teams work with both the HIV infected well and with the dying. In the former case, the person may be well enough to start planning for his or her illness and death, to start planning for their children's future, to start to pass on their knowledge to others. There is an urgent need, in Africa in particular, to help people to start talking about all these things, to ensure that they have access to voluntary counselling and testing services, so that the testimony of the infected and well can be heard, their needs addressed and the quality and length of their life lengthened so that they can continue to nurture and raise their children and to contribute productively to the economy. Apart from anything else, Africa cannot afford to lose prematurely their knowledge and skills and their children need them to be there with them for as long as possible.

The other issues that you raise are ones that concern me deeply. The terrible pain, loss and grieving associated with this epidemic and the fact that it is cumulative and that the future will be much worse than the already often unbearable present. And the deep need to be able to continue to love and to express that love, even if the loved one is infected. Remember Berlin. Although we must do everything in our power to try to ensure that loving someone is not an inevitable death sentence for the spouse and a curse for the children of this love. We must make sure that such people can talk through this choice, have access to good quality and affordable condoms and that the psychological and emotional problems associated with using them in every act of lovemaking during the relationship can be talked through. (I revised and expanded some of my Berlin thoughts on this recently, in Mombasa, at the first conference of the Network of African People with HIV and AIDS. The reaction of those attending, men and women each in their own way, has given me much food for thought).

Your words and insights on hope are, again, critically important. This, and the associated emotions of empathy, compassion, laughter, respect, love, empowerment, etc., that is, the will to live, are all that will carry people through the terrifying trauma and pain that this epidemic carries within itself.

How much ofthe afternoon (and evening?) of June 8 can you and Alison give to me/us? There is so much to discuss. If the Regional Bureau is in agreement, I would also like you and Alison to meet with the team doing the evaluation of the Africa Regional Project which will be in town that week for their briefing. For these are the ends of the Project. How can one evaluation progress towards them?

I am very much looking forward to seeing you. Thanks for writing down your thoughts and reflections and sending them to me. I was touched. Some of your observations brought tears to my eyes.

Being in Australia, by the way, is wonderful. Love,

Elizabeth

## 9. Regional Inclusion

The Salvation Army international team co-ordinated a series of regional workshops focused on "concept analysis ", beginning in November 1993 in Zambia (for Africa), September 1994 in the Philippines (for East Asia and the Pacific), Bangladesh in February 1995 (for South Asia) and Bolivia in August 1995 (for Latin America).

With each of these workshops, it was possible for UNDP (New York) to allocate a small funding grant to support the work of the international team which, in most cases, was the catalyst to other organizations giving funding sufficient to meet the needs (e.g. a $5,000 grant for the meeting in the Philippines stimulated other donors to provide the rest of the funding amounting to $75,000). Perhaps of more significance was the inclusion of people from other organisations and locations.

For example, the inclusion of people from Bulgaria, Poland and Russia (2 from each location, representing national and non-government responses) proved to be a major creative element stressing the process of inclusion at a meeting attended by people responding to AIDS and HIV from villages in Papua New Guinea, from the Marshall Islands, and from Salvation Army administration levels in other countries of the region.

But the *conceptual foundations of care, community, change, hope and sustainability* were shared effectively, across culture and language, and so it was possible to find convergence as well as to acknowledge divergence. The programme development culture of eastern Europe superficially appeared to jar with the ethos of the meeting; and yet the necessary struggle to find common ground was probably key to accelerated learning by all the participants.

Of significance was the recognition of the *value of spirituality and faith* in motivating people to respond, within organisations, to the challenges of the epidemic. There is a strong faith tradition in Eastern Europe and in South-East Asia. This congruency, itself a reflection of the congruency of respectful recognition of identity between the Salvation Army International Headquarters and UNDP New York, was a strengthening feature of the meeting.

Madu Balu Nath, of the UNDP HIV & Development project in Delhi, acknowledged similar values in her participation in the Bangladesh meeting. She spoke of the need to work from the inside out, of participation with community spirit, and of listening to community voices as a means of guidance in the response to the epidemic.

For example, Juan Jacobo Hernandez of Colectivo Sol was able to say, at a moment of crisis and creative development involving a former Salvation Army officer who is HIV positive and who was also a participant, "The Church has AIDS. The Salvation Army has AIDS. Thank you God." He prefaced his comment by saying he had never prayed before.

Around this time Elizabeth began to speak of the need for a gathering of religious leaders and the Salvation Army team is supportive of that approach, willing to participate and facilitate— a future challenge.

It is a sobering thought to recognise that the intimacy of life is expressed through relationship, which in turn is expressed sexually, emotionally, and through the exploration of the meaning of 'soul' which finds its expression in various forms of prayer.

There is a language of hope forming—based, for example, on the acknowledgment of the need for intimacy and health of relationship; and of terrible loss that is not just happening now but awareness as to the awful knowledge that the past and the future are being lost in the present. This is loss of community memory. Yet hope is yearned for, sensed, claimed, and expressed in the poorest of circumstances. People feel it in caring with each other; in working together for change now; in simply being able to talk in new ways; and in still believing in a future, unseen and unfelt, yet it is there.

## 10. National and Local Interaction

The horror and hope of Rwanda is unmatched. In April 1995, it was possible for the International Salvation Army team to support the Salvation Army work in development through agriculture, health and pastoral care by advising on how that work could be interlinked with response to HIV and AIDS.

It was recognised that HIV/AIDS is an entry point to the fragility and capacity of life and this is no more true anywhere than in Rwanda which is searching for its "soul" through the visible process of reconciliation.

As in other countries, a visit to the UNDP office, encouraged through correspondence from Mina Mauerstein-Bail to the UNDP Resident Representative in Kigali (as had happened previously with Bangladesh, Uganda, etc.), paved the way for mature interactive mutual learning between the two organizations, ... at country level.

*The values represented* included recognition of the role of an international structure to help facilitate within the organisation so as to make it receptive to the "stranger" at the doorway. Cultivation of a spirit of inclusion and mutual learning was the service of UNDP, New York, and the result was affirmation in the mind of the Salvation Army team in Rwanda that HIV/AIDS is a development and reconciliation issue.

## Summary

Inter-organisational sharing is not just about sharing information and holding on to personal identity no matter what—effectiveness is determined by *shared values*, that embrace respect; affirmation of the other identity given that it is founded in genuine compassion, and a capacity for strategic action embracing both care and change; a culture of mutual learning, of facilitation, of service, of listening in to community voices, of sitting within the suffering without ever believing it is possible to provide for it entirely; and participation in the search for hope. These values are crucial to the "common ground" of conceptual reflection for effective programme development.

The key concepts for the Salvation Army include the interlinkage of care to prevention, belief that change is possible, community as circles of belonging and participation; sustainability depending on the interlinkage of the person in community to care and prevention. Hope is related to all these factors.

There is an obvious congruencey with UNDP's ongoing exploration and reflection on conceptual foundations. Different language may be used, but there are nevertheless similar foundations.

These are based, perhaps for both organizations, in a mixture of organisational identity, experience, instinct, and the personal values of those involved. These are related to personality, character and experience, yet they alone do not provide a common ground for learning—it is their linkage to conceptual definition and, in turn, to patterns of action that helps draw the organisations together informally and formally in a continuing exploration of the unknown, the unfelt and the unseen.

Perhaps the most powerful, positive, interlinking factor is the mutual recognition that the epidemic has outstripped us in its negative impact. There is a curiously powerful common background for people of the Salvation Army International Headquarters technical assistance team and the people involved in HIV and Development, New York—experiences of suffering, of participation, of positive change; and a capacity for conceptual reflection indivisibly linked to these experiences. These are the elements that are most important to forming the common ground that is essential for effective organizational sharing.

This Case Study was prepared by Captain Dr. Ian Campbell and Alison Rader of the Salvation Army, HIV and Health Programme Development Team.

## 7. SOME ISSUES RELATING TO THE NATURE OF CHANGE WITHIN DEVELOPMENT PRACTICE

Recent practices of technical co-operation used by UNDP and others have an inclusive, process oriented approach. This approach is characterised by use of the concepts of partnership, shared reflection on lived experiences, the gradual evolution of people's understanding and ability to act, and a collective development of effective responses which cannot be pre-determined but which are, almost by definition, relevant to the lives of the people who develop them and are thus more likely to be sustainable.

The dominant model of development which guides development and HIV-related practice generally uses an approach characterised by use of analysis of situations through externally designed research, and programming based on interventions or disseminations. These programmes aim to change people's behaviour and determine the possible range of effective responses according to pre-conceived and measurable predictions of outcomes.

The evaluation found that the proponents of the effectiveness of the new human development paradigm, and those who are most able to explain how it works, are most often those whose lives are directly affected by the epidemic and who have themselves been through transformative experiences. They often expressed a quiet yet confident hope that the processes with which they are working will continue to result in effective responses to the challenges of HIV and development.

Those working within a less process-oriented approach expressed the most pessimism and the least belief in forward movement. In the absence of finding effective "models" which work and which are replicable, they were unable to capture the sense of forward movement which was evident amongst people who were acting within a paradigm of inclusion and participation.

## 7.1 Key Lessons Learnt

This section is based on the results of interactive discussions held in the field between evaluation team members, partners of the Programme and others who have been involved in using similar approaches. It explains some implications arising from the way in which changes are occurring in development practice. These changes affect what is happening in the field, as described here from the perspectives of those whose lives are affected.

While discussions take place amongst high level international organisations about the need for new approaches to development practice, and changes take place in the field within specific development projects, many individuals and organisations now feel caught between two paradigms: the traditional approaches of technical co-operation, which still dominate the understanding of many middle level bureaucrats in funding and programming agencies, and the newer approaches of sustainable human development, which are being applied in ways which make sense in their daily practice.

Thus, there are important difficulties which arise from the experience of being caught between two very different, and often seemingly irreconcilable, approaches. Such difficulties are intensified because even some agencies which are involved in the development of new approaches, including UNDP, are not yet reorienting their programme planning, management and evaluation processes in ways which clearly support such changes.

## 7.2 Problems with Interaction Between Different Types of Development Practice

The fact that process-oriented approaches to HIV and development are taking place within an international climate in which most programming responses to HIV and development are still based on practices derived from a more directive paradigm presents problems. These problems include the following:

(i) Since the approaches of the sustainable human development and capacity building are still being developed and explored through processes of social learning, it follows that they are not widely understood, not clearly articulated even by those adopting them, not accepted by all UN or donor agencies, and not consistently applied.

(ii) For this reason, many people are using one approach amongst the people who are affected by the epidemic and whose understanding and action they are supporting, but having to account to funding agencies, or donor countries, using the language and appearing to use the practices of the other paradigm.

(iii) The sustainable human development approach requires changes to many current practices of technical co-operation. It requires important shifts in the roles and practice of many individuals and organizations, both in donor and recipient countries. Many individuals and organizations are resistant to such change.

## 8. CONCLUSIONS AND RECOMMENDATIONS

The UNDP HIV and Development Programme (HDP) used the Special Programme Resources (SPR) to explore and enhance understanding of the ways in which the approaches of sustainable human development can be applied towards building capacity to understand, and to effectively respond to, the HIV epidemic. The evaluation process was exploratory and forward-looking, aiming to generate further and deeper understanding of the nature and approach of this type of programming.

Key findings of the evaluation were:

— that there are many people now engaged enthusiastically in what they themselves consider to be effective and sustainable responses to the HIV epidemic within their own contexts;

— that these people themselves affirm that the approaches used within the Programme, and similar approaches used by others, have enhanced their understanding and responses to the epidemic within the context of human development; and

— that the way these approaches have been described, developed and articulated by the HDP have validated and enhanced their own capacity, and thus helped answer the central question of, "How can we, together, move forward?"

In essence, it could be said that the work of the Programme

was based on an inter-related series of active and reflective processes which were used to catalyse further active and reflective processes in responding to the HIV epidemic. Using approaches which evolve from its understanding of development practice, the Programme worked with people committed to responding compassionately and effectively to the epidemic to help catalyse such reflective processes. Those processes began to challenge commonly held assumptions about what drives the epidemic and what may work to slow it down, and to shift the focus of attention onto the processes of social change which will lead to effective community and national responses.

The types of process-oriented approaches explored through the HDP are:

- based on human interaction, and the facilitation of processes;
- necessarily slow at first because they must grow from shared understanding and consensus building which, in turn, must evolve as real human relationships evolve within the context of lived experience; but
- lead to more effective, adaptable and sustainable responses in the long term because they build on capacity which already exists and thus create strategic effects which continue beyond the participation of the Programme, without resulting in dependency relationships with donors or technical advisers.

In effect, the processes of inclusion and partnership draw out people's understanding of both what is occurring within their own contexts and of their capacity to respond. An important strategic effect of these approaches, as described by evaluation participants, is that the people who are involved as direct partners of UN or donor agencies which use these types of development practice themselves use similar approaches in their interaction with others in their own countries and in regional networks addressing specific concerns. Thus, their own practice extends the effects of the individual programme under consideration. The evaluation was, in effect, another component of this ongoing evaluative and action-focussed approach.

Understanding of sustainable human development is still evolving as the nature of effective development practice is being explored on many fronts. The HIV epidemic, varying in its evolution and its effects in different countries, and at different stages of the epidemic within countries, presents particular challenges to any fixed understanding of what may work to catalyse effective responses to it. The problems addressed with certain responses today will be different tomorrow, or in different contexts. Therefore, new processes must continually be created to enhance understanding and to develop effective responses to new problems based on processes of social learning *which arise from within* communities and nations.

Such processes do not end with the drawing together of lessons learnt through one programme such as the SPR. This is important because, even though many of the practices of the Programme are now being adopted by other agencies, approaches based on the need to enhance understanding of the nature of effective processes and partnerships are not. While it is important that the lessons learnt through the Programme are shared and disseminated, it is equally important that the processes which led to these lessons themselves continue, both in UNDP and elsewhere. This is very different from the nature of lessons learnt through many other types of research or programming: in this case, understanding and practice must continue to evolve simultaneously through use of inclusive processes and continual questioning.

The evaluation has highlighted that approaches consistent with the principles of sustainable human development are taking place within a world in which development practice is often characterized by the mores of traditional technical co-operation. Approaches for the achievement of sustainable human development which include shared reflection, inclusion, and the conscious use of processes to allow scope for a range of possible outcomes, are beginning to be adopted. Traditional technical co-operation is driven by donor preferences, and characterised by use of external experts and use of quantitative measures to ascertain effectiveness in meeting predetermined objectives or outcomes. It is less concerned with capacity building or with the discourse of partnership or participation.

The differences between these two approaches lead to different types of practice. However, the differences are not often acknowledged, as highlighted by some reported experiences of evaluation participants. The result is that many people seek to promote social learning through using the project design processes, reporting, measuring procedures and language systems of traditional forms of technical co-operation. Conversely, it is possible for people to change their use of language but not practice. However, both the Programme and the evaluation process found that it is possible for people and agencies to shift their understanding and practices from traditional approaches to those described in Section 5. This occurs more easily when the reasons for, and the approaches of, sustainable human development are articulated, explained and communicated interactively, allowing people space to consider the relevance of these approaches within their own contexts.

That this is necessary was highlighted through one of the

findings of the evaluation process: those people approaching the HIV epidemic using approaches consistent with the framework of sustainable human development demonstrated more hope, confidence and forward movement than those working within alternative approaches.

It is important now to ensure that the lessons learnt through the HDP are shared amongst the people whose lives are affected, and disseminated within UNDP, other UN agencies and the international development assistance community. What is required is a more widespread *understanding and adoption of the approaches of sustainable human development* within the context of the HIV epidemic.

Thus, there is a need to share the lessons learnt within the HDP using approaches consistent with the Programme itself. That is, in ways which enable a wider variety of people affected by HIV and development to be involved, and which facilitate reflection about the relevance of these approaches in various contexts and the sharing of ideas about possibilities for changes in development practice.

For the people directly affected, this requires use of approaches to sharing what has been learnt in ways which are inclusive, and which create space for such sharing and further network development. The very nature of what has been learnt leads not to a set of ideas to be disseminated so much as a series of processes to be invoked.

For UN and donor agencies, this requires that approaches to sharing what has been learnt incorporate processes which enable critical reflection on the possibilities for changes within current development practice. Changes are required, for example, in the processes used for research, training, policy and strategy development, programme design, reporting procedures, and evaluation methods. These changes, in turn, require changes in skills required, and therefore in methods used for staff development and for future selection and training of staff and consultants. Ultimately, changes will be required in the management practices of UN and donor agencies, particularly changes which will enable the inclusion of the people whose lives are affected in determining priorities and aproaches to be used in programming.

UNDP has a particular role within the new joint co-operative programme, UNAIDS, and the current evaluation process indicates two key challenges:

1. There is a need to ensure ongoing association between the evolving understanding of effective approaches in sustainable human development and the evolving understanding of effective responses to the HIV epidemic. This

will be most likely if there is an ongoing direct association of UNDP with development of responses to the HIV epidemic.

2. In order that UN Resident Co-ordinators can effectively undertake their function of co-ordinating the support of UN agencies to national responses to the HIV epidemic, there is a need to ensure that UNDP in-country staff, the Resident Representatives and staff of other agencies understand the ways in which the approaches of sustainable human development can enhance understanding and lead to more effective action in response to the HIV epidemic.

Recommendations are based on the lessons learnt through the HDP and the deeper understanding of the approach which has arisen through the evaluation. They are based on the need to ensure that the processes of social learning generated through the SPR continue amongst individuals, communities and nations affected, and also within the UN system. The adoption of these recommendations will enable ongoing sharing of what has been learnt amongst other people and agencies who are, or who are interested in, developing similar approaches. Such sharing will ensure more widespread adoption of approaches which promote responses to the HIV epidemic which are grounded in people's lived experiences and evolve in ways which build upon existing capacities.

*Recommendation 1:* That UNDP share what has been learnt through the HDP with the people whose lives are directly affected by the challenges of HIV and development. This sharing must take place using processes which enable and encourage the involvement of people who are not normally part of development networks, and using processes such as workshops and network development which enable inclusion, reflection, sharing and the development of ongoing partnerships within nations and within regions.

*Recommendation 2:* That UNDP share what has been learnt through the HDP with UNAIDS, other UN agencies and with bilateral and NGO donor agencies. This sharing must take place using processes, such as workshops, which enable interactive discussion and reflection on current development practice within the HIV epidemic, and which lead to the development of new approaches in project design, management and evaluation practices. This sharing must not be limited to those staff or agencies already engaged in responding to the HIV epidemic.

*Recommendation 3:* That UNDP take active steps to ensure an ongoing association between evolving understanding of approaches in sustainable human development and evolving understanding of effective responses to the HIV epidemic. This could commence with a series of related planning workshops at country, regional and global levels, in which UNDP staff and others develop means to ensure such an ongoing association. These methods may include new approaches to staff development and new methods for interaction between UNDP staff and others engaged in responding to the challenges of HIV and development.

*Recommendation 4:* That UNDP, in association with UNAIDS, support UN Resident Co-ordinators in co-ordinating UN agency support for national responses to the HIV epidemic, by ensuring that Resident Representatives are educated about both the association between HIV and development and the nature of approaches to sustainable human development which facilitate enhanced understanding of, and effective responses to, the HIV epidemic.

## REFERENCES

Banuri T. Hyden G. Juma C. Rivera M. Sustainable human development: from concept to operation, a guide for the practitioner. New York, UNDP, 1994

Benbouali A. Evaluating success and assessing performance: a draft discussion paper. UNDP Office of Evaluation and Strategic Planning. Internal paper, New York, UNDP, July 1995.

Denzin N K. *Interpretive interactionism.* Sage, *1989,* Newbury Park, California.

Chambers R. Poverty and livelihoods: whose reality counts? An overview paper prepared for the UNDP Stockholm Roundtable on Global Change, 22-24 July 1994.

Joy L. and Bennett S. Process consultation: systemic improvement of public sector management. New York, UNDP, 1994.

Lakoff G. The contemporary theory of metaphor. In: Ortony A (ed.). Metaphor and thought. Second edition. New York, Cambridge University Press, 1993.

OECD/UNDP/World Bank. Report of the High-Level Development Assitance Committee/UNDP/World Bank Seminar 1994: "Improving the effectiveness of technical co-operation in the 1990s". OECD/UNDP/World Bank, 1994.

OECD. Development Assistance Committee: principles for new orientations in technical co-operation. Organisation for Economic Co-operation and Development, 1991.

Patton M. Q. Qualitative evaluation research and methods. Sage, 1990, Newbury Park, California.

Patton M Q. Developmental evaluation. Evaluation Practice, 15(3), 1994, 311-319.

Peavey F. Strategic questioning, an approach to creating personal and social change. In: By life's grace: musings on the essence of social change (pp.86-111). New Society Publishers, 1994, Philadelphia, Pennsylvania

Reid E. Approaching the epidemic: the community's response. AIDS Care, 6(5), 1994, 551 -557

Schon D. A. Beyond the stable state: public and private learning in a changing society. Temple Smith, 1971, London.

Speth J. G. Foreword by the administrator. In: Banuri, *et al.* Sustainable human development: from concept to operation: a guide for the practitioner, New York, UNDP, 1994.

de Vylder S. Sustainable human development and macro economics: strategic links and implications. UNDP, 1995.

Weiss C. H. Evaluation research: methods of assessing programme effectiveness. Prentice Hall, 1972, Englewood Cliffs, New Jersey.

# 45

# HIV Co-ordination at the United Nations

Ms. Elizabeth Reid
Director, HIV and Development Programe, UNDP
to the Co-ordination Segment of ECOSOC relating to HIV and AIDS

---

*13 July, 1992*

Mr. President, Distinguished Delegates, Colleagues,

On behalf of the Administrator of UNDP, Mr. William Draper, I welcome this opportunity to address you.

The UNDP statement on this agenda item is available and was circulated in advance as requested by delegations last week. This statement directly addresses the issues relating to the co-ordination of HIV-related policies and prograrnmes from UNDP's perspective. Since it is available and because Dr. Merson's forceful statement has also covered many similar issues, I will not directly summarize the statement. Rather I would like to take this opportunity to respond to the request of the delegations of the United Kingdom, Argentina, Canada and others to identify some of the relevant issues and problems and to outline possible strategies to address them.

Mr. President,

There are, I believe. two important characteristics of the HIV epidemic which need to be acknowledged and understood for they affect and determine the nature of the response to the epidemic.

Firstly, the epidemic is at one and the same time both a crisis and an endemic condition. It is a crisis because the speed of spread of this virus can be so awesome. Infection rates in adult populations can, and have, increased from two per cent to 25 per cent in only a small number of years, before people are even aware that they are surrounded by infected family and friends, before they are aware that their communities have been invaded. This fact alone should be sufficient for it to be viewed as a disaster, albeit too often invisible in its early stages, as much in need of an immediate response as the invasion of one country by another. For war nowadays rarely has the toll in human lives that this virus is causing.

That it is an endernic condition may best be simply illustrated by the fact that, even if in seriously affected countries there were to be no further cases of infection as from today, the pain and trauma of the deaths of those already infected will continue for the next twenty years and the social and economic repercussions of their deaths will continue on for decades and generations after that. We know thav nowhere in the world is the spread abating or even slowing down. Each day of continuing spread adds to the duration ot its devastating impact.

Both dimensions, the epidemic as crisis and the epidemic as endemic, need to be recognised. Each has its own appropriate responses.

Secondly, the epidemic manifests itself both as a specific problem out also as a pervasive one. Its specificity is revealed in increasing numbers of people, mostly healthy, productive young men and women, getting sick and dying. The response of the first decade of the epidemic addressed this quality of the epidemic.

However, as is argued in the UNDP statement, the repercussions of these deaths will permeate and affect every facet of human life and national development, more so in seriously affected countries where men and women are infected in more or less the same numbers. The causes and the consequences of the spread of the virus embrace poverty and wealth, disempowerment and influence, deprivation and development, trust and bad taste; the very way we are as human beings.

Both of these dimensions of the epidemic, its particularity and its ubiquity, must also be recognised. Each of these too has its own appropriate responses.

Thus this epidemic is conceptually slippery: at once a crisis and an endemic condition; at once a specific issue and a permeating one.

Mr President,

These two characteristics of the HIV epidemic impose a set of imperatives upon us:

* the imperative of an effective response;
* the imperative of a sustainable response; and
* the imperative of a co-ordinated response.

The prerequisite of an effective response is a common understanding of the nature of the epidemic, which takes into account its above two characteristics, and a shared vision of the way forward. This we do not yet have. This should not surprise us for the epidemic is a new and complex phenomenon for which there is no likeness in living memory, not one drawn from war, not from disease, not from natural disasters nor from man-made ones, including poverty.

This is not to say that we are blindly groping. As the Secretary-General's report (E/1992/67) states, we are doing what we know needs to be done while we search for new and more effective ways to respond. The more we share a vision of an effective way forward, the more co-ordination will naturally follow.

Both WHO and UNDP have placed high priority on this quest: through expert group meetings, informal consultations, the exchange of experiences, the documentation of successes and through informal exchanges between communities and governments, among donors and within the United Nations system. UNDP has developed and piloted a workshop designed to reach a common understanding at country level of the nature of the epidemic and of effective approaches to its many facets. Such an understanding is an antecedent condition for co-ordination.

At global level, the recent proposal for a Global HIV/AIDS Co-ordination Forum was born from the same analysis.

The second imperative, that of a sustainable response, means that while the required human and financial resources must be available for identified effective responses, these responses must also be ranked in order of effectiveness since resources, whether of individuals, communities, nations or of external support agencies, are limited.

The commitment and contributions of affected individuals and communities have yet to be recognized or valued but they are extensive. They lie at the heart of a sustainable response to this epidemic but in most cases they need to be supplemented by further human and financial resources. The closeness of these individuals and communities to the problems and needs created by the epidemic ensures that the responses are appropriate. Similarly, governments are increasingly allocating resources to the epidemic.

Thus priority must be given to strengthening national capacity to ensure that these resources, and that of the external support agencies, are used in the most effective manner. There is not time and there are not sufficient resources for ill-conceived, inappropriate and ineffective responses. The selection must be ruthless for the demand on resources will continue and increase inexorably for decades. Communities and governments must have the ability to monitor assess and evaluate their interventions and to modify, redesign and expand them.

Where the response to the epidemic is effective and sustainable, hope is brought into being that the desolation and distress of this epidemic can be restrained, a hope that can turn back the tides of fatalism and despair.

Mr. President,

Only one other requirement then remains for a co-ordinated response: there is a need for mechanisms to ensure that the search for affective and sustainable policies and interventions is an ongoing process. Such mechanisms are needed among the community groups responding to the epidemic, between such groups and government, among government ministries, between the public and the private sectors, among external support agencies, especially within the UN system, and between donors and countries.

These mechanisms must be flexible for different countries have different capacities and different needs. A variety of approaches to co-ordination have been established. They need to be rationalised and strengthened. The United Nations Resident Co-ordinator has a critical role to play in ensuring that this occurs at country level.

Mr. President,

UNDP, with its understanding of the complex dynamics of human development, can assist in bringing about a common understanding of the nature of the epidemic and a common vision of the way forward.

Further, UNDP, with its relation to the United Nations Resident Co-ordinator, will be a critical player in the process of creating mechanisms for dialogue, collaboration and co-ordination.

Finally, UNDP, with its extensive presence at country level, its neutrality and its experience in a broad range of sectors and programmes, is a resource to be mobilized for national capacity building to ensure that this imminent threat to human survival, human rights and human development can be overcome.

Mr. President, Distinguished Delegates, Colleagues,

On behalf of the Administrator of UNDP, Mr. William Draper, I welcome this opportunity to address you under this agenda item designed to provide an overview of trends and prospects for the world economy and their implications for development.

The UNDP statements on agenda item 3 (b) touched briefly on the characteristics which distinguish this epidemic from other diseases but also from war and from natural and man-made disasters. T. refer the distinguished delegates to this statement and will not take up this aspect of the epidemic now.

This epidemic is occurring at a time in history when not only economic and political trends are causing concern but also i a period of quite unsettling social change itself affected by current economic trends.

Firstly, the structures of family life are changing. In all regions of the world, fewer women marry today than in 1970 and fewer women are having children. More than 30 per cent of households in the world are headed by women but at least a quarter of the women heading households in developing regions are elderly.

Secondly, since the 1970s, women's share in the labour force has been rising and it is anticipated that it will continue to rise. Almost everywhere women are working more outside of the household while at the same time the household remains a major place of work for women. The proportion of men who are economically active is down everywhere. Whilst women's share in the labour force is rising, the proportion of women and of women headed households below the poverty line is increasing.

While women's lives in families are changing, there is little evidence that men are undergoing comparable change.

This weakening of family structures is occurring at the same time that in most countries of the world investment in social support systems to families and employees has dropped significantly.

Women's survival is increasingly an issue of serious concern. Women outlive men almost everywhere but they are still in the minority in many developing regions because of higher rates of female mortality. There are not as many women as men in the world. Indeed in many countries, there are fewer than 95 women for every 100 men. Women's survival is already threatened by gender selective abortion, female infanticide, the criminal neglect and abuse of young girl children, the unacceptable extent of the death of women during pregnancy and in childbirth and other threats to women's lives. These deaths are avoidable; the social and economic distress caused by them should not be being borne.

These socio-economic trends pre-date the HIV epidemic. The epidemic will exacerbate them and in turn will itself be fed by them. The structures of family life will be further and radically changed as parents die dcattering households. Extended family support systems may have burdens placed on them that they are unable to bear. Yet families provide nurturing, care, companionship and security to their members. They act as buffers against crises and form an important part of the basis of community coping strategies. It is imperative that social policy frameworks be established so that these family structures are strengthened and supported if we are to live through this epidemic.

The survival of women is being further threatened by their increasing rates of HIV infection. Already, one in every 21 women in Africa die from childbirth related causes. Add to this the current estimate of one in every 40 women in Africa being HIV infected. Both these causes of death are preventable wherever they occur in the world. The economic and social dislocation caused by this wanton slaughter or women will not be able to be home either by households or by nations.

None of these trends can be addressed in isolation. They are interwoven and interrelated. Perhaps this epidemic will be the catalyst which will force us to action. However, for our response to be effective and sustainable, we will need to forge a number of social contracts or partnerships.

The first social contract must be between men and women.

This epidemic and its impact will never be overcome unless men and women can forge a true partnership of mutual respect and trust and of equitable sharing of the burdens caused by this epidemic, the burdens of sadness, pain, care and support. Women alone cannot stop the spread of the virus and women alone cannot bear the burden of its personal, social and economic consequences. Men must be involved. A social contract must emerge, and soon, to face these challenges together, as husband and wife, brother and sister and as partners, friends and colleagues.

Secondly, there must be a social contract between the affected and the not yet directly affected.

The infected and those close to them are amongst the most powerful agents of change in the world today. They can give us glimpses of how we can peacefully co-exist with the virus, of how we can become empowered through the trauma and the tragedy of the epidemic. Within the desolation of this epidemic, they give us snatches of laughter and happiness. They can help us explore and better understand the nature of intimacy, desire and sexuality in the age of the virus.

But these insights of the affected will not be shared, this gift will remain ungiven, if, in the sharing, the affected are stripped of their self esteem and dignity, subjected to humiliation and discrimination, left alone in a hostile limelight without support and companionship.

This is a critical social contract: the opposite of the Them/Us mentality which has sadly too often characterized perceptions of and responses to the epidemic. There is not other in the shadow of the epidemic. We are all there.

The social contract, therefore, must enable the creation of a supportive milieu that encourages the affected to speak out, tell their stories, reflect on their lives and hopes and help us all to live peacefully with this epidemic.

The third social contract must be between communities and government.

The responses of affected communities provide us with the hope that the epidemic can be overcome and the inspiration as to how this can come about. These responses are universal. Wherever the virus has spread, communities have responded, to provide care and support to stop further infection, to assure the rights of the affected, to minister to spiritual, emotional and physical needs.

But individuals, families and communities cannot carry this epidemic alone. There must be a social contract, a partnership between governments and affected communities. Governments must provide an enabling environment that will noursh and sustain these responses. This enabling environment must include national policies that acknowledge the centrality of community responses, a body of legal and human rights laws that respect the principles of non-discrimination and respect for the rights and dignity of affected individuals, mechanisms for interaction between government and communities, and assistance, as required, for programme design, delivery and financing by communities.

The need for additional resources for this epidemic is frequently mentioned. Whilst it is clear that external resources are needed, it is important to stress that the first financial resources that are mobilized to respond to this epidemic are those of individuals, families and communities. This remains unrecognized and unquantified. We must name this and quantify it for sadly this is the way that most people recognize value.

These resources-peoples' volunteered time, the food, meals and insights they share, the transport provide, the labour contributed, the funds raised- lie at the heart of a sustainable response.

Yes, the resources must be supplemented. They are not without end; they themselves are depleted by the epidemic; they are not, always or usually, sufficient. The communities know what additional resources, human or financial, they need for sustenance and growth. They need to be empowered to be able to define their external support requirements, select them, manage them and account for them in appropriate ways whether these resources come from national or international sources.

Mutual trust and respect is a sine qua non for a social contract between communities and their government. This may not be easy for either but it must come about.

The fourth social contract must be a global economic contract.

As the epidemic deepens, its devastating impact on all aspects of human life and national development is becoming better understood. Certain nations may be brought towards the threshold of destitution. Will there be a global economic contract? Will the world community provide the foreign direct investment in the education and health of people and in the technological development of these nations? Will there be global social safety nets to allow nations rendered poor by this epidemic, and the poor within them,. to survive.

The free working of the global market tends to increase the disparities between rich and poor nations and rich and poor individuals. At the national level, governments try to offset such tendencies by redistributing income through systems of progressive income tax and by supplementing this with social safety nets to prevent people from falling into poverty and absolute destitution. No such systems exist at present at the global level.

The closest the world comes to a global safety net is the current system of development assistance. However, this system is fatally flawed, firstly in the inadequacy of its extent. Secondly because its allocation at present is unrelated to levels of poverty. South Asia, for example, receives $ 5 per person. India has 34 per cent of the world's absolute poor, yet receives only 3.5 per cent of total aid flows. Countries that invest more heavily in military expenditure receive more aid than those with modest investments.

If overseas aid is to be able to serve as a social safety net for the world's poor, it will have to be based on principles requiring that aid should be directed to priority concerns for human survival and human development.

These four social contracts or partnerships are essential to an effective sustainable response to this epidemic.

We now know well the main areas for programme focus in response to the epidemic. These are behaviour change, the care, support and treatment of those affected and, as the epidemic deepens, the maintenance of the basic infrastructure of communities and nations: water supply, electricity, road maintenance, financial institutions, education and health systems and so on.

Our strategy for the immediate future must be to bring about the social contracts or partnerships which will enable us to achieve these programme ends.

UNDP is committed to helping forge these social contracts and to working actively with communities, nations and the international community to identify and strengthen effective, sustainable policies and interventions.

# 46

# World AIDS Day, 1 December

Today, the international community rededicates itself to fighting the world-wide scourge of HIV/AIDs, to combating fear, ignorance and prejudice, and to providing new hope for the millions of people around the world living with HIV.

HIV/AIDS is a global problem. No country or region is immune Today, some 22 million people are living with HIV/AIDS, while the total number of world-wide AIDS related deaths has reached 6 million. These are appalling statistics, but there is nothing inevitable about the global spread of HIV.

In the developed world, the success of prevention and sex education programmes, and awareness campaigns among intravenous drug users have demonstrated that rates of HIV infection can begin to be arrested and addressed with positive results.

In the developing world, the challenge remains greater. Over ninety per cent of all new HIV infections occur here, and programmes to prevent the spread of the infection have so far met with limited success. In addition, new anti-virus therapies and treatments remain extremely costly and beyond the means of the vast majority of AIDS sufferers in the developing world.

The United Nations has taken a lead in promoting vital education and prevention programmes, and is working closely with Member States and local populations on the ground. The Joint United Nations Programme on AIDS, launched on 1 Janurary 1996, marks an important step forward in the global fight against HIV/AIDS. The Programme, in partnership with Member States, is working hard to promote greater co-operation and co-ordination in the field, and to develop new policy initiatives and mobilise new resources at the global, regional and country levels.

Above all, this initiative emphasises the growing partnership between the United Nations system and individual people living with HIV. The Programme seeks to be inclusive in its dealings with affected communites and individuals throughout the world.

The challenge of World AIDS Day is to translate understanding and awareness of HIV/AIDS into positive action and more effective and co-ordinated public policy response around the world. Today, more than ever, the global challenge of HIV/AIDS demands an informed, considered and generous response from us all.

# 47

# Challenges for UNDP in A Changing World 1990-2000: Social Trends

**Ms. Elizabeth Reid**
UNDP, New York

The last two decades have seen the emergence of a number of social trends which will converge in the coming decade, fomenting a period ot rapid social change. This decade may well become known as the white water decade with the development community at times feeling that it is being swept out of control down its rapids.

If people are to be placed at the centre of development during these changing times, the social context of development will be as important as its political, economic and administrative contexts.

I wish to look briefly at some social trends relating to family structures, gender and the HIV epidemic, which I believe, will affect the fabric of our societies.

## THE STRUCTURES OF FAMILY LIFE ARE CHANGING?[1]

Families provide nurturing, care, companionship and security to their members. They act as buffers against crises and form an important part of the basis of communities' coping mechanisms.

In all regions, fewer women marry today than in 1970 and those who do spend less of their lives married and fewer having children.

In Africa, the proportion of women in the 20 to 24 age group who have never married increased between the 1970s and the early

'80s from 25 to 33 per cent. A similar but less pronounced trend occurred in all other regions except Asia.

In all regions, similar but less pronounced trends occurred among:

* teenage women
* men 20-24 years
* women and men 25-44 years.

This trend for both women and men may be significantly reinforced during the 1990s by the HIV epidemic.

**Up to 30 per cent of households are headed by women. At least a quarter of the women heading households in developing regions are elderly.[2]**

The Latin American and Caribbean region has the highest number of countries where more than 20 per cent of households are headed by women:

Barbados (44), Chile (22), Cuba (28), Dominica (38), El Salvador (22), French Guiana (31), Grenada (45), Guadeloupe (34), Guyana (24), Honduras (22), Jamaica (34), Martinique (35), Netherlands Aptilles (30), Panama (22), Peru (23), Puerto Rico (25), St. Kitts & Nevis (46), St. Lucia (39), St. Vincent/Grenadines (42), Trinidad and Tobago (25), Uruguay (21) and Venezuela (22). Africa has 8 such countries; Asia and the Pacific, one.

The proportion of both women headed households and households headed by elderly women and men could significantly increase in the 1990s in countries seriously affected by the epidemic.

**Extended family support systems may have burdens placed on them that they are unable to bear in high incidence areas.**

Infection is clustered in families. It is highly likely that both husband and wife may die, leaving the elderly, children and other household members without means of support. Where the adult population is seriously affected, the reliability of traditional support systems may be threatened.

The proportion of women and women-headed households below the poverty line is increasing. Poverty accelerated the spread of the HIV epidemic, particularly for women for whom sex work is often the only available coping strategy. In turn, the epidemic deepens poverty, destitution and homelessness.

**Increasingly divorce is instigated by women.**

In Europe three-quarters of all divorces are instigated by women.

**Since the 1970s, women's share in the labour force has been rising and it is anticipated it will continue to rise.**

Almost everywhere women are working more outside of the

household while at the same time the household remains a major place of work for women.

Women everywhere retain primary responsibility for household work, even when they have economic responsibilities inside and outside the household. Men in developing regions generally do even fewer household chores than men elsewhere. The proportion of men who are economically active is down everywhere.

**While women's lives in families are changing, there is little evidence that men are undergoing comparable change.**

This weakening of family structures is occurring at the same time that in most countries of the world investment in social support systems to families and employees has dropped significantly. If these trends continuez alternative sources of nurturing, care, companionship and security will have to be found for we cannot live or develop as human beings without them.

## WOMEN'S SURVIVAL WILL INCREASINGLY BE AN ISSUE OF SERIOUS CONCERN THROUGH THE 1990s

Women now outlive men almost everywhere but they are still in the minority in many developing regions because of higher female mortality.

There are not as many women as men in the world (2.65b out of a total 5.3b—1990). Indeed in many countries, there are fewer than 95 women for every 100 men. All of these countries except two are in the Asia and Pacific and West Asia regions.[2]

Women's survival is threatened by:

— Gender selective abortion, female infanticide and the criminal neglect and abuse of young girl children. The Indian economist, Amartya Sen, argues that there are 100 million missing women in Asia in our generation.

— Maternal deaths and disability. One million women die each year of reproduction related causes, mainly illicit and unsafe abortions and obstetric complications. Over 100 million women become disabled or suffer a disabling illness each year as a result of complications in pregnancy.[3]

— Ninety eight per cent of all maternal deaths and disabilities occur in the developing world.

— In Africa one in 91 women will die in pregnancy or childbirth.

In Asia: 1:54
In Latin America: 1:73
In Northern Europe: 1:10,000

Other threats to women's lives include: bride burning, dowry deaths (estimated at 1 every 12 minutes in India) domestic violence and the HIV epidemic.

These deaths and disabilities arc wanton and avoidable. The extent of the loss of productively active women is unaffordable. The social cost and distress caused by these mother's deaths and women's disabilities are unbearable. The demand for changes will increase throughout the 1990s.

## FOR THE REMAINDER OF THE 1990s, THE SURVIVAL OF PEOPLE, BOTH MEN AND WOMEN, AND THEIR SOCIAL, POLITICAL AND ECONOMIC INSTITUTIONS WILL BE OF INCREASING CONCERN.

The HIV epidemic has been visible now for over 10 years. However, our understanding of the epidemic and its implications for human survival and human development is still in its infancy.

**Yet this epidemic has totally permeated our societies.**

WHO/GPA estimates:

— globally, one in every 250 adults is infected;

— in sub-Saharan Africa, 1 in every 40 adults, women and men, is infected.

**The epidemic spreads with alarming rapidity wherever the conditions for spread are present.**

In one African country, the incidence of HIV infection in the urban adult population has doubled each year in the last four years:

1987: 0-3 per cent adults infected
1988: 6-8 per cent
1989: 10-12 per cent
1990: 22-24 per cent

A similar rate of spread has been identified in Thailand where infection rates among compulsorily drafted military recruits have risen from 2 per cent in 1989 to 6 per cent in 1990.

**The incidence of modes of transmission varies with the social context.**

WHO/GPA estimates:

* Globally, 60 per cent occurs between women and men
15 per cent between men
15 per cent through injecting drug use
10 per cent all others

* In Africa, 80 per cent between men and women
10 per cent perinatally
10 per cent all others

These figures indicate where programming priorities must lie if the epidemic is to be stemmed.

**The characteristics which distinguish it from other diseases include:**

- the long period between infection and onset of illness, on average 10 years in developed countries, possibly less in developing countries;
- the majority of those infected are adult men and women; people with significant numbers of dependents and in their economically most productive years;
- the associated epidemics, tuberculosis, for example, which is now a serious problem in most affected communities:
- the fact that once a person is infected, and the overwhelming majority of people are unaware that they are infected, he or she is infectious for life and unless precautions are taken can transmit the virus to others.

**The epidemic is not randomly distributed. It is clustered in households, geographically and occupationally.**

In Thailand, the highest number of known cases of infection occurs among construction site workers (36 per cent). In the Central African Republic, 22 per cent of those infected are students.

**Whenever people move, the virus moves, particularly where the movement is of single people.**

Thus, spread of the virus is facilitated by:

- transport systems
- labour markets
- formal and informal teaching patterns
- seasonal labour
- warfare, destabilization, mandatory and other forms of civil unrest.

The conditions of spread are exacerbated by urbanisation poverty, and migration.

This epidemic will, as it spreads and deepens, force us to rethink approaches to national planning and development assistance. At the same time, the epidemic will undermine national capacity to plan, manage and deliver in countries with high infection rates in urban areas.

Virtually everything we do as planners and agents of development will be affected. The epidemic and its impact will have to be factored into everything we do.

Both economic growth and the mechanisms for redistribution will be undermined. The epidemic will reduce private and public savings. At the same time, demands for public interventions and expenditures will rise, for example, in health, housing, social security and food subsidies. Productivity will be reduced through illness and deaths, particularly of skilled and experienced personnel.

Redistributive mechanisms such as credit and social investment schemes, employment creation schemes, education and training will need to be rethought as mechanisms to address critical needs and to improve the human condition.

There will be immense costs to communities and nations. The early illness and death of the active labour force will generate a need for replacement social investment at a time of shrinking public and national resources. The anguish of the illness and deaths of so many young adults will be difficult to bear. However, an understanding of the extent of the personal, social and economic costs will strengthen the demand for effective prevention programmes, the most effective way of minimising the adverse impact of the epidemic.

We cannot assume that there will be sustained large scale resources transferred to seriously affected countries. The resources and responses will need to come from within communities and nations.

If the 1990s is a period of rapid social change with many trends amplifying the adverse consequences of other trends, then our programming and procedures will need the flexibility to respond and there will be an even stronger imperative for effective programmes. We will be held to account and judged on the extent to which we contribute to human survival find human development.

We need to learn to apply research findings directly to programming. Let me give a few brief illustrative examples, conscious that the brevity will distort the complexity of social situations.

Studies show the following:

— There is no correlation between improving women's socioeconomic status and reducing maternal death and disability.

An improvement in women's social and economic lives is essential for human development. Howevers maternal death and disability can be reduced only by an analysis of direct causes and the establishment of a programme to address them. The methodology for this and the range of direct causes are known.[4]

— The return on investment in women's education is consistently higher than the return on educating men.

Studies in Malaysia show that the net return to education at all levels of wages and productivity is consistently 20 per cent higher for girls and young women than for boys and young men.[2]

The World Bank is now reflecting this in its programming in certain countries by offering financial assistance to parents who allow their female children to go to school.

— Increasing women's income leads to a spread of benefits to all other household members, which does not occur with increases to men's income.

These data have been available for some time but have not, to my knowledge, been taken into account in programme development. Investing more in opportunities for women in education and in formal and informal opportunities for work is far more than an investment in women. It is an investment in their families and communities. It is an effective way to assist people out of poverty. It is a *sine qua* non for human development.

— Women are assiduous and prompt with credit repayments.

Experience with credit schemes in all regions show that defaults in repayments by women are consistently held to less than 2 per cent. One study of women's loan repayment behaviour in Ahmedabad, India, showed that most defaults were because of maternal deaths and disability.[4]

— Information alone rarely changes sexual behaviour.

Information, education and communication (IEC) are necessary but not sufficient to change behaviour. An evaluation of a well designed IEC programme for the prevention of further transmission of the HIV virus showed that 98 per cent of the sexually active population knew accurately how the virus is transmitted and how transmission can be prevented but only 5 per cent had in fact changed their behaviour to prevent themselves from becoming infected.

— Securing the blood supply will have only a slight impact on reducing the rapid spread of the HIV epidemic.

A secure blood supply is critical to retaining people's faith in modern medical services. However, a number of approaches to modelling the epidemic have shown that the resultant impact on the spread of the epidemic under most known circumstances is minimal.

It should be noted that today's data are not necessarily tomorrow's. The social context must be monitored since the situation is not static. For example, Jamaican data indicate decreasing participation of boys in secondary education. Such trends should trigger the establishment of a monitoring system and a response to prevent the range of possible serious consequences of such a trend.

The convergence of these social trends has implications for

the restructuring of the United Nations system. We cannot afford any longer to assume that knowledge and technology can be transferred or technical advice given without regard for the cosial context. Just as they cannot be divorced from the economic and political context. Social analysis must form an integral part of the situational analysis upon which all forms of assistance are based. Diarrhoeal diseases cannot be addressed outside of the context which gives rise to the problem and within which the solutions will be found. Grain storage technology must be accepted by the communities within which it is being introduced and must be suitable to their needs and circumstances. There are many such examples and they are all familiar to us.

Yet the system as presently structured does not facilitate achieving these basic necessities. The context of change is best known by nationals and national capacity must be strengthened to demand a multi-disciplinary and integrated approach. The UN system must be able to respond. This will require a change in the way of the Specialised Agencies or a new role for DIESA. UNDP's advantage is that because of its network of field offices, it is close to and better placed to understand the social context within which human development takes place.

## NOTES

1. Coote, A. et. al. *Changing Family Structures.* Report of the Institute of Policy Studies, London 1991.
2. United Nations Statistical Office. *The World's Women 1970-1990: Trends and Statistics.* United Nations, New York, 1991.

   2. Op. cit.
3. Jacobsen, Jodi L. Women's Reproductive Health... *The Silen Emergency,* World Watch Paper 102, June 1991. World Watch Institute, Washington, 1991.
4. Forward Looking Assessment of the Prevention of Maternal Mortality and Morbidity in the Context of the Safe Motherhood Initiative, UNDP, 1991.

   2. Op. cit.

   4. Op. cit.

###